Statins

The HMG-CoA Reductase Inhibitors in Perspective

Second edition

Statins

The HMG-CoA Reductase Inhibitors in Perspective

Second edition

Edited by

ALLAN GAW MD PhD
Director
Clinical Trials Unit
Glasgow Royal Infirmary
Glasgow, UK

CHRISTOPHER J PACKARD FRCPath DSc
Professor of Pathological Biochemistry
University of Glasgow, and
Top Grade Biochemist,
Department of Pathological Biochemistry
Royal Infirmary, Glasgow, UK

JAMES SHEPHERD PhD FRCPath FRCP(Glasg) FRSE
Professor of Pathological Biochemistry
University of Glasgow, and
Honorary Consultant Biochemist
Department of Pathological Biochemistry
Royal Infirmary
Glasgow, UK

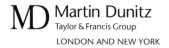
Martin Dunitz
Taylor & Francis Group
LONDON AND NEW YORK

© 2000, 2004 Martin Dunitz, an imprint of the Taylor & Francis Group plc

First published in the United Kingdom in 2000 by
Martin Dunitz Ltd

Second edition published in 2004
by Martin Dunitz, an imprint of the Taylor & Francis Group plc, 11 New Fetter Lane, London
EC4P 4EE

Tel.:   +44 (0) 20 7583 9855
Fax.:   +44 (0) 20 7842 2298
E-mail: info@dunitz.co.uk
Website: http://www.dunitz.co.uk

Although every effort has been made to ensure that all owners of copyright material have
been acknowledged in this publication, we would be glad to acknowledge in subsequent
reprints or editions any omissions brought to our attention.

Although every effort has been made to ensure that drug doses and other information are presented accurately in this publication, the ultimate responsibility rests with the prescribing
physician. Neither the publishers nor the authors can be held responsible for errors or for any
consequences arising from the use of information contained herein. For detailed prescribing
information or instructions on the use of any product or procedure discussed herein, please
consult the prescribing information or instructional material issued by the manufacturer.

A CIP record for this book is available from the British Library.

ISBN 1-84184-292-3

Distributed in the USA by
Fulfilment Center
Taylor & Francis
10650 Toebben Drive
Independence, KY 41051, USA
Toll Free Tel.: +1 800 634 7064
E-mail: taylorandfrancis@thomsonlearning.com

Distributed in Canada by
Taylor & Francis
74 Rolark Drive
Scarborough, Ontario Canada, M1R 4G2
Toll Free Tel.: +1 877 226 2237
E-mail: tal_fran@istar.ca

Distributed in the rest of the world by
Thomson Publishing Services
Cheriton House
North Way
Andover, Hampshire SP10 5BE, UK
Tel.: +44 (0)1264 332424
E-mail: salesorder.tandf@thomsonpublishingservices.co.uk

Printed and bound in Spain by Grafos SA

Contents

Contributors

Christie M Ballantyne
Associate Professor and Clinical Director
Section of Atherosclerosis
Department of Medicine
Baylor College of Medicine
6565 Fannin Street, MS A-601
Houston, TX 77030
USA

Gerard Jan Blauw
Leiden University Medical Centre
Albinusdreef 2
2333 ZA Leiden
The Netherlands

Albert VG Bruschke
Professor of Cardiology
Leiden University Medical Center
Albinusdreef 2
2333 ZA Leiden
The Netherlands

Brendan M Buckley
Department of Pharmacology and Therapeutics
University College Cork
2200 Cork Airport Business Park
Cork
Ireland

Robert P Byington
Professor, Section on Epidemiology
Department of Public Health Sciences
Wake Forest University School of Medicine
Medical Center Boulevard
Winston-Salem, NC 27157-1063
USA

J Jaime Caro
Caro Research Institute
336 Baker Avenue
Concord, MA 01742
USA

Mehmet Cilingiroglu
Cardiology Fellow
Section of Cardiology
Department of Medicine
Baylor College of Medicine
6550 Fannin Street, MS A-601
Houston, TX 77030
USA

Akira Endo
Department of Applied Biological Science
Faculty of Agriculture
Tokyo Noko University
Fuchu-Shi,
Tokyo 183
Japan

Ole Faergeman
Department of Medicine and Cardiology
Aarhus Amtssygehus University Hospital
Tage-Hansens Gade 2
DK-8000 Aarhus
Denmark

Curt D Furberg
Professor, Department of Public Health Sciences
Wake Forest University School of Medicine
Medical Center Boulevard
Winston-Salem, NC 27157-1063
USA

Allan Gaw
Director, Clinical Trials Unit
4th Floor, Walton Building
Glasgow Royal Infirmary
Glasgow G4 0SF
UK

Krista F Huybrechts
Caro Research Institute
336 Baker Avenue
Concord MA 01742
USA

J Wouter Jukema
Associate Professor of Cardiology
Head, Cardiac Catheterization
Laboratory/Interventional Cardiology
Department of Cardiology, C5-P
Leiden University Medical Center
PO Box 9600
2300 RC Leiden
The Netherlands

William B Kannel
Professor of Medicine and Public Health
Boston University School of Medicine
Framingham Heart Study
73 Mt Wayte Avenue
Framingham, MA 01702
USA

Philippine Kiès
Department of Cardiology
Leiden University Medical Center
Albinusdreef 2
2333 ZA Leiden
The Netherlands

Michael B Murphy
Department of Pharmacology and Therapeutics
University College Cork
Clinical Sciences Building
Cork University Hospital
Wilton
Cork
Ireland

Christopher J Packard
Department of Pathological Biochemistry
Glasgow Royal Infirmary
4th Floor, Queen Elizabeth Building
10 Alexandra Parade
Glasgow G31 2ER
UK

James Shepherd
Head, University Department of Pathological Biochemistry
Glasgow Royal Infirmary
Castle Street
Glasgow G4 0SF
UK

Gilbert R Thompson
Emeritus Professor
Division of Investigative Science
Imperial College, Faculty of Medicine
Hammersmith Hospital
Du Cane Road
London W12 0NN
UK

Andrew M Tonkin
National Heart Foundation of Australia
411 King Street
West Melbourne
Victoria 3003
Australia

J Wayne Warnica
Professor of Medicine
University of Calgary
Department of Cardiology
Director, Cardiac ICU
Foothills Provincial General Hospital
1403 29 Street NW
Calgary, Alberta
Canada T2N 2T9

Peter WF Wilson
Framingham Heart Study
73 Mt Wayte Avenue
Framingham, MA 01702
USA

Preface to the first edition

The first studies using lipid-lowering drugs, such as the early fibrates or the bile acid sequestrant resins, provided, at best, equivocal results, which fuelled the arguments for inaction or procrastination among physicians. When the statins were introduced into clinical practice and, more importantly, when they were tested in the fire of the randomized controlled clinical trial, these arguments disappeared. The statins were proven to provide clinical benefits in terms of reduction in all-cause mortality and coronary morbidity in a wide spectrum of patients.

Now that the question of whether we can reduce the risk of atherosclerotic disease in our patients has been answered, we face new challenges. What targets, if any, should we strive for in cholesterol lowering? What is the significance of the non-lipid effects of the statins? Which statins should we use? Can we afford to use any?

The clinical trials that have taught us so much about the statins were not designed to answer these new questions. How could they have been? When the trials were set up, a moratorium was being called for on all lipid-lowering drug prescribing. Therefore, it was essential to answer the fundamental questions of safety and efficacy before we could allow ourselves the relative luxury of considering the detail. And, it is the continued study of this detail that makes the story of the statins alive and, as yet, incomplete.

This book tells the story of the statins, for the most part in the words of those who lived this story. The background, describing the lipid world before the statins, is told by the Framingham investigators. Akira Endo, working with his team in Japan, discovered the early statins and describes his breakthrough. The major clinical trials from Scandinavia, North America, Australia and New Zealand and, of course, Scotland are detailed by those who conducted them. The book is completed by other chapters on the pharmacology and mechanisms of action of the statins, the statin angiographic trials, the use of statins after vascular surgery, guidelines for the use of the statins in clinical practice and the cost-effectiveness of statin therapy. The concluding chapters detail the future statin trials, of which there are many, and we take a look into the future of lipid-lowering therapy beyond statins.

We would like to thank Alan Burgess, Rebecca Hamilton and the team of Martin Dunitz Publishers without whose encouragement this book would not have been completed. We also acknowledge the hundreds of investigators, the tens of thousands of trial subjects, and the millions of patients receiving statin therapy throughout the world today, for without them there would have been no story to tell.

Allan Gaw, Christopher J Packard and
James Shepherd

Preface to the second edition

Statins have become a global phenomenon in terms of both the market value of prescribed drugs and the spectrum of attributed clinical benefit. They are at the core of coronary prevention programmes, and are also under investigation for their impact on other diseases such as osteoporosis and rheumatoid disease. The evidence base underpinning their use in a wide range of patients has expanded year on year. Trial experience continues to show that the drugs are safe and effective in all patients tested. Yet further studies are planned to explore new aspects of statin pharmacology, pleiotropic effects and the limits of clinical effectiveness. Against this background of ever-expanding knowledge of this class of drugs, we felt it appropriate to update the previous edition of this book. The success of the first edition of this book – its breadth of coverage and appropriate depth of information – prompted us only to make changes where necessary. That said, major advances in this field required substantial rewrites of several chapters and the introduction of new ones. What we have produced represents an up-to-date and in-depth review of statins from both a scientific and a clinical perspective.

We are indebted to our authors who have produced excellent reviews of their subjects and have presented these in a format that can be easily read by specialist and generalist alike. We would also like to thank Drs Jane Kent, Eleanor Dinnett and Moira Mungall for their valuable help and comments on the manuscripts. Lastly, we would like to acknowledge our editorial and production team at Martin Dunitz, principally Pete Stevenson and Giovanna Ceroni. Sticks and carrots were used in equal and appropriate measure and they have allowed us to produce what we believe is a very valuable addition to the literature in this increasingly important field.

Allan Gaw
Christopher J Packard
James Shepherd

1

Hyperlipidaemia as a risk factor for vascular disease

Allan Gaw

INTRODUCTION

Enormous resources are put into the study of human lipid and lipoprotein metabolism. Similarly, great efforts are made to develop and test drugs that alter the lipid profile. The reason for these endeavours is a simply stated hypothesis: that a raised blood cholesterol concentration causes atherosclerotic vascular disease and by lowering the blood cholesterol level we can prevent this disease.

Coronary heart disease (CHD) is the main clinical manifestation of atherosclerosis and is the major cause of death in modern, industrialized countries and an increasing cause in developing countries.[1] Atherosclerosis may also affect the peripheral arteries and the cerebral circulation, leading to other debilitating or life-threatening conditions. It is not surprising therefore that given the possibility that such a prevalent disease may be preventable, we have seized upon the opportunity. In recent years, the hypothesis outlined above has been proven and we now enter a new era in medicine where we are armed with an unsurpassed portfolio of evidence upon which to base our clinical practice. This book focuses specifically on the statins, a group of drugs that indisputably have had the most important impact in this field. However, before these drugs are discussed in detail it is important to understand the background to this subject. In this introductory chapter we shall examine the evidence for hyperlipidaemia as a risk factor, review the pathogenesis of atherosclerosis, look at lipid and lipoprotein metabolism in detail, and discuss the classification of the dyslipidaemias.

RISK FACTORS FOR CHD

A risk factor is a characteristic that predisposes an individual to the development or progression of the condition in question. Risk factors are defined on the basis of epidemiological studies, but a distinction must be made between characteristics that are simply associated with CHD and those that actually cause it. For causation to be established the following criteria must be fulfilled:

- There must be a strong, temporal correlation between the existence of the characteristic and the incidence of CHD.
- This correlation must be consistent, dose-responsive and predictive.
- There must be a possible mechanism of action by means of which the risk factor can exert its influence.
- The association must be reversible.

There have been many studies undertaken to identify CHD risk factors. One of the best known and earliest is the Framingham Study, which started in 1948 as a long-term epidemiological analysis of CHD and continues today. This study clearly identified the link between raised blood cholesterol and increased CHD risk.[2] A second important study – the Multiple

Table 1.1 Risk factors for CHD	
Modifiable	*Non-modifiable*
Smoking	Age
Raised blood pressure	Male sex
Raised LDL cholesterol	Family history of
Low HDL cholesterol	CHD
Raised triglyceride	Personal history
Diabetes mellitus	of CHD
Obesity	
Diet	
Thrombogenic factors	
Lack of exercise	
Excessive alcohol consumption	

Risk Factor Intervention Trial (MRFIT), which screened a total of 356 662 men and followed them up for six years – supported these findings.[3]

There are now a large number of characteristics or traits that have been identified as risk factors for CHD. A small number of these function as independent risk factors; that is, they exert their influence independently of the presence of any other risk factor. There are many others that are secondary; that is, they have a positive correlation with CHD but require the presence of other risk factors for this to be manifest. It is useful to consider risk factors in the clinical setting as those that can be modified, either by lifestyle changes or therapeutic intervention, and those that are not modifiable. A list of the major risk factors is shown in Table 1.1.

It is important to realize that risk factors do not generally occur in isolation but tend to cluster in an individual. This is significant because, when risk factors coexist, they interact and their combined effect is much greater than would be expected from the sum of their individual effects.

The concept of multiple CHD risk factors is of great practical importance because it means that the patient at greatest risk is not necessarily the individual with a single serious risk factor such as severe hypercholesterolaemia. Instead the individual with a poor profile of risk factors such as the male smoker with moderate hyper-

tension and moderately elevated lipids is at relatively greater risk. This is illustrated in Fig. 1.1.

While this chapter focuses on hyperlipidaemia as a risk factor for vascular disease, it is important to recognize that other risk factors are equally important. In clinical terms, any attempt to modify a patient's vascular disease risk profile must attend to all the major correctable risk factors, especially hyperlipidaemia, smoking and hypertension. For balance, we shall briefly examine the roles of smoking and hypertension as CHD risk factors within the context of controlling hyperlipidaemia.

Smoking

Smoking is probably the greatest preventable cause of death in developed countries. It accounts for 50% of all avoidable deaths and, of these, one half are due to cardiovascular disease.[4,5] The risk associated with smoking is related to the amount of tobacco smoked daily and the length of time over which the individual has smoked.[6]

The exact mechanism by which smoking exerts its influence is unclear. It is apparent, however, that it enhances the development of atherosclerosis in addition to increasing the occurrence of thrombotic events. The latter are thought to be the most important, as stopping smoking leads to a quicker reduction in CHD risk in patients with established disease than in those who are asymptomatic. In patients with established CHD, the risk in those who stop smoking approaches that of those who have never smoked in approximately two or three years.[7] Asymptomatic individuals, however, require ten years or more before reaching the risk levels of those asymptomatic individuals who have never smoked.[8,9]

Hypertension

CHD risk increases with increasing blood pressure but it is not possible to identify a threshold value below which a patient is safe from CHD. For this reason, the diagnosis of hypertension is somewhat arbitrary and there is not a universally agreed method of classification.

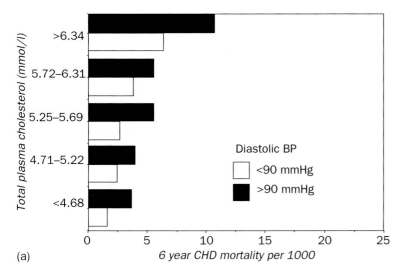

(a)

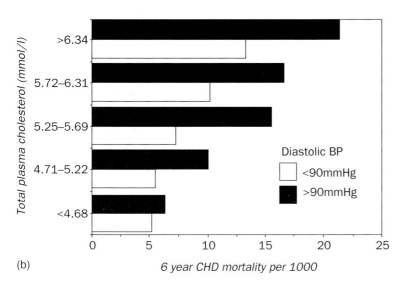

(b)

Fig. 1.1 (a) CHD mortality for non-smokers by plasma cholesterol and blood pressure. (b) CHD mortality for smokers by plasma cholesterol and blood pressure. (Adapted with permission from ref. 3.)

Treatment of mild hypertension by lifestyle modification has been evaluated by a number of randomized controlled trials such as that carried out by Stamler et al.[10] It has been demonstrated that changes such as a reduction in dietary salt intake, weight loss and reduced alcohol intake together with increased exercise can successfully reduce blood pressure. However, trials have been too short and too small to say, as yet, what these effects would be on CHD morbidity.

Much evidence does exist concerning the reduction of CHD mortality and morbidity effected by the use of anti-hypertensive drugs. The meta-analysis by Collins et al.[11] showed a reduction in CHD risk of 14%. This is smaller than predicted from epidemiological data and contrasts with the reduction in stroke risk of 42%, which was just as predicted from epidemiological studies. The reasons for this discrepancy are not yet clear but may be due to the very slow development of coronary atherosclerosis. For the full clinical benefit to become apparent, these trials may have to be much longer.

The greatest benefit of blood pressure reduction is obtained by those with high overall risk.

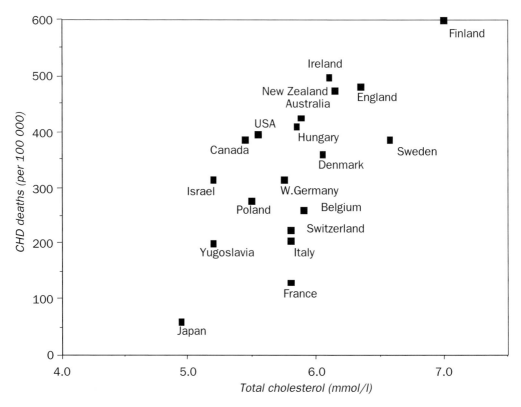

Fig. 1.2 International relationship between CHD mortality and total serum cholesterol. (Adapted with permission from ref. 13.)

Consequently, even modest reductions in blood pressure will be worthwhile in those with multiple risk factors and/or pre-existing vascular disease or severe hypertension.

Once hypertension has caused target organ damage the CHD risk associated with a particular blood pressure level is much higher. Left ventricular hypertrophy carries a particularly poor prognosis. Management should therefore be aimed at preventing target organ damage and should be initiated without delay. While there is still debate about the choice of initial treatment for hypertensive patients, the recent Antihypertensive and Lipid-Lowering Treatment to Prevent Heart Attack Trial (ALLHAT) supports the use of thiazide diuretics.[12]

DYSLIPIDAEMIA

Cholesterol and LDL

The identification of cholesterol as a possible risk factor for CHD was first made after the recognition that in countries with a high mean blood cholesterol the mortality from CHD was also high. Figure 1.2 gives the results from one such study, showing the relationship between mean total cholesterol and number of CHD deaths.[13] The country with the highest cholesterol levels in this study, Finland, also experiences the highest CHD mortality. The position of Japan on this graph (Fig. 1.2) is significant, as it experiences a relatively low CHD mortality. This is in keeping with its generally low

Table 1.2   Ni-Hon-San study: CHD rates and risk factors in Japanese men in three societies

	Japan	Hawaii	California
Acute MI rate/1000	7.3	13.2	31.4
Hypertensive heart disease/1000	9.3	1.4	4.6
Non-smokers (%)	26.0	57.0	64.0
Serum total cholesterol (mmol/l)	4.7	5.6	5.9

Adapted with permission from ref. 11.

cholesterol levels but occurs in spite of high population rates of smoking and hypertension, two other important risk factors for CHD.

This relationship has been studied further in the Ni-Hon-San study, which looked at CHD rates and risk factors in Japanese men in three societies.[14] The results of this are summarized in Table 1.2. It is clear from this that serum cholesterol level is one of the most important factors in predicting CHD risk in the population.

Cholesterol is directly involved in atherogenesis and it has been shown that the severity of atherosclerosis is directly proportional to the concentration of cholesterol in the blood.[15] It is also clear that diet is important, as studies such as the Seven Countries study[16] have shown that CHD is inversely related to the ratio of polyunsaturated to saturated fats in the diet.

The above studies have identified the association between CHD and cholesterol, but in order to quantify the risk it was necessary to design prospective cohort studies. The results of three such studies are illustrated in Fig. 1.3.[17] In these studies the relationship between CHD risk and cholesterol level is curvilinear. This was reinforced by the much larger MRFIT study, which was able to show that the relationship between cholesterol and CHD was not one of threshold, i.e. there is a graded and continuous risk and

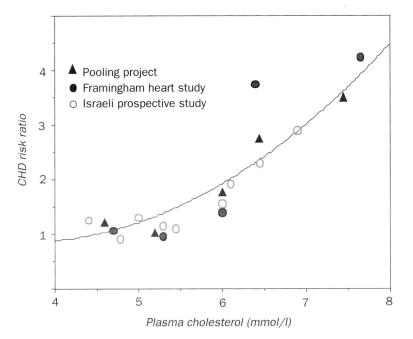

Fig. 1.3 Relation between plasma cholesterol level and relative risk of CHD in three prospective studies. (Adapted with permission from ref. 17.)

there is probably no cholesterol level which can be considered completely safe in terms of cardiovascular risk.[3]

There has been some concern over the risks of low cholesterol, as MRFIT demonstrated a J-shaped relationship between total cholesterol and total mortality. This increase in total mortality occurring at cholesterol levels below 4 mmol/l has been duplicated in other studies and it has been suggested that low cholesterol causes cancer. However, international comparative data do not support this hypothesis. For example, in Japan, where 90% of men have cholesterol levels below 4.4, the overall risk of cancer is no greater than that experienced by American or Northern European men.[18] A more likely explanation is that a low plasma cholesterol concentration is an effect of cancer rather than a cause.

Concerns have also arisen with regard to low plasma cholesterol levels and stroke resulting from intracranial haemorrhage. This risk is small and, as suggested by Iso et al.,[19] is far outweighed by the cardiovascular risks (including thrombotic stroke) of raised plasma cholesterol levels.

Our discussion so far has centred on total cholesterol as a risk factor, but since 60–70% of plasma cholesterol is transported in the form of low-density lipoprotein (LDL), the effects of total cholesterol reflect the effects of LDL cholesterol.

HDL cholesterol

There is considerable evidence to support an inverse relationship between plasma high-density lipoprotein (HDL) and CHD risk. The British Regional Heart Study is one such source of evidence and their results concerning HDL and CHD risk are shown in Fig. 1.4.[20] This inverse relationship exists for both men and women and is equally strong in patients with established heart disease as well as those who are asymptomatic. Pre-menopausal women have levels of HDL cholesterol that are 0.2–0.3 mmol/l higher than those of their male counterparts. After the menopause this difference diminishes with increasing age and may partly explain the relative protection of women from CHD.

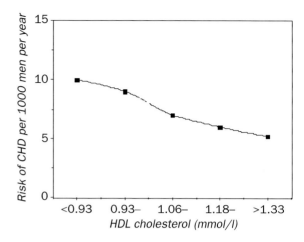

Fig. 1.4 Risk of CHD events according to concentration of HDL. (Adapted with permission from ref. 20.)

Plasma HDL is lowered by:

- smoking
- obesity
- physical inactivity.

Modification of these factors may reverse this HDL lowering effect. Diets containing high polyunsaturated fat levels have been shown to decrease LDL cholesterol while simultaneously lowering HDL cholesterol. However, it is possible to lower LDL cholesterol while maintaining HDL cholesterol levels by reducing saturated fat and substituting moderate amounts of monounsaturated and polyunsaturated fats in the diet.

The importance of HDL as a risk factor is related to LDL levels, and the ratio of total cholesterol to HDL cholesterol is a better predictor of CHD risk than either of the variables alone. A ratio of five or less appears to be desirable and is of particular importance when considering treatment options for patients whose cholesterol levels are in the 5–6.5 mmol/l range.

Lp(a)

This is an LDL-like lipoprotein whose plasma concentration is related to CHD risk.[21] It may be of importance only when total cholesterol levels are high. Its plasma level is genetically determined and these levels are resistant to most conventional lipid-lowering strategies. As yet it does not have a clear role in the assessment of CHD risk.

Triglyceride

The plasma triglyceride level is related to the risk of CHD. This effect is more marked in patients with raised plasma cholesterol levels. A raised triglyceride is also commonly associated with low HDL and increased levels of small, dense LDL, which is regarded as particularly atherogenic. Many subjects with hypertriglyceridaemia also produce increased levels of a particularly atherogenic type of LDL (small, dense LDL).

It has been noted by Assman et al.[22] that the combination of:

- hypertriglyceridaemia (plasma triglyceride >2.3 mmol/l)
- total cholesterol/HDL cholesterol ratio >5
- low HDL (<1.0 mmol/l men or 1.1 women) is a predictor of particularly high CHD risk.

Another condition associated with abnormal triglyceride levels is the 'insulin resistance syndrome'.[23] This consists of hypertriglyceridaemia, usually occurring with low HDL cholesterol levels, and may constitute an additional link between triglyceride and CHD.

ATHEROSCLEROSIS

Atherosclerosis is the most important underlying disease process in the industrialized world, leading to a variety of clinical manifestations, namely CHD, cerebrovascular disease and peripheral vascular disease. Atherosclerosis may be thought of as a focal, fibroproliferative, inflammatory response to endothelial injury. This 'response to injury' hypothesis for the pathogenesis of atherosclerosis was proposed by Ross.[24] There are other hypotheses that try to explain the complex pathogenesis of the atherosclerotic plaque but none have been so widely accepted as that of a normal repair process gone awry – where the healing process becomes the disease itself.

The term is derived from the Greek *athere* meaning porridge and *skleros* meaning hard. Together these terms aptly describe the pathological changes that take place inside affected blood vessels.

Atherosclerosis affects large and medium-sized arteries, producing changes in the intima and media of the vessel wall. The disease is not uniformly distributed throughout the arterial tree – some vessels, such as the internal mammary artery, are usually spared whereas the coronaries are highly susceptible. Veins are not affected unless they are subjected to arterial blood pressures, as is seen in the saphenous vein when used for coronary artery bypass grafting.

Atherosclerotic lesions develop throughout life and have been found in children[25] and in apparently healthy young men, such as soldiers killed in the Korean war.[26]

The significance of lipids in the development of atherosclerosis has long been recognized. As far back as 1845, the pathologist Vogel[27] observed the presence of cholesterol in atheromatous tissue and in 1913 Anitschkov[28] demonstrated experimentally the link between dietary cholesterol and atherosclerosis in rabbits. The more recent epidemiological evidence linking cholesterol and CHD has been discussed above.

The normal arterial wall

Before considering the pathophysiology of atherosclerosis it is necessary to remind ourselves of the normal arterial structure. The intima is the innermost layer of the vessel. It is composed of a single layer of endothelial cells, which have a number of important functions:

- forming a non-thrombogenic, non-adherent surface
- acting as a semi-permeable barrier
- synthesizing and releasing chemical regulators of vascular tone, growth factors and cytokines
- maintaining the basement membrane
- modifying lipoproteins as they cross into the artery wall.

The media, or middle layer, is made up of vascular smooth muscle cells. They are separated from the intima by the internal elastic membrane and from the adventitia by the external elastic membrane. Vascular smooth muscle cells can exist in a contractile form or a synthetic form. They can only proliferate in the synthetic form but they can be induced to adopt this form by the action of cytokines and growth factors. Their functions include:

- regulating blood pressure and blood flow by producing vasodilatation or vasoconstriction
- synthesizing growth factors and cytokines
- synthesizing extracellular matrix proteins – collagen, elastin and proteoglycans.

The adventitia is the outermost layer, which contains the nerves and small blood vessels that supply the artery itself.

Endothelial injury

As mentioned above, endothelial injury is thought to be the primary event in atherogenesis but it is clear that gross changes, such as the loss of endothelial cells with exposure of the underlying matrix, do not necessarily occur at the sites of early lesions. Injury is a term that extends in meaning from cellular damage to more subtle effects such as loss of function. The arterial endothelium serves several key functions listed above. When endothelial cells are injured by exposure to mechanical trauma or other injurious agents such as viruses or toxins, one way that they manifest their dysfunction is to become sticky. Elegant scanning electron microscopy studies have revealed that injured endothelium allows the adherence of monocyte/macrophages and T lymphocytes.[24]

One of the principal forms of injury believed to initiate atherogenesis is increasingly thought to be mediated by lipoproteins. However, the main problem with the acceptance of this hypothesis has been that normal lipoproteins are unable to induce atherogenic changes *in vitro*. Although lipoproteins certainly do enter the subendothelial space of arteries, they are not phagocytosed by macrophages there, nor does their presence initiate any form of immune/inflammatory reaction.

A major breakthrough was made when it was recognized that when lipoproteins are chemically modified by oxidation their atherogenic potential is switched on.[29] In this state they are actively ingested by macrophages. These cells possess cell surface scavenger receptors and may even have a specific receptor for oxidized LDL (oxLDL). Unlike lipoprotein uptake mediated via the LDL receptor, uptake via these scavenger receptors is not down-regulated as the cell acquires sufficient lipids for its metabolic and synthetic needs. Instead, the ingestion of oxLDL goes on unchecked to the point where the macrophage is overladen by lipids and due to its vacuolated appearance is referred to as a foam cell. oxLDL is also chemotactic for monocytes and induces their transmigration across the arterial endothelium from the circulation into the subendothelial space. Perhaps attracted by the entrapped oxLDL, these cells invade the subendothelial space by squeezing between endothelial cells. This event has even been photographed both in hypercholesterolaemic non-human primate aortae and in human coronary arteries.[24] It is then that macrophages begin their terminal path towards foam cells by phagocytosing the modified lipoproteins.

Fatty streaks

The endothelial injury that initiates atherosclerosis may only be apparent microscopically. The first readily visible sign of the disease process is the appearance of fatty streaks. This term is applied to the small, flat, yellow dots that are visible on gross inspection of the intimal surface of affected arteries. These streaks are the necessary first step in the process of atherosclerosis but do not always progress to mature lesions. They may remain static or even disappear. The fatty streak lesions may be the precursor of larger atherosclerotic plaques but they are viewed by most workers in the field as entirely reversible phenomena. This is evident from the work of Freedman et al., who examined the hearts of adolescents from populations who experience low levels of CHD and found they demonstrated a similar

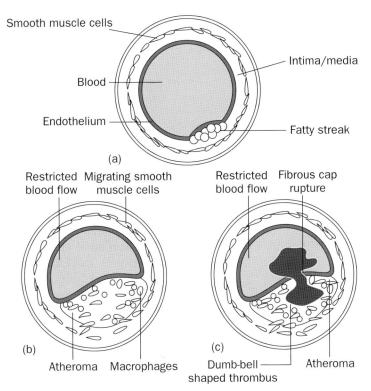

Fig. 1.5 (a) Development of a fatty streak. (b) The development of a raised fibrolipid plaque. (c) Diagram of a histological cross-section of a major atheromatous plaque rupture. The plaque has a large defect in the fibrous cap, through which a dumb-bell-shaped mass of thrombus has formed, part being within the plaque and part virtually occluding the lumen. (Adapted with permission from ref. 31.)

number of fatty streaks to those young people from population groups with high levels of CHD.[30] It is also believed that new fatty streaks are continually forming throughout adult life.

Fatty streaks are the result of an accumulation of lipid-filled macrophages, called foam cells, in the intima. This is illustrated in Fig. 1.5.

Raised fibrolipid plaque

The progression of the fatty streak to the characteristic atherosclerotic plaque takes place in two stages:

- Firstly, the foam cells, engorged with lipid, begin to die and rupture in the centre of the fatty streak. Release of their cytoplasmic contents leads to the presence of extracellular lipids and the release of many chemical mediators of the inflammatory response.
- Secondly, the vascular smooth muscle cells migrate and proliferate. Smooth muscle cells push into the lipid-rich plaque, where they divide and begin to elaborate a connective tissue matrix.

The increase in cell numbers and the laying down of collagenous matrix both serve to increase the bulk of the plaque, which now protrudes into the artery lumen and is referred to as a raised fibrolipid or advanced plaque (see Fig. 1.5). These plaques appear yellow or white on gross examination because their core predominantly contains lipids or connective tissue. Such plaques are difficult to age but necropsy studies suggest that they take 10–15 years to develop.

Plaque rupture and thrombosis

The dangers of the atheromatous plaque lie in its size and its tendency to fissure and ulcerate. The final pathway to a major clinical event, such as an acute myocardial infarction, is not clear but haemorrhage into an atheromatous plaque, rupture or fissuring of a plaque or thrombosis on the surface of a plaque are mechanisms that are likely to be involved (see Fig. 1.5).

In studies by Davies and Thomas, the role of the atheromatous plaque and thrombus formation were clarified in patients with acute coronary syndromes.[31] Thrombus formation was seen as a rapidly changing, dynamic process and of major importance in these conditions.

In fatal cases of myocardial infarction, postmortem studies have shown that coronary thrombi in nearly all cases are related to the fissuring of the atheromatous plaque. The factors that determine whether thrombus does occur within the lumen are partially local, including:

- the size and geometry of the intimal tear
- whether lipid is extruded into the lumen itself
- the degree of stenosis
- the blood flow rate at the site.

Systemic factors such as the thrombotic or thrombolytic potential at the time will also play a part. Not all plaque fissuring will result in these dire consequences, as the plaque may restabilize and heal over although the healed plaque will often be larger than before.

Regression of the plaque

The concept of therapeutic intervention producing reversal or regression of atherosclerotic lesions originated in the 1940s. Post-mortem examinations of individuals who had suffered great weight losses prior to their death revealed that the extent of plaque development in the aorta and coronary arteries was much less than expected. In response to these findings, many studies have been conducted to confirm and evaluate these observations.

Recently, the results from randomized, controlled clinical studies using different treatments for lowering cholesterol have been reported. In the Familial Atherosclerosis Treatment Study, middle-aged men who had moderately elevated LDL, a family history of CHD and angiographic evidence of CHD had reduced frequency of progression of coronary lesions and increased frequency of regression and reduced incidence of CHD events if prescribed lipid-lowering therapy.[32]

In the Lifestyle Heart Trial, the objective was to determine if lifestyle changes in diet, exercise, smoking and stress could affect coronary atherosclerosis.[33] Patients with angiographically documented CHD were assigned to an experimental group or to a usual care control group. The experimental group patients were prescribed a regimen that included a low-fat vegetarian diet, smoking cessation, stress management training, moderate aerobic exercise and group support. After only a year, patients in the experimental group showed significant overall regression of coronary atherosclerosis in contrast to the control group, who, having made less comprehensive lifestyle changes, showed significant overall progression of coronary atherosclerosis.

LIPOPROTEIN METABOLISM

Lipids and lipoproteins

A lipid is any substance that is insoluble in water but soluble in apolar solvents such as ether. In the body, lipids have a number of important functions, by providing:

- an energy source
- synthetic precursors, e.g. for hormone metabolism
- raw materials for cellular components, e.g. membranes.

In order to utilize these lipids, the body has developed a transportation system via the aqueous medium of the plasma. It has overcome the inherent difficulties of this by packaging lipids in lipoproteins.

Lipoproteins are multimolecular packages. Their hydrophobic, non-polar core of cholesteryl ester and triglyceride is surrounded by a surface layer of phospholipids, proteins and some free cholesterol. The phospholipids are arranged with their non-polar end pointing in towards the core while their polar end points outwards and is in contact with the aqueous environment. This is represented in Fig. 1.6.

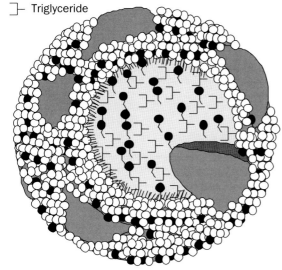

● Cholesteryl ester

▬ Apolipoprotein

● Free cholesterol

⊖ Phospholipid

⅂⊢ Triglyceride

Fig. 1.6 Diagram of a lipoprotein. This represents the basic structure of all lipoproteins although the proportion of the various components which make up the particle vary between lipoprotein classes, as do the types of proteins which are present.

Classification and function of the lipoproteins

The most widely used classification defines four main classes of lipoprotein on the basis of their density These are chylomicrons, very low-density lipoprotein (VLDL), LDL and HDL. These are shown in Table 1.3 together with a summary of their functions.

Apolipoproteins, enzymes and receptors

Apolipoproteins (apo) are the protein constituents of lipoproteins and have three main functions:

- They facilitate lipid transport by helping to make cholesteryl esters and triglyceride soluble through their interaction with phospholipids.
- They regulate the interaction of these lipids with the enzymes lecithin-cholesterol acyltransferase (LCAT), lipoprotein lipase (LPL) and hepatic lipase.
- They bind to cell surface receptors.

There are five broad groups of apolipoproteins, apoA to apoE, but this is a very active area of research and new additions are frequently being made to the list. Since a major function of the apolipoproteins is in regulating enzymes and binding to receptors, it would be useful to examine these more closely.

Table 1.3 The plasma lipoproteins	
Lipoprotein	*Function*
Chylomicrons	Largest lipoprotein. Synthesized by gut after fatty meal. Main carrier of dietary lipid. Rapid clearance, undetectable after 12-hour fast
Very low-density lipoprotein (VLDL)	Similar in structure to chylomicrons but smaller. Synthesized in liver. Main carrier of endogenously produced triglyceride
Low-density lipoprotein (LDL)	Generated from VLDL in the circulation. Main carrier of cholesterol, accounting for 60–70% plasma cholesterol
High-density lipoprotein (HDL)	Smallest but most abundant. Protective function. Returns cholesterol to liver for excretion from peripheral tissues. Carries 20–30% of plasma cholesterol

Lipoprotein lipase (LPL)
This is a triglyceride lipase found principally in the capillaries of adipose tissue, skeletal and cardiac muscle, and is involved in the metabolism of chylomicrons. Women have relatively higher levels of LPL in adipose tissue (as opposed to skeletal muscle) than men and this correlates with their higher HDL cholesterol levels.

Hepatic lipase
This is also a triglyceride lipase but it is found on the hepatic endothelium and is thought to play an important role in the metabolism of the remnant particles which result from the action of lipoprotein lipase on VLDL and chylomicrons. Hepatic lipase is also thought to be involved in HDL metabolism.

Lecithin-cholesterol acyltransferase (LCAT)
This enzyme is produced by the liver but acts in the plasma to esterify cholesterol with fatty acids derived from lecithin.

LDL receptor
This is a single-chain transmembrane protein which recognizes apoB100 and apoE and thereby binds LDL and other apoB-containing lipoproteins. Its function is to ensure a constant supply of cholesterol throughout the body for cell membrane and steroid synthesis. Its discovery was a breakthrough as it provided a mechanism for understanding the genetic disease familial hypercholesterolaemia.[34]

HMG-CoA reductase
All cells that can synthesize cholesterol express this glycoprotein in their endoplasmic reticulum. It is found especially in the liver, small intestine, adrenal glands and gonads. The enzyme catalyses the conversion of the simple molecule 3-hydroxy-3-methylglutaryl coenzyme A (HMG-CoA) to mevalonic acid, in the endogenous cholesterol pathway. Its activity is downregulated by the end-product cholesterol and its metabolites such as 26-hydroxycholesterol. Therefore, endogenous cholesterol synthesis is decreased by exposing cells to lipoproteins such as LDL, which facilitate delivery of exogenous cholesterol to the cell.

Cholesterol homeostasis is thus ensured by the co-ordinated interaction of LDL receptor expression and HMG-CoA reductase activity. Pharmacological agents that block endogenous cholesterol synthesis stimulate LDL receptor activity, thereby causing a reduction in plasma levels of LDL cholesterol.

Exogenous lipoprotein metabolism

Human lipoprotein metabolism may be thought of as three interconnected and interdependent cycles. All three pathways are centred on the liver, which is the key organ in lipoprotein metabolism although all organs in the body are in some way involved, either as consumers or producers of the plasma lipoproteins and the regulatory factors that control their metabolism.

We shall consider firstly the exogenous lipid pathway which deals with the transport and utilization of dietary lipids. Each day we eat about 0.5 g of cholesterol and about 100 g of triglyceride. Under normal circumstances, most dietary triglyceride is absorbed but only about half of the dietary cholesterol is taken up, the remainder being lost in faeces.[35]

Dietary lipids are packaged into large chylomicrons within the intestinal mucosal cells. These are then secreted into lacteals within the wall of the small bowel, where they travel to the bloodstream via the thoracic duct. In the circulation their triglyceride is gradually removed by the action of the enzyme LPL. As the chylomicron loses its triglyceride core the particle becomes smaller and deflated with folds of redundant surface material. These particles, now called chylomicron remnants, are taken up by the liver, where their cholesterol content may be used for cell membrane synthesis, as the building blocks for bile salts, or may be excreted into the bile. The liver provides the only route by which cholesterol leaves the body in significant amounts.

Endogenous lipoprotein metabolism

The endogenous pathway deals with the transport and utilization of lipids produced in the liver. Lipids synthesized in the liver have several fates.[35,36]

- Cholesterol and triglyceride are exported in VLDL, which is the major vehicle for endogenous triglyceride transport.
- Surplus lipid may be stored, temporarily, within the hepatocyte.
- Cholesterol may be eliminated into the bile, either unchanged or following oxidation to bile acids.[37] This enterohepatic circulation of bile acids may be interrupted by medical or surgical means with profound effects for hepatic lipid metabolism. Such therapeutic manoeuvres can therefore be used to advantage in the management of hypercholesterolaemia.

After secretion into the bloodstream the VLDL synthesized by the liver undergo the same form of delipidation as chylomicrons by the action of LPL. This results again in the formation of smaller triglyceride-poor particles, and the VLDL remnants are called intermediate-density lipoprotein (IDL). After further delipidation these particles become LDL. LDL may be removed from the circulation by the high-affinity LDL receptor route or by other less well-defined scavenger receptor routes.

Reverse cholesterol transport

This pathway serves to return cholesterol from the peripheral tissues to the liver where it can be excreted in the bile. The key lipoprotein in this cycle is the HDL particle. With the discovery that plasma HDL levels are associated with protection from CHD[38] came the concept that this lipoprotein acts as a vehicle to transport cholesterol from peripheral tissues to the liver. Some such mechanism is essential since cholesterol cannot be broken down to any significant extent in humans or animals and must therefore be excreted intact via its major organ of elimination, the liver. HDL begins as a lipid-deficient precursor and is transformed into a lipid-rich lipoprotein. It then transfers its cholesterol directly to the liver, or indirectly to other circulating lipoproteins, which then return it to the liver.

As stated above, these three pathways do not function independently but are closely interrelated, governing the complex process of cholesterol utilization by the body.

LABORATORY ASSESSMENT OF DYSLIPIDAEMIA

Lipid profiles: what to measure

The most common aberrant lipid profile linked with atherogenesis and an increased risk of vascular disease is an elevated plasma LDL cholesterol level, but increasingly it is being recognized that individuals with low plasma HDL cholesterol and hypertriglyceridaemia are also at increased risk.

The units used for cholesterol and triglyceride are either mg/dl or mmol/l The conversion factors for these are:

$$Cholesterol\ mg/dl = mmol/l \times 38.67$$
$$Triglyceride\ mg/dl = mmol/l \times 88.57$$

Blood for lipid analysis may be collected into plain containers, which will give the serum level, or into containers with the anticoagulant, ethylenediamine tetraacetic acid (EDTA), which will allow plasma levels to be measured. Tubes containing heparin should not be used for lipid analyses. Some laboratories prefer to measure plasma levels, the advantage being that the EDTA enhances lipoprotein stability during storage; furthermore the buffy white coats of the white cells can be kept for subsequent DNA analysis.

A range of different analyses may be performed on the blood sample by the biochemistry laboratory, increasing in complexity from a simple total cholesterol measurement to a full lipoprotein analysis and perhaps even DNA analysis.

Most commonly a total cholesterol and triglyceride will be measured and in addition an HDL cholesterol may be provided. As well as these measured values, the LDL cholesterol may be calculated, provided these three other parameters are known. This is done by using the Friedewald formula:

Friedewald formula

LDL cholesterol (mmol/l) = total cholesterol − HDL cholesterol − [0.45 × triglyceride (mmol/l)]

The accuracy with which the LDL cholesterol is estimated using this formula is relatively poor due to the summation of different analytical errors but it does provide some useful information. It is important to note, however, that the Friedewald formula should not be used if the plasma triglyceride concentration is greater than 4.0 mmol/l.

The most comprehensive (and expensive) analysis is known as a beta quantification, where the total cholesterol, triglyceride, VLDL cholesterol, LDL cholesterol and HDL cholesterol will be provided. In most circumstances this full lipoprotein profile is not necessary and patients can be adequately managed with a total cholesterol, triglyceride and HDL cholesterol with or without a calculated LDL.

Timing of samples: when to measure

If a total cholesterol measurement is all that is required, then fasting is not necessary. For plasma triglyceride or lipoprotein cholesterol levels to be measured accurately, the patient should have been instructed to fast. It is very important to give explicit instructions regarding fasting to ensure that the patient neither eats nor drinks anything, except water, for 12 hours prior to the blood sampling.

As with all blood chemistries, there are a number of factors that affect the results of plasma lipid levels reported from the biochemistry laboratory:

- biological variation, which might give different results from one day to the next

- analytical imprecision, which may produce slightly different values even if the same blood sample is measured in the same laboratory but on different days.

Because of these sources of variation, it is important to obtain more than one sample for lipid analysis before any action is taken. International guidelines often recommend that at least three measurements should be carried out on three separate samples before management decision are made.[39]

Interpretation of results

There is probably no level of cholesterol below which an individual is completely safe from the development of vascular disease. However, it is still useful to have an idea of the statistically normal range of lipid measurements that occur in the population, as the people who exist at the upper limit of these distributions are prime candidates for risk factor modification. The results obtained by the Lipid Research Council in their prevalence study to ascertain the distribution of various lipid and lipoprotein levels are shown in Tables 1.4 and 1.5.[40] The influences of sex and age are clearly demonstrated in these tables.

CLINICAL DISORDERS OF LIPID METABOLISM

Disorders of lipoprotein metabolism are among the commonest metabolic diseases seen in clinical practice. In addition to their important role in the development of CHD, some lipid disorders have other consequences, most notably acute pancreatitis, failure to thrive in infants, neurological disorders and the development of cataracts. There is currently no satisfactory comprehensive classification of dyslipidaemia. The simplest means of dividing them is into primary and secondary disorders.

Primary hyperlipidaemia

The primary hyperlipidaemias are the result of underlying metabolic defects, which have a genetic basis. Not all of the primary forms have been fully characterized at a molecular level.

Table 1.4   Plasma lipid levels in American white males (mmol/l)

Total cholesterol

Age	Mean	5–95 percentiles
0–19	4.0	3.0–5.2
20–24	4.3	3.2–5.4
25–29	4.7	3.5–6.3
30–34	4.9	3.6–6.6
35–39	5.2	3.7–7.0
40–44	5.3	3.9–7.0
45–69	5.6	4.0–7.1
70+	5.3	3.9–7.0

Triglyceride

Age	Mean	5–95 percentiles
0–9	0.6	0.3–1.1
10–14	0.7	0.3–1.4
15–19	0.9	0.4–1.6
20–24	1.1	0.5–2.3
25–29	1.3	0.5–2.8
30–34	1.5	0.5–3.0
35–39	1.7	0.6–3.6
40–54	1.7	0.6–3.6
55–64	1.6	0.6–3.3
65+	1.5	0.6–2.9

Adapted with permission from ref. 40.

Table 1.5   Plasma lipid levels in American white females (mmol/l)

Total cholesterol

Age	Mean	5–95 percentiles
0–19	4.1	2.8–5.2
20–24	4.4	2.9–5.5
25–34	4.5	3.3–6.1
35–39	4.8	3.6–6.3
40–44	5.0	3.7–6.6
45–49	5.3	3.9–6.7
50–54	5.7	4.2–7.3
55+	5.9	4.4–7.6

Triglyceride

Age	Mean	5–95 percentiles
0–9	0.7	0.4–1.2
10–19	0.8	0.4–1.5
20–34	1.0	0.4–1.9
35–39	1.1	0.4–2.2
40–44	1.2	0.5–2.4
45–49	1.2	0.5–2.6
50–54	1.3	0.6–2.7
55–64	1.4	0.6–2.8
65+	1.5	0.7–2.7

Adapted with permission from ref. 40.

Secondary hyperlipidaemia

Hyperlipidaemia is a well-recognized consequence of a number of conditions and in some cases may be the presenting feature. Most patients presenting with hyperlipidaemia will have the secondary type, the most common cause being dietary. Of course, patients with secondary hyperlipidaemia may also have an underlying genetic defect and primary hyperlipidaemia may be exacerbated by secondary causes.

Secondary hyperlipidaemia may be encountered in diabetes mellitus,[41,42] obesity,[43] nephritic syndrome,[44] post renal transplantation,[45] alcohol abuse and hypothyroidism.[46] A number of commonly prescribed drugs may also affect the lipid profile. Sex steroids[47] are well known to influence lipid levels but thiazide diuretics, beta-blockers and immunosup-pressants may result in a variety of lipid changes.

CLASSIfiCATION OF DYSLIPIDAEMIA

The Fredrickson or World Health Organization classification is the most widely accepted. This classification, shown in Table 1.6, relies on the findings of analysis of the patient's plasma, rather than genetics. It is therefore a phenotypic rather than genotypic classification. This has a number of consequences. Patients with the same underlying genetic defect may fall into different groups or may change grouping as their disease progresses or is treated. However, the major advantage of using this classification is that it is very widely known and gives some guidance to management. It is also important to realize that the six different classes of hyper-lipoproteinaemia defined in the Fredrickson

Table 1.6   Fredrickson (WHO) classification of hyperlipoproteinaemia

	Normal	Type I	Type IIa	Type IIb	Type III	Type IV	Type V
Lipoprotein	N	+CM	+LDL	+LDL +VLDL	+IDL	+VLDL	+CM +VLDL
Total cholesterol	N	N or +	+	+	+	N or +	N or +
Triglyceride	N	++	N	+	+	+	++
LDL cholesterol	N	N or −	+	+	N or −	N	N

CM, chylomicrons; N, normal; +, increased; −, decreased.
This system is based on the appearance of a fasting plasma sample after standing for 12 hours at 4°C and analysis of its cholesterol and triglyceride content

classification are not equally common in the population. Types I and V are rare, while types IIa, IIb and IV are very common. Type III hyperlipoproteinaemia, also known as familial dyslipoproteinaemia, is intermediate in frequency, occurring in about one in 5000 of the population.

Genetic classifications have been attempted but are becoming increasingly complex as different mutations are discovered. Some of the recognized genetic causes of hyperlipidaemia are shown below in Table 1.7. Until the advent of gene therapy and/or specific substitution therapy, genetic classifications, while biologically sound, are unlikely to prove very useful in clinical practice.

CONCLUSION

There is clearly an impressive portfolio of epidemiological evidence to support the role of hyperlipidaemia as an independent risk factor for atherosclerotic vascular disease. In recent years there have been further complementary studies, which have proven the lipid hypothesis. These studies, utilizing powerful lipid-lowering drugs, have consistently shown that changing the lipid profile has an impressive beneficial effect on the risk of an individual suffering from the clinical consequences of atherosclerotic disease. These large clinical studies have used the statins. The remainder of this book will focus on the discovery, pharmacology and clinical utility of this group of drugs.

Table 1.7   Some examples of specific genetic causes of hyperlipidaemia

Disease	Genetic defect	Fredrickson	Risk
Familial hypercholesterolaemia	Reduced numbers of functional LDL receptors	IIa or IIb	Increased risk of CHD
Familial hypertriglyceridaemia	Possibly single gene defect	IV or V	? Increased risk of CHD
Familial combined hyperlipidaemia	Possibly single gene defect	IIa, IIb, IV or V	? Increased risk of CHD
Lipoprotein lipase deficiency	Reduced levels of functional lipoprotein lipase	I	Increased risk of pancreatitis

REFERENCES

1. Murray CJL, Lopez AD. Mortality by cause for eight regions of the world. Global Burden of Disease Study. *Lancet* 1997; **349**: 1269–76.
2. Kannel WB, Castelli W, Gordon T et al. Serum cholesterol lipoproteins and risk of coronary heart disease: the Framingham Study. *Ann Intern Med* 1971; **74**: 1–12.
3. Stamler J, Wentworth D, Neaton JD. Is relationship between serum cholesterol and risk of premature death from coronary heart disease continuous and graded? *JAMA* 1986; **256**: 2823–8.
4. Bartechi CE, MacKenzie TD, Schrier RW. The human costs of tobacco use (first of two parts). *N Engl J Med* 1994; **330**: 907–12.
5. MacKenzie TD, Bartechi CE, Schrier RW. The human costs of tobacco use (second of two parts). *N Engl J Med* 1994; **330**: 975–80.
6. Wilhelmsen L. Coronary heart disease: epidemiology of smoking and intervention studies of smoking. *Am Heart J* 1988; **115**: 242–249.
7. Manson JE, Tosteson H, Ridker PM et al. The primary prevention of myocardial infarction. *N Engl J Med* 1992; **326**: 1406–16.
8. Kawachi J, Colditz GA, Stampfer MJ et al. Smoking cessation in relation to total mortality rates in women. *Ann Intern Med* 1993; **119**: 992–1000.
9. Hammond EC, Garfinkel L. Coronary heart disease, stroke and aortic aneurysm: factors in etiology. *Arch Environ Health* 1969; **19**: 167–82.
10. Stamler R, Stamler Y, Grimm R et al. Nutritional therapy for high blood pressure. Final report of a four year randomized controlled trial. The Hypertension Control Program. *JAMA* 1987; **257**: 1484–91.
11. Collins R, Peto R, MacMahon S et al. Blood pressure, stroke and coronary heart disease. Part 2. Short term reductions in blood pressure: overview of randomised drug trials in their epidemiological context. *Lancet* 1990; **335**: 827–38.
12. The ALLHAT Officers and Coordinators for the ALLHAT Collaborative Research Group. Major outcomes in high-risk hypertensive patients randomised to angiotensin-converting enzyme inhibitor or calcium channel blocker vs diuretic: the Antihypertensive and Lipid-lowering Treatment to Prevent Heart Attack Trial (ALLHAT). *JAMA* 2002; **288**: 2981–97.
13. Simons LA. Interrelations of lipids and lipoproteins with coronary artery disease mortality in 19 countries. *Am J Cardiol* 1986; **57** (Suppl G): 5–10.
14. Marmot MG, Syme SL, Kagan A et al. Epidemiologic studies of coronary heart disease and stroke in Japanese men living in Japan, Hawaii and California: prevalence of coronary and hypertensive heart disease and associated risk factors. *Am J Epidemiol* 1975; **102**: 514–25.
15. Solberg LA, Strong JP. Risk factors and atherosclerotic lesions: a review of autopsy studies. *Arteriosclerosis* 1983; **3**: 187–98.
16. Keys A. *Seven Countries: A Multivariate Analysis of Death and Coronary Heart Disease.* Cambridge, Massachusetts: Harvard University Press, 1980.
17. Grundy SM. Cholesterol and heart disease: a new era. *JAMA* 1986; **256**: 2849–58.
18. Katan MB. Effects of cholesterol lowering on the risk for cancer and other non-cardiovascular diseases. *Atherosclerosis* 1986; **7**: 657–61.
19. Iso H, Jacobs DR, Wentworth D et al. Serum cholesterol levels and six year mortality from stroke in 350,977 men screening for the Multiple Risk Factor Intervention Trial. *N Engl J Med* 1989; **320**: 904–10.
20. Gaw A, Hobbs HH. Molecular genetics of Lp(a) – new pieces to the puzzle. *Curr Opin Lipidol* 1994; **5**: 149–55.
21. Pocock SJ, Shaper AG, Phillips AN. Concentrations of high density lipoprotein cholesterol, triglycerides and total cholesterol in ischaemic heart disease. *BMJ* 1989; **298**: 998–1002.
22. Assman G, Schulte H. Relation of high density lipoprotein cholesterol and triglyceride to incidence of atherosclerosis coronary artery disease (the PROCAM experience). *Am J Cardiol* 1992; **70**: 733–7.
23. Reaven GM. Banting Lecture 1988. Role of insulin resistance in human disease. *Diabetes* 1988; **37**: 1595–607.
24. Ross R. The pathogenesis of atherosclerosis: a perspective for the 1990s. *Nature* 1993; **362**: 801–9.
25. Pathological Determinants of Atherosclerosis in Youth (PDAY) Research Group. Natural history of aortic and coronary atherosclerotic lesions in youth. Findings from the PDAY study. *Arterioscler Thromb* 1993; **13**: 1291–8.
26. Enos WF, Holmes RH, Beyer J. Coronary disease among United States soldiers killed in action in Korea. *JAMA* 1953; **152**: 1090–3.
27. Vogel J. *Patholog. Anat. Des menschlichen Korpers,* Leipzig. (*The Pathological Anatomy of the Human Body.*) London: H. Balliere, 1845.

28. Anitschkov N. Uber die Veranderungen der Kaninchenaorta bei experimenteller Cholesterinsteatose. *Beitrage zur pathologisten Anatomie und zur allgemeinen Pathologie* 1913; **56**: 379–404.

29. Steinberg D, Parthasarathy S, Carew TE et al. Beyond cholesterol: modifications of low density lipoprotein that increase its atherogenicity. *N Engl J Med* 1989; **320**: 915–24.

30. Freedman DS, Newman WP 3rd, Tracy RE et al. Black–white differences in aortic fatty streaks in adolescence and early adulthood: the Bogalusa Heart Study. *Circulation* 1989; **77**: 856–64.

31. Davies MJ, Thomas AC. Plaque fissuring – the cause of acute myocardial infarction, sudden death, and crescendo angina. *Br Heart J* 1985; **53**: 363–73.

32. Brown G, Albers JJ, Fisher LD et al. Regression of coronary artery disease as a result of intensive lipid-lowering in men with high levels of apolipoprotein B. *N Engl J Med* 1990; **323**: 1289–98.

33. Ornish D, Brown SE, Scherwitz LW et al. Can lifestyle changes reverse coronary heart disease? The Lifestyles Heart Trial. *Lancet* 1990; **336**: 129–33.

34. Brown MS, Goldstein JL. The LDL receptor. In: Gallo LL, ed. *Cardiovascular Disease*. New York: Plenum Press, 1987: 87–91.

35. Norum KR, Berg T, Helgerud P, Drevon CA. Transport of cholesterol. *Physiol Rev* 1983; **63**: 1343–97.

36. Packard CJ, Shepherd J. Cholesterol 7α hydroxylase: involvement in hepatobiliary axis and regulation of plasma lipoprotein levels. In: Fears R, Sabine JR, eds. *Cholesterol 7α Hydroxylase*. Boca Raton, Florida: CRC Press, 1986: 147–65.

37. Dietschy JM, Wilson JD. Regulation of cholesterol metabolism. *N Engl J Med* 1970: **282**: 1128–38.

38. Gordon DJ, Probstfield JL, Garrison RJ et al. High-density lipoprotein cholesterol and cardiovascular disease. Four prospective American studies. *Circulation* 1989; **79**: 8–15.

39. Pyörälä K, de Backer G, Graham I et al. (1994) Prevention of coronary heart disease in clinical practice. Recommendations of the Task Force of the European Society of Cardiology, European Atherosclerosis Society and European Society of Hypertension. *Eur Heart J* 1994; **15**: 1300–31.

40. Rifkind BM, Segal P. Lipid research clinics program reference values for hyperlipidemia and hypolipidemia. *JAMA* 1983; **250**: 1869–72.

41. Howard BV. Lipoprotein metabolism in diabetes mellitus. *J Lipid Res* 1987; **28**: 613–28.

42. Steiner G. Diabetes and atherosclerosis: an overview. *Diabetes* 1981; **30** (Suppl 2): 1–7.

43. Angel A, Roncari DAK. (1978) Medical complications of obesity. *Can Med Assoc J* 1978; **119**: 1408–11.

44. Jungst D, Caselmann WH, Kutschera P, Weisweiler P. Relation of hyperlipidemia in serum and loss of high density lipoproteins in urine in the nephrotic syndrome. *Clin Chim Acta* 1987; **168**: 159–67.

45. Nicholls AJ, Cumming AM, Catto GRD et al. Lipid relationships in dialysis and renal transplant patients. *Q J Med* 1981; **50**: 149–60.

46. Series JJ, Biggart EM, O'Reilly DStJ et al. Thyroid dysfunction and hypercholesterolemia in the general population of Glasgow, Scotland. *Clin Chim Acta* 1988; **172**: 217–22.

47. Wallace RB, Hoover J, Barrett-Connor E et al. Altered plasma lipid and lipoprotein levels associated with oral contraceptive and oestrogen use. *Lancet* 1985; **ii**: 111–15.

2

Lipid control in the pre-statin era

William B Kannel and Peter WF Wilson

INTRODUCTION

Incontrovertible evidence indicates that dyslipidaemia is intimately involved in atherogenesis and that correcting disordered lipid metabolism slows progression of lesions, stabilizes them and reduces coronary morbidity and mortality.[1,2] The mechanisms of lipid-induced atherogenesis are now better understood, involving oxidative modification of low-density lipoprotein (LDL) cholesterol, small-dense LDL, reverse cholesterol transport in high-density lipoprotein (HDL) and platelet activation.[3–6] Modification of diet, weight control, exercise and a number of pharmaceutical agents can interfere with various elements of this atherogenic process. Currently available agents include statins, fibric acid derivatives, resins that sequester cholesterol in the bowel, antioxidants and niacin. Rapid, convenient and economical techniques are currently available for measuring blood lipids, and guidelines have been promulgated for the evaluation and treatment of dyslipidaemia.[1] However, it is still not determined whether therapy tailored to the pattern of dyslipidaemia is more efficacious than therapy focused primarily on lowering LDL cholesterol.

The positive relationship of serum total and LDL cholesterol and inverse relationship of HDL cholesterol to the rate of development of coronary disease is well established by numerous prospective epidemiological investigations.[1,6–9] Large-scale controlled trials have consistently shown that lowering serum total and LDL cholesterol in otherwise healthy adults can reduce the incidence of initial coronary events.[1,2] Few trials specifically examined the efficacy of raising HDL cholesterol or lowering triglycerides but subgroup analysis of existing trials suggested that risk reduction is also related to the degree to which HDL cholesterol is raised and triglyceride is lowered.[10,11] One recent trial has shown benefit for secondary coronary heart disease prevention of raising reduced HDL cholesterol (and lowering the accompanying triglyceride) where these were the primary lipid abnormalies.[11] Many, but not all, investigations found that the serum total cholesterol is an indicator of the likelihood of recurrent coronary events.[12–16] Nevertheless, pre-statin trials conducted in middle-aged men with coronary disease did show that lowering lipids reduces coronary events and mortality and slows progression of atherosclerotic lesions.[17–19] Reductions in overt coronary events and mortality achieved exceeded expectations based on the amount of regression of lesions observed, suggesting that therapy of dyslipidaemia may also stabilize lesions.

PREVALENCE OF DYSLIPIDAEMIA

The range of serum cholesterol, and LDL cholesterol in particular, varies widely both in the general population and in patients who develop coronary disease (Fig. 2.1). Framingham Study data indicate that the prevalence of hypercholesterolaemia in the range recommended for evaluation or treatment by current guidelines is substantial at all ages and in both sexes (Table 2.1). The prevalence of cholesterol values characterized as definitely elevated (>240 mg/dl) is about 30–45%. About half of the original

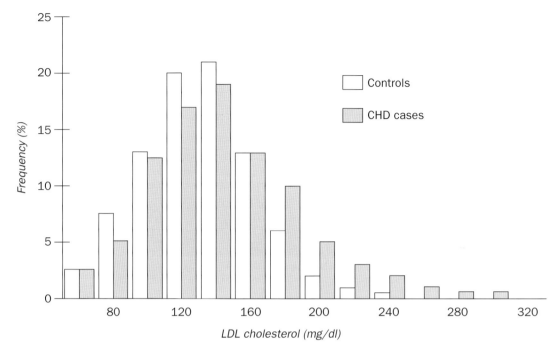

Fig. 2.1 LDL cholesterol distribution in cases of coronary heart disease and controls. (Adapted with permission from ref. 20.)

Table 2.1   Prevalence of mild and definite hypercholesterolaemia in the general population by age and sex: Framingham Study

	Percent prevalence			
	Mild		Definite	
	(200–239 mg/dl)		(>240 mg/dl)	
	(5.2–6.2 mmol/l)		(>6.2 mmol/l)	
Age (yrs)	**Men**	**Women**	**Men**	**Women**
35–44	37	37	38	24
45–54	39	35	44	50
55–64	39	29	44	50
65–74	40	29	34	61
75–84	41	35	19	47
85–94	32	41	11	21

cohort would be eligible for treatment based on their serum total cholesterol values alone or in combination with other risk factors. In the offspring cohort, cholesterol levels were found to be substantially lower at all ages, with only 20% of men and women aged 30–69 years having cholesterol values >240 mg/dl (6.21 mmol/l).[20] In this offspring sample LDL cholesterol >160 mg/dl (4.14 mmol/l) occurred in about 20% of men and 22% of women.

Table 2.2   Mean serum cholesterol of persons developing coronary heart disease in the Framingham Study by decade (1950s–1980s)

| Decade | Average cholesterol level | |
	Men	Women
1950s	246 mg/dl	281 mg/dl
	6.4 mmol/l	7.3 mmol/l
1960s	243 mg/dl	246 mg/dl
	6.3 mmol/l	6.4 mmol/l
1970s	229 mg/dl	244 mmol/l
	5.9 mmol/l	6.3 mmol/l
1980s	228 mg/dl	248 mg/dl
	5.9 mmol/l	6.4 mmol/l

The prevalence of such abnormal cholesterol values among persons who sustained myocardial infarctions was about 50% overall: 66% of women and 35–52% of men, in whom the prevalence of hypercholesterolaemia decreased in advanced age. Although the risk of coronary disease is distinctly greater in persons with such high cholesterol values, it is important to recognize that 20% of myocardial infarctions in the Framingham Study occurred in persons with cholesterol values <200 mg/dl, which is considered safe.[20] Most of these low cholesterol patients had HDL cholesterol levels <35 mg/dl, emphasizing the importance of the total/HDL cholesterol ratio as the determinant of the atherogenic potential of dyslipidaemia. The risk of coronary disease has been shown to increase with the ratio even in persons with serum total cholesterol values below 240 mg/dl (6.2 mmol/l).[20] The average total and LDL cholesterol at which coronary events occurred in the Framingham Study were well below those recommended for treatment in men and barely above them in women.[21] The average serum total cholesterol at which coronary disease occurs diminishes with advancing age. Assessment of the average cholesterol at which coronary events occurred in the Framingham

Study in the 1950s to the 1980s revealed a steady decline, largely reflecting the ageing of the cohort and the declining average cholesterol of the general population (Table 2.2).

NUTRITIONAL COUNSELLING

In the pre-statin era there were many studies that attempted to demonstrate the utility of controlling blood lipids with dietary measures. There is ample evidence that a diet consisting of too much fat, cholesterol and calories and too little fibre is the major determinant of the level of blood lipids in the general population.[22] The decline of average total cholesterol value in the general population over the past five decades is almost certainly a consequence of changes in the saturated fat and cholesterol intake in the national diet of the USA.[22,23] Migrants from low to high coronary incidence parts of the world experience a rise in their cholesterol values and along with it an increase in their coronary mortality rate.[24] Thus, for the general population, attention to nutrition is the best means for improving the population burden of atherogenic dyslipidaemia. The required alteration in the national diet is feasible, and even small shifts in the population's blood lipid distribution can produce a substantial impact on coronary mortality. However, it is doubtful that a dietary approach is sufficiently efficacious for the high-risk coronary candidate with a major dyslipidaemia. Studies of the efficacy of nutrition counselling for controlling blood lipids that were undertaken showed unimpressive results.[25–27] These discouraging results should not be taken to indicate that a dietary approach to prevention of coronary disease is without merit, as alterations to the national diet appear to have had a significant impact on the prevalence of dyslipidaemia in the general population, and this in turn has been accompanied by a substantial reduction in coronary mortality.[22] NHANES surveys of the serum total cholesterol of the US population for 1979 to 1991 found that the average had declined, and that the prevalence of elevated cholesterol (>240 mg/dl) fell from 26% to 20% (Fig. 2.2). Also, in the Framingham Study, comparison of serum lipids

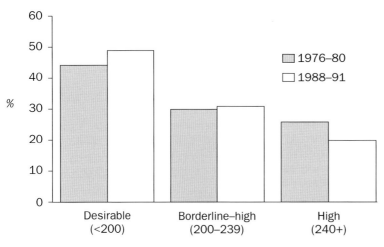

Fig. 2.2 Age-adjusted serum total cholesterol in a US population aged 20–74 years. NHANES II and NHANES III experience.

Table 2.3   Results of cholesterol reduction on lesion regression and progression in diet trials

| | | Percent of patients | | | |
| | | Progressing | | Regressing | |
Diet trial	Duration	Control	Treatment	Control	Treatment
LHT[1]	1 year	53%	18%	42%	82%
STARS	3 years	46%	15%	4%	38%
Heidelberg[2]	1 year	–	–	10%	21%
SCRIP[3]	4 years	39%	28%	6%	39%
STARS[4]	3 years	46%	12%	4%	33%

1. Also had smoking cessation, exercise and stress reduction.
2. Also had exercise.
3. Also had multiple drugs.
4. Also had cholestyramine.
Adapted with permission from ref. 62.

in the original cohort with their offspring of the same age 18 years later found that total and LDL cholesterol levels, but not HDL or triglycerides, were lower in the offspring. In both the Framingham Study and the USA in general, coronary death rates declined substantially during this period.[28] Furthermore, serum cholesterol values of coronary cases also declined from an average of 246 mg/dl to 228 mg/dl in men and from 281 mg/dl to 248 mg/dl in women (see Table 2.2).

However, the population-based nutrition-related benefits are not apparent for dietary treatment implemented for high-risk dyslipidaemic candidates for coronary disease.[29] Even intensive expert nutritional counselling was found to have a disappointingly small effect on blood lipids, and even this was probably unsustainable for any length of time. Nevertheless, regression and a slowing of the progression of lesions were shown to occur in several diet trials (Table 2.3). Diet therapy alone does not appear to be appropriate for the majority of patients who already have overt coronary heart disease, or for those who have more than mild dyslipidaemia. Diet therapy does not achieve the sizeable LDL reductions observed in statin trials (26–35%) that have been accompanied by substantial reductions in coronary events and all-cause mortality.[30,31] However, when drugs are used, their effects are greater when combined with diet, and nutritional counselling can reduce the amount of drug therapy required.

For the high-risk dyslipidaemic candidate for coronary disease, medication is usually required to substantially reduce the risk of coronary disease. In patients with moderate dyslipidaemia, the need for drug treatment can best be ascertained by using multivariate risk assessment. Risk profiles based on Framingham Study data, which are available from the American Heart Association, enable assessment of the conditional probability of a coronary event based on the total burden of major risk factors.[32] This makes it possible to better evaluate the need for aggressive drug therapy and avoid needlessly alarming or falsely reassuring the moderately dyslipidaemic patient.

WEIGHT CONTROL

Attempts to control dyslipidaemia by reducing weight in obese persons were also undertaken in the pre-statin era. This was logical because obesity and weight gain were shown to raise total cholesterol and triglycerides and to reduce HDL cholesterol. For this reason, weight control was advocated as a means for correcting dyslipidaemia.[33,34] Correction of abdominal obesity, which appears to be particularly disadvantageous as it promotes the insulin-resistance syndrome, still seems logical. Obesity-promoted insulin resistance induces lipoprotein lipase deficiency, elevated triglyceride, small-dense LDL and reduced HDL cholesterol, and is also often accompanied by glucose intolerance and hypertension.[35,36] About one-quarter of the dyslipidaemia in the general population may be a component of this insulin-resistance syndrome. Although weight reduction can significantly improve the lipid profile, it has proved difficult to sustain this advantage because of our inability to achieve *sustained* weight control in obese patients.

EXERCISE

Exercise was also promoted to combat dyslipidaemia because physical activity and fitness was associated with a reduced incidence of coronary disease in many epidemiological studies, and this protection was attributed to exercise-induced increase in HDL cholesterol and improvement in insulin resistance.[37] However, its influence on lipids is debated. The majority of longitudinal studies have shown that exercise improves the lipid profile but some studies have been negative.[38,39] Some believe the benefit is confined to obese men.[40] A recent well-conducted study reported that men who increased their regular exercise levels increased their HDL cholesterol by 4.76 mg/dl (0.1 mmol/l) and decreased their total/HDL ratio by 0.72 mg/dl (0.02 mmol/l) and their triglyceride by 18.2 mg/dl (0.2 mmol/l).[40]

ESTIMATING THE EFFICACY OF LIPID LOWERING

Meta-analysis of randomized trials evaluating the efficacy of cholesterol lowering prior to the WOSCOP and 4S statin trials demonstrated clear reductions in coronary mortality and events, but equivocal impacts on all-cause mortality.[41] This was either because drugs other than statins were used or because earlier trials evaluated treatments that had rather modest effects on cholesterol and LDL and were of only short duration. Also, trials selected for these meta-analyses varied and yielded somewhat conflicting conclusions about the size of the effect and the population subgroup to which the benefit might apply. Because these meta-analyses were done retrospectively there is an inherent *post-hoc* selection of studies to include and treatment questions to be answered. Also, only in recent statin trials has it been shown that lipid correction reduces the risk of stroke events.

REGRESSION TRIALS

Coronary angiographic findings were used as a surrogate endpoint in early lipid-lowering trials

Table 2.4   Weighted percent change in lipids achieved in angiographic trials

Therapy	LDL cholesterol	HDL cholesterol	Triglyceride
Diet–lifestyle	−16.3%	−6.3%	+22.6%
Resins	−23.6%	+2.4%	+12.4%
Statins	−30.7%	+6.9%	−14.6%
Combination drugs	−28.7%	+20.%	−24.9%
All drug trials	−29.6%	+10.8%	−15.9%
Partial ileal bypass	−37.3%	+2.4%	+21.6%
All trials	**−25.7%**	**+6.8%**	**−3.9%**

Diet trials: LHT; Heidelberg; STARS. Statin trials: CCAIT; MARS; MAAS; REGRESS. Resin trials: NHLBI; STARS. Combination drug trials: CLAS; FATS; SCOR; SCRIP; HARP. Surgery: POSCH.
Adapted with permission from ref. 42.

because this required a smaller sample to explore the efficacy of the lipid-correcting agents employed. However, the small number of patients within the trials limited the ability to examine the relation of the treatment-induced angiographic change to clinical outcomes. Fourteen such trials were compiled in a meta-analysis by Rossouw including the following studies: NHLBI; CLAS; POSCH; FATS; Lifestyle Heart; SCOR; STARS; SCRIP; CCAIT; Heidelberg; MARS; HARP; PLAC-1; and MAAS.[42] This meta-analysis confirmed that lowering LDL cholesterol inhibits progression and induces some regression with similar efficacy whether the intervention was by diet, drugs or surgery. Cardiac events were significantly reduced and trends for cardiovascular and all-cause mortality were favourable. Most individual randomized angiographic trials of blood lipid interventions showed favourable trends, with only three of 14 analysed failing to show a statistically significant benefit.[41] Interventions in these trials ranged from diet and lifestyle modification to drugs and surgery (Tables 2.3 and 2.4). There were differences in medications used singly and in combination, the amount of lipid modification achieved, baseline lipid values and the way the angiographic outcomes were classified. Only one study was designed with the power to examine treatment effects on cardiovascular event rates.[43] All interventions reduced LDL cholesterol (by an average of 26%) whereas

effects on HDL cholesterol and triglyceride varied by type of intervention (see Table 2.4).[44]

Meta-analysis of these trials indicated that treatment reduced the odds of progression by 49% and increased the odds of regression more than two-fold (Fig. 2.3).[42] Of those untreated, lesion progression was observed in 50%, and 9% appeared to regress, whereas in those actively treated only 34% showed progression and 18% regressed (Table 2.5). All types of intervention significantly reduced progression and the regression observed was similar for all interventions. Statins did not appear to be superior to diet, lifestyle, resins or other combinations of drugs for regressing lesions (see Fig. 2.3) despite the greater reduction of LDL cholesterol achieved. Compared with the modest improvement in angiographic findings, cardiovascular event rates were disproportionately reduced by 47%. Drugs, lifestyle and surgery were all favourable for both angiographic and clinical outcomes. Partial ileal bypass produced the most favourable angiographic outcome, which was probably attributable to longer duration of therapy.[43] Trials with higher baseline LDL cholesterol appeared to have a more favourable angiographic outcome. LDL lowering by 30 mg/dl (0.8 mmol/l) appeared to be sufficient to modify angiographic outcomes, with only modest additional gains from further LDL reductions.[42] The trials mainly achieved a slowing of lesion progres-

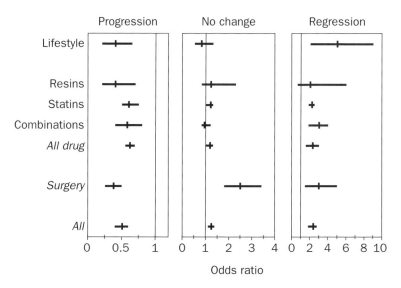

Fig. 2.3 Odds ratios for angiographically determined disease progression. No disease change and disease regression by type of intervention. (Adapted with permission from ref. 42.)

Table 2.5   Angiographic outcomes in trials by type of intervention

Intervention	Percent regressing		Percent progressing	
	Treated	Controls	Treated	Controls
Lifestyle	33%	9%	17%	39%
Resin	11%	6%	24%	46%
Statins	17%	10%	35%	47%
Drug combinations	23%	10%	35%	48%
All drugs	18%	10%	34%	47%
Surgery	13%	5%	37%	65%
All trials	**18%**	**9%**	**34%**	**50%**

Trials: LHT; STARS; NHLBI; CCAIT; MARS; MAAS; REGRESS; CLAS; FATS; SCOR; SCRIP; HARP; POSCH.
Adapted with permission from ref. 42.

sion; compared with controls, the rate of progression was halved. Despite the small differences in artery obstruction achieved, they appeared to prevent future clinical coronary events,[44] leading to the suspicion that treatment stabilizes small, dangerous lipid-rich lesions.[45,46] It appears from the meta-analysis of Rossouw that a certain minimum (perhaps 20%) reduction in LDL cholesterol is needed to slow coronary artery lesion progression and, however achieved, this produces similar benefits in retarding lesion progression.[42]

Trials that achieved a greater than 20% reduction in LDL cholesterol were particularly successful in demonstrating inhibition of progression. Probably due to small numbers, this benefit could not be conclusively shown for patients with LDL cholesterols less than 130 mg/dl (93.4 mmol/l) but was clear for higher LDL values. It appears that angiographic trials were useful for testing the efficacy of lipid interventions in reducing the size of lesions but it is interesting that the reduction in clinical events observed in these trials was far greater than would be expected from the haemodynamically trivial amount of lesion regression observed. These trials indicate that intensive treatment may substantially reduce cardio-

Table 2.6   Reduction in occurrence of clinical events in angiographic trials by type of therapy

| Trial | No. of patients | | % CV events | | Percent |
	Treated	Controls	Treated	Controls	Difference
Lifestyle	88	95	8%	12%	33%
Resins	83	81	8%	25%	68%
Statins	752	753	11%	17%	35%
Combination drugs	353	326	12%	17%	29%
All drug trials	1188	1160	11%	17%	35%
Ileal Bypass	333	301	30%	52%	42%
All trials	**1609**	**1532**	**15%**	**24%**	**37.5%**

Lifestyle trials: LHT; Heidelberg; STARS. Resin trials: NHLBI; STARS.
Statin trials: CCAIT; MARS; MAAS; REGRESS. Combination drug trials: CLAS;
FATS; SCOR; SCRIP; HARP. Surgical trial: POSCH.
Adapted with permision from ref. 42.

vascular events in as little as two years. Trial results are consistent with recommendations to reduce LDL cholesterol to below 100 mg/dl (2.6 mmol/l), although any amount of lowering appears to be beneficial.

CLINICAL ENDPOINT TRIALS

Numerous clinical trials testify to the efficacy of cholesterol lowering in reducing coronary heart disease incidence using a variety of interventions, including drugs, diet and lifestyle modification (Table 2.6). However, the early trials left some important issues unresolved. They varied as to whether they were single- or multifactor trials. Early trials of cholesterol lowering were hampered by their inability to succeed in reducing the serum total cholesterol by more than 5–15%. Nevertheless, meta-analysis of these trials showed a statistically significant benefit for cardiovascular and coronary morbidity but was unable to demonstrate more than borderline effects on all-cause mortality despite the reduction in coronary mortality, the leading cause of death.[47–49] However, some individual studies, such as the Stockholm Ischaemic Heart Disease Secondary Prevention Study and the Coronary Drug Project, utilizing niacin and clofibrate, reported statistically significant reductions in overall mortality.[17]

Effects were also unclear for women, the elderly and persons with lower coronary risk.[48]

These uncertainties appear to have been largely due to the modest cholesterol reductions achieved in the pre-statin trials, the short duration of these trials, their small sample sizes and the varied selection of different trials to be included in the meta-analyses.[49,50] A meta-analysis based on only six primary prevention trials suggested that treatment was associated with a significant increase in accidental and violent deaths, whereas a more comprehensive analysis based on 25 trials failed to show any significant increase in any kind of non-coronary mortality.[51] A recent meta-analysis now reports a significant *reduction* in total mortality in secondary prevention trials.[52] However, some conclude that such a benefit may be confined to those at very high risk for recurrent coronary disease.[48] The advent of trials using the more powerful LDL-lowering therapies such as the statins has provided more reliable estimates of the effects of treatment in the elderly, in diabetics, in women and in low-risk persons.[53]

The earlier regression trials were able to demonstrate modest regression of lesions but at first failed to appreciate the disproportionately great reduction in clinical coronary events they were achieving (Fig. 2.4). The early trials also did not specifically examine the influence of

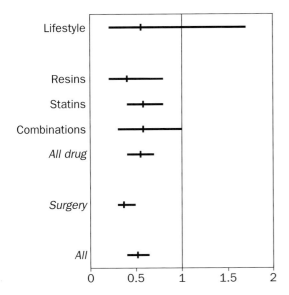

Fig. 2.4 Odds ratios for cardiovascular disease events by type of intervention and for all trials. (Adapted with permission from ref. 42.)

raising HDL cholesterol or lowering triglycerides. Further, the efficacy of therapy in the elderly and in women was not given enough attention.

The older secondary prevention trials failed to examine the benefits of treatment in those with the moderate cholesterol and LDL values that characterize most coronary cases. All the trials, past and present, have failed to directly address the issue of whether therapy tailored to the pattern of dyslipidaemia present is superior to indiscriminate therapy without regard to the pattern. Even with all these limitations, examination of the efficacy of treatment in these early studies indicate benefits that compare favourably for coronary mortality (20–25% declines) with those evaluating other medical interventions such as beta-blockade or aspirin. A meta-analysis by Rossouw including more recent trials confirms a highly significant 47% reduction in cardiovascular events with no obvious advantage of the more potent LDL-lowering properties of statins (see Fig. 2.4).

Data from the early trials suggest that fibrate and niacin treatment confer more benefit in those whose dyslipidaemia is characterized by elevated triglyceride and reduced HDL cholesterol,

whereas resins and, later on, statins might be more efficacious in dyslipidaemias that are predominantly characterized by elevated LDL cholesterol.[17,54] Probucol, a potent antioxidant, which had the disadvantage of reducing HDL cholesterol, proved unrewarding in earlier trials, and trials of vitamin E also proved inconclusive.[55]

A troublesome feature of the early studies was their inability to demonstrate a significant improvement in overall mortality despite a reduction in coronary events and deaths. An important consideration in examining this issue is the level of risk in the control group in the meta-analysis carried out to examine the mortality experience. It is important to adjust for this because the risk level is highly correlated with both the degree of cholesterol reduction and the total mortality, confounding the cholesterol–mortality relationship and analysis; adjusting for the risk level in the control group provided no statistically significant indication that fibrate trials had results inferior to other drug trials.[56]

Earlier trials suggested that there might be an increase in non-cardiovascular mortality or non-fatal disease. More recent meta-analysis of randomized cholesterol-lowering trials indicates that there is no excess of all-cause mortality when adjustment is made for the degree of cholesterol reduction and treatment modality. However, it seems possible that excess mortality from non-cardiovascular causes could have been due to specific effects of some of the hormonal or fibrate drug treatments used to reduce cholesterol.[57]

Examination of the reduction in clinical events achieved in angiographic trials by the type of intervention gives no indication of superiority of any particular lipid-controlling therapy. In particular, as for retarding progression of lesions, there is no indication of obvious advantage of statins over the other modes of therapy (see Table 2.6). Lipid management in primary prevention appears to be just as effective as for secondary prevention in terms of the percent reduction in risk achieved compared with controls, although the absolute reduction in risk achieved is greater in those who have already had an event (Table 2.7).

Table 2.7 **Large-scale drug and surgical trials of clinical outcome benefits of treating dyslipidaemia**

		Percent change in lipids			Percent reduction
Primary prevention	**Treatment**	**LDL**	**HDL**	**Chol**	**CV death & MI**
LRC–CPPT	Resin	−12%	+4%	−8%	19%*
Helsinki	Fibrate	−10%	+12%	−10%	33%*
WOSCOP	Statin	−16%	+3%	−12%	31%***
AFCAPS/TexCAPS	Statin	−28%	+6%	−18%	37%**
Secondary prevention					
CDP–Niacin	Niacin	NA	NA	−10%	14%*
POSCH	Ileal bypass	−38%	+4%	−23%	35%***
4S	Statin	−35%	+8%	−25%	34%***
CARE	Statin	−28%	+5%	−20%	24%**
LIPID	Statin	−25%	+5%	−18%	26%***

* $p < 0.05$; ** $p < 0.01$; *** $p < 0.001$.
Adapted with permission from ref. 63.

CONCLUSIONS

Lipid regulation, by drugs or other means, has been shown, both in earlier non-statin trials and in more recent trials employing statins, to reduce the morbidity and mortality promoted by dyslipidaemia. The percentage reduction in risk achieved with LDL cholesterol reduction appears to be similar in primary and secondary prevention. Because of the fivefold greater risk of patients with overt coronary disease, secondary prevention trials have reported larger absolute reductions in events than primary prevention studies. Because of the lower event rates in primary prevention trials they were unable to demonstrate a significant reduction in overall mortality and benefit for women, diabetics or the elderly.

The disproportionately great reduction in clinical cardiovascular events achieved for the amount of regression of lesions induced in the lipid-correcting trials strongly suggests that the therapy also stabilizes lesions and retards thrombogenesis. This bonus of therapy appears to occur with all types of therapy and is poorly correlated with the degree of reduction in blood lipids achieved.

The importance of primary prevention by correction of dyslipidaemia should not be underestimated, because of the large attributable risk imposed by dyslipidaemia in the general population. Also, about a third of initial coronary attacks are acutely fatal and therefore not amenable to secondary prevention. As noted in the ATPIII NCEP report, the greatest potential for decreasing the population burden of coronary disease lies in primary prevention, both in high-risk coronary candidates by drug therapy and in the general population by nutritional changes, weight control and more exercise.

There is a suggestion that the more effective medical therapy now available for dyslipidaemia may be at least as effective as revascularization for coronary disease.[58] Unstable lesions that cause myocardial infarctions are not necessarily severely stenotic and stenotic lesions are not necessarily unstable. Revascularization is chiefly directed at severe coronary artery stenosis and does not treat the dangerous smaller unstable lesions. Although mortality rates are more favourably influenced by surgery, it does not appear to greatly influence the likelihood of occurrence of a myocardial infarction.[59,60] In contrast to revascularization, therapy of dyslipidaemia reduces myocardial infarction rates by about 30% over five years and appears to favourably influence the smaller unstable lesions that are overlooked by revascularization procedures.[58] The relative efficacy of therapy for dyslipidaemia and revascularization, alone and in combination, needs to be evaluated.

The NCEP guidelines of 1987–2001 led to increases in the proportion of hypercholesterolaemic persons treated by physicians and increased awareness of the importance of controlling elevated serum cholesterol among both physicians and the general population. However, the overall levels of treatment and control remain too low.[61] Only 42% of hypercholesterolaemic persons are now aware of their condition and only 4% are treated and controlled. Hypercholesterolaemia awareness was reported to be increasing from 31% to 50% between 1987 and 1989 and the prevalence of hypercholesterolaemia decreased from 30% to 25%. However, black people were less likely to be either aware or treated.

ACKNOWLEDGEMENT

The authors are from the National Heart, Lung and Blood Institute's Framingham Heart Study, National Institutes of Health. Framingham Heart Study research is supported by NIH/NHLBI Contract No.01-HC-25195 and the Visiting Scientist Program which is supported by Serviér Amerique.

REFERENCES

1. Expert Panel on Detection, Evaluation and Treatment of High Blood Cholesterol in Adults (Adult Treatment Panel III). Executive Summary of the Third Report of the National Cholesterol Education Program (NCEP). *JAMA* 2001; **285**: 2486–97.
2. Pyorala K, DeBacher G, Graham I et al. Prevention of coronary heart disease in clinical practice. Recommendations of the Task Force of the European Society of Cardiology, European Atherosclerosis Society and European Society of Hypertension. *Eur Heart J* 1994; **15**: 1300–31.
3. Crouse JR, Parks JS, Schey HM, Kalil FR. Studies of low density lipoprotein molecular weight in human beings with coronary artery disease. *Lipid Res* 1985; **26**: 566–74.
4. Austen MA, Breslow JL, Hennekens CH et al. Low density lipoprotein subclass patterns and risk of myocardial infarction. *JAMA* 1988; **260**: 1917–21.
5. Steinberg D, Witzum JL. Lipoproteins and atherogenesis: current concepts. *JAMA* 1990; **264**: 3047–51.
6. Kannel WB, Castelli WP, Gordon T. Lipoprotein cholesterol in the prediction of atherosclerotic disease: new perspectives based on the Framingham Study. *Ann Intern Med* 1979; **90**: 85–91.
7. Rhoads GG, Gulbrandsen CL, Kagan A. Serum lipoproteins and coronary heart disease in a population study of Hawaiian Japanese men. *N Engl J Med* 1976; **294**: 293–8.
8. Stampfer MJ, Sacks FM, Salvini S et al. A prospective study of cholesterol, apolipoproteins and risk of myocardial infarction. *N Engl J Med* 1991; **325**: 373–381.
9. Stamler J, Wentworth D, Neaton JD. Is the relationship between serum cholesterol and risk of premature death from coronary heart disease continuous or graded? Results in 356,222 primary screenees of the Multiple Risk Factor Intervention Trial (MRFIT). *JAMA* 1986; **256**: 2823–8.
10. Frick MH, Elo O, Haapa K et al. Primary prevention trial with gemfibrozil in middle-aged men with dyslipidemia. Safety and treatment, changes in risk factors and incidence of coronary disease. *N Engl J Med* 1987; **317**: 1237–45.
11. Rubins HB, High density lipoprotein and coronary heart disease. Lessons from recent intervention trials. *Prev Cardiol* 2000; **3**: 33–9.
12. Wong ND, Wilson PWF, Kannel WB. Serum cholesterol as a prognostic factor after myocardial infarction: the Framingham Study. *Ann Intern Med* 1991; **115**: 687–93.
13. Ulvenstam G, Bergstrand R, Johansson S et al. Prognostic importance of cholesterol levels after myocardial infarction. *Prev Med* 1984; **13**: 355–66.
14. Aronow WS, Herzig AH, Etienne F et al. 41 month follow-up of risk factors correlated with new coronary events in 708 elderly patients. *J Am Geriatr Soc* 1989; **37**: 501–6.
15. Khaw KT, Barrett-Connor E. Prognostic factors for mortality in a population based study of men and women with a history of heart disease. *J Cardiopulm Rehab* 1986; **6**: 474–80.
16. Heliovaara M, Karvonen JM, Punsar S, Haapakoski J. Importance of coronary risk factors in the presence or absence of myocardial ischemia. *Am J Cardiol* 1982; **55**: 325–9.

17. Carlson LA, Rosenhamer G. Reduction in mortality in the Stockholm Ischemic Heart Disease Secondary Prevention Study by combined treatment with clofibrate and nicotinic acid. *Acta Med Scand* 1988; **223**: 405–18.

18. Blankenhorn DH, Nessim SA, Johnson RL et al. Beneficial effects of combined colestipol–niacin therapy on coronary atherosclerosis and coronary venous by-pass grafts. *JAMA* 1987; **257**: 3233–40.

19. Brown G, Alliers JJ, Fisher LD et al. Regression of coronary artery disease as a result of intensive lipid-lowering therapy in men with high levels of apolipoprotein B. *N Engl J Med* 1990; **323**: 46–55.

20. Genest J Jr, McNamara JR, Ordovas JM et al. Lipoprotein cholesterol, apolipoprotein A-I and B and lipoprotein (a) abnormalities in men with premature coronary artery disease. *J Am Coll Cardiol* 1992; **19**: 792–802.

21. Kannel WB. Range of serum cholesterol values in the population developing coronary artery disease. *Am J Cardiol* 1995; **76**: C69–C77.

22. LaRosa JC, Hunninghake D, Bush D et al. The cholesterol facts: a summary of the evidence relating dietary fats, serum cholesterol and coronary heart disease: a joint statement of the American Heart Association and the National Heart Lung and Blood Institute. *Circulation* 1990; **81**: 1721–33.

23. Johnson CL, Rifkind BM, Sempos CT et al. Declining serum total cholesterol levels among US adults: the National Health and Nutrition Examination Surveys. *JAMA* 1993; **269**: 3002–8.

24. Kagan A, Harris BR, Winkelstein W Jr et al. Epidemiologic studies of coronary heart disease and stroke in Japanese men living in Japan, Hawaii and California: demographic, physical, dietary and biochemical characteristics. *J Chronic Dis* 1974; **27**: 345–64.

25. Caggiula AW, Watson JE, Kuller LH et al. Cholesterol-Lowering Intervention Program: effect of the step 1 diet in community office practices. *Arch Intern Med* 1996; **156**: 1205–13.

26. Ims DG, Kuller LH, Traver ND. Use and outcomes of a cholesterol-lowering intervention for rural elderly subjects. *Am J Prev Med* 1993; **9**: 274–81.

27. Hunninghake DB, Stein EA, Dujorne CA et al. The efficacy of intensive dietary therapy alone or combined with lovastatin in outpatients with hypercholesterolemia. *N Engl J Med* 1993; **328**: 1213–19.

28. Sytkowski PA, Kannel WB, D'Agostino RB. Changes in risk factors and the decline in mortality from cardiovascular disease: the Framingham Heart Study. *N Engl J Med* 1990; **322**: 1635–46.

29. Kannel WB. Preventive efficacy of nutritional counseling. *Arch Intern Med* 1996; **156**: 1138–9.

30. Shepherd J, Cobb SM, Ford I et al., for the West of Scotland Study. Prevention of coronary heart disease in men with hypercholesterolemia. *N Engl J Med* 1995; **333**: 1301–7.

31. Scandinavian Simvastatin Survival Study Group. Randomized trial of cholesterol lowering in 4444 patients with coronary heart disease: the Scandinavian Simvastatin Survival Study (4S). *Lancet* 1994; **344**: 1383–9.

32. Wilson PWF, D'Agostino RB, Levy D et al. Prediction of coronary heart disease using risk factor categories. *Circulation* 1998; **97**: 1837–47.

33. Dattilio AM, Kris-Etherton PM. Effects of weight reduction on blood lipids and lipoproteins: a meta-analysis. *Am J Clin Nutr* 1992; **56**: 320–8.

34. Denke MA, Sempos CT, Grundy SM. Excess body weight, an under-recognized contributor to dyslipidemia in white American women. *Arch Intern Med* 1994; **154**: 401.

35. Reaven GM. Syndrome X: 6 years later. *J Intern Med* 1994; **236** (Suppl 736): 13–22.

36. Bouchard C, Bray GA, Hubbard VS. Basic and clinical aspects of regional fat distribution. *Am J Clin Nutr* 1990; **52**: 946.

37. Berlin JA, Colditz GA. A meta-analysis of physical activity in prevention of coronary heart disease. *Am J Epidemiol* 1990; **132**: 612–28.

38. Marti B, Suter E, Riesen WF et al. Effects of long term, self monitored exercise on serum lipoprotein and apolipoprotein profile in middle-aged men. *Atherosclerosis* 1990; **81**: 19–31.

39. Sedgwick AW, Thomas DW, Davies M. Relationships between change in aerobic fitness and changes in blood pressure and plasma lipids in men and women: the Adelaide 1000 4-year follow-up. *J Clin Epidemiol* 1993; **81**: 19–31.

40. Wei M, Macera CA, Hornung CA, Blair SN. Changes in lipids associated with change in regular exercise in free living men. *J Clin Epidemiol* 1997; **50**: 1137–42.

41. Gould AL, Rossouw JE, Santanello NC et al. Cholesterol reduction yields clinical benefit. A new look at old data. *Circulation* 1995; **91**: 2274–82.

42. Rossouw JE. Lipid-lowering interventions in angiographic trials. *Am J Cardiol* 1995; **76**: C86–C92.

43. Buchwald H, Varco RL, Matts P et al. and the POSCH Group. Effect of partial ileal bypass surgery on mortality and morbidity from coronary artery disease in patients with hypercholesterolemia. *N Engl J Med* 1990; **323**: 946–55.

44. Waters D, Craven TE, Lesperance J. Prognostic significance of progression of coronary atherosclerosis. *Circulation* 1993; **87**: 1067–75.

45. Fuster V, Badimon L, Badimon J, Cheseboro J. The pathogenesis of coronary artery disease and the acute coronary syndromes. I. *N Engl J Med* 1992; **326**: 242–50.

46. Fuster V, Badimon L, Badimon J, Cheseboro J. The pathogenesis of coronary artery disease and the acute coronary syndromes. II. *N Engl J Med* 1992; **326**: 310–18.

47. Muldoon MF, Manuck SB, Matthews KA, Lowering cholesterol concentration and mortality: a quantitative review of primary prevention trials. *BMJ* 1990; **301**: 309–14.

48. Davey-Smith G, Song F, Sheldon TA. Cholesterol lowering and mortality: importance of considering initial level of risk. *BMJ* 1993; **306**: 1367–8.

49. Law MR, Thompson SG. Assessing possible hazards of reducing serum cholesterol. *BMJ* 1994; **308**: 373–9.

50. Keech AC. Does cholesterol lowering reduce total mortality? *Postgrad Med J* 1992; **68**: 870–1.

51. MacMahon S. Lowering cholesterol: effects on trauma death, cancer death and mortality. *Aust NZ J Med* 1992; **22**: 580–2.

52. Law MR, Wald MJ. By how much and how quickly does reduction in serum cholesterol concentration lower risk of ischaemic heart disease? *BMJ* 1994; **308**: 367–72.

53. Sacks FM, Rouleau JL, Moye LE et al., for the CARE Investigators. Baseline characteristics in the Cholesterol and Recurrent Events (CARE) trial of secondary prevention in patients with average serum cholesterol. *Am J Cardiol* 1995; **75**: 621–3.

54. Frick MH, Elo O, Haapa K et al. Helsinki Heart Study: primary prevention trial with gemfibrozil in middle-aged men with dyslipidemia: safety of treatment, changes in risk factors and incidence of coronary heart disease. *N Engl J Med* 1987; **317**: 1237–45.

55. Stephens NG, Parsons A, Schofield PM et al. Randomized controlled trial of vitamin E in patients with coronary disease. Cambridge Heart Antioxident Study (CHAOS). *Lancet* 1996; **347**: 781–6.

56. Holme I. Relation between total mortality and cholesterol reduction as found by meta-regression analysis of randomized cholesterol-lowering trials. *Control Clin Trials* 1996; **17**: 13–22.

57. Holme I. Effects of lipid-lowering therapy on total and coronary mortality. *Curr Opin Lipidol* 1995; **6**: 374–8.

58. Forrester JS, Shah PK. Lipid lowering versus revascularization. An idea whose time has come. *Circulation* 1997; **96**: 1360–2.

59. Muhlbaier L, Pryor D, Rankin J et al. Observational comparison of event-free survival with medical and surgical therapy in patients with coronary artery disease: 20 years of follow-up. *Circulation* 1992; **86** (Suppl 5): II198–II204.

60. Mark D, Nelson C, Califf R et al. Continuing evolution of therapy for coronary artery disease: initial results from the era of coronary angioplasty. *Circulation* 1994; **89**: 2015–25.

61. Nieto FJ, Alonso J, Chambless LE et al. Population awareness and control of hypertension and hypercholesterolemia. The Atherosclerosis Risk in Communities Study. *Arch Intern Med* 1995; **155**: 677–84.

62. Spagnoli LG, Mauriello A, Orlandi A et al. Age-related changes affecting atherosclerotic risk. Potential for pharmacological intervention. *Drugs Aging* 1996; **8**: 275–98.

63. Simes RJ, Baker J, MacMahon S et al., on behalf of the LIPID Study Group. Pravastatin reduces total mortality in patients with coronary heart disease and average cholesterol levels: relationship of baseline cholesterol and treatment effect in the LIPID trial. *J Am Coll Cardiol* 1998; **31**: A281.

3

The discovery and development of the statins

Akira Endo

INTRODUCTION

By 1970, epidemiologic studies had shown that increased levels of blood cholesterol were causally related to an increased risk of coronary heart disease.[1,2] The Framingham Study,[2] the most famous of these surveys, which started in 1949, showed that the risk of coronary heart disease (CHD) rose progressively with an increase in the level of blood cholesterol. Several clinical studies suggested that the lowering of cholesterol levels by the ingestion of low-fat diets or by treatment with lipid-lowering drugs would reduce the incidence of coronary heart disease.[3–5] At the beginning of the 1970s, there were some reasons to believe that levels of blood cholesterol could be reduced by inhibiting 3-hydroxy-3-methylglutaryl coenzyme A (HMG-CoA) reductase, the rate-controlling enzyme in the cholesterol synthetic pathway.[6,7]

In 1971, we began our search for microbial products that would inhibit HMG-CoA reductase and that might therefore reduce levels of plasma cholesterol in humans. We postulated that some micro-organisms would produce such novel compounds, and this possibility fascinated us because such products had not been isolated previously. These studies led to the discovery of a potent, low-toxicity reductase inhibitor, named mevastatin (formerly called compactin or ML-236B),[8] the prototype of the statins. Subsequently, we elucidated the biochemical mechanisms of action of mevastatin,[9,10] and by the end of the 1970s we had

shown that mevastatin markedly reduced levels of total and low-density lipoprotein (LDL) cholesterol in both experimental animals and patients with primary hypercholesterolaemia.[11–13] These findings apparently stimulated the worldwide development of mevastatin analogs (statins) in the 1980s and, by 1991, three statins – lovastatin (formerly called mevinolin or monacolin K), simvastatin and pravastatin – had been approved and marketed in the USA and many other countries.[14,15] Since then, three statins that were chemically synthesized have also been introduced to the market.[16] All of these statins have been well established as effective and safe cholesterol-lowering agents and have been used by millions of patients.[17,18] Several landmark clinical trials with statins have recently demonstrated that lipid-lowering therapy reduces cardiovascular morbidity and mortality in both primary and secondary prevention.[19–21] This chapter will primarily focus on the history of the discovery and development of mevastatin, the prototype of the statins, and lovastatin, the first to be marketed.

BACKGROUND

In the 1950s and 1960s, several lipid-lowering drugs were reported and introduced to clinical use. Large doses of nicotinic acid reduce plasma levels of triglycerides by between 20–80% and LDL cholesterol by 10–15%.[22,23] Nicotinic acid produces an intense cutaneous flush and pruritus, involving the face and the upper part of the body. Other adverse effects include rash, gastrointestinal upset, hyperuricaemia, hyperglycaemia and hepatic dysfunction.[23] Cholestyramine, an insoluble anion exchange resin, decreases levels of plasma LDL cholesterol by up to 30%.[24,25] This drug is probably one of the safest drugs for the treatment of hypercholesterolaemia. Nevertheless, large doses (usually 12–16 g per day) are unpleasant to take. The most frequent adverse effects are bloating, mild nausea and constipation.[23] Clofibrate is effective in reducing plasma levels of triglycerides and cholesterol.[26] It was used widely for the treatment of hypertriglyceridaemia. In most patients, its cholesterol-lowering effects are minimal to moderate. Adverse effects include mild gastrointestinal distress, skin rash, alopecia and impotence. In the late 1970s, clofibrate was shown not to be effective in the prevention of atherosclerosis.[27,28] Plant sterols such as β-sitosterol are poorly absorbed and are thought to compete with cholesterol for absorption sites in the intestine. Their cholesterol-lowering effects are variable.[29] Oestrogens are unsuitable as lipid-lowering agents in men, because of their feminizing effects and because they elevate very low-density lipoprotein (VLDL) and triglycerides.[23,30] Neomycin reduces plasma levels of LDL cholesterol; effects on VLDL cholesterol are variable.[31,32] Ototoxicity and nephrotoxicity may occur in patients with impaired renal function.[23] Dextrothyroxine moderately reduces plasma levels of LDL cholesterol.[33] However, use of this drug may cause serious cardiac toxicity. Thus, none of the lipid-lowering drugs available at the beginning of the 1970s could be considered to be ideal.

Cholesterol can be derived either from the intestinal absorption of dietary cholesterol or from *de novo* synthesis within the body. In the 1960s, studies with animals showed that when cholesterol was removed from the diet, the liver increased its capacity to synthesize cholesterol and accounted for about 80% of all detectable sterol synthetic activity in the body.[6] On the other hand, when cholesterol was added to the diet, cholesterol synthesis in the liver was nearly completely suppressed. Feedback suppression of hepatic cholesterol synthesis by dietary cholesterol is mediated through changes in the activity of HMG-CoA reductase, a microsomal enzyme that catalyses the conversion of HMG-CoA to mevalonate.[7,34] In addition to regulation by dietary cholesterol, reductase activity in the liver is regulated by hormonal or environmental conditions.[6] Under these conditions, changes in reductase activity in the liver are closely related to changes in the overall rate of cholesterol synthesis. The control mechanism for cholesterol synthesis is partially or completely lost when liver cells become malignant.[7] Further, it was suggested that in humans, much more cholesterol is synthesized than is absorbed from the intestine, even when a large quantity of cholesterol is ingested.[6,35] Thus, at the time that our study began in 1971, it seemed reasonable to believe that the level of blood cholesterol might be lowered by inhibiting hepatic activity of HMG-CoA reductase.

In 1928, Alexander Fleming discovered penicillin from a mould belonging to the genus *Penicillium*.[36] A decade later, penicillin was developed as a systemic therapeutic agent by a research group at Oxford University headed by Florey, Chain and Abraham.[37] Stimulated by the discovery of penicillin, Waksman et al. conducted a well-planned scientific search for antibacterial substances, and in 1940 they isolated streptomycin, an antibiotic active against the tubercle bacillus, from *Streptomyces griseus*.[38] Since then, hundreds of antibiotics have been isolated from a variety of micro-organisms, and some of them have been shown to inhibit many different kinds of metabolic pathways, not only in bacterial cells but also in mammalian cells.[39] Although no microbial metabolites that inhibited any enzymes involved in cholesterol synthesis had been isolated previously, in view of the versatility of micro-organisms, we hoped that some of them would produce novel compounds that would inhibit HMG-CoA reductase.

From 1966 to 1968, I was in New York as a research associate at the Albert Einstein College of Medicine. During this stay, while I studied

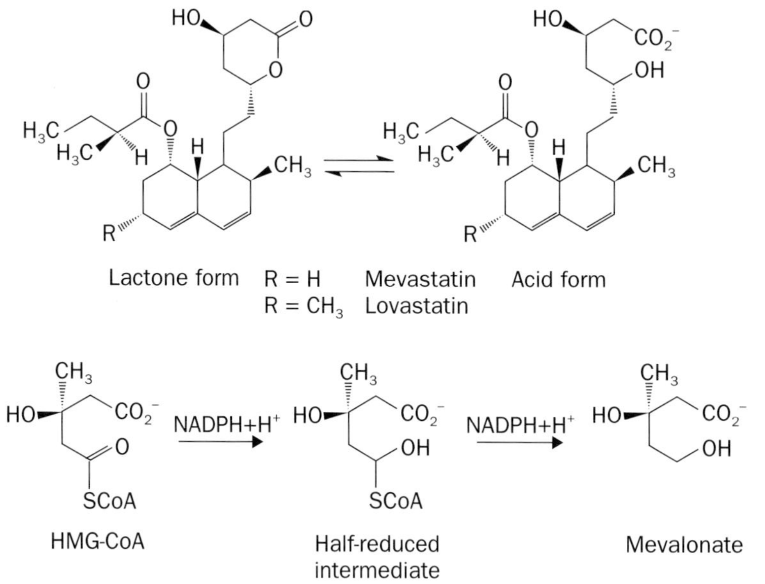

Fig. 3.1 Structural formulae of natural statins and the conversion of HMG-CoA to mevalonate by HMG-CoA reductase.

the biosynthesis of bacterial lipopolysaccharide, I learned that CHD was the leading cause of death in the USA and other Western countries and that high levels of blood cholesterol were a major cause of atherosclerosis and CHD. This experience was the major motive for conducting the project on HMG-CoA reductase inhibitors.

ISOLATION OF MEVASTATIN

In mid-1971, we began our work in Tokyo by collecting and growing microbial strains. Over a two-year period, 6000 microbial strains were tested for their ability to block lipid synthesis. Consequently, a strain of *Penicillium citrinum* was found to produce active compound(s) that inhibited HMG-CoA reductase. To isolate the active component(s), culture filtrate (600 l) was extracted with organic solvents and applied to repeated silica gel chromatography, followed by crystallization, giving crystals (23 mg) of mevastatin. In November 1973, the structure of mevastatin was determined by a combination of spectroscopic, chemical and X-ray crystallographic methods (Fig. 3.1).[8] Mevastatin has a decalin (hexahydronaphthalene) ring substituted with a β-hydroxy-δ-lactone moiety, which is converted into the water-soluble 3,5-

dihydroxy acid by treatment with alkali or in the liver (see Fig. 3.1).[9] Mevastatin was independently isolated as an antibiotic from *Penicillium brevicompactum* by Brown et al.[40] The search for additional active compounds by my group was continued for another ten years, and led to the isolation of several statins, including lovastatin (monacolin K) (see Fig. 3.1).[41–43]

MECHANISM OF ACTION

The water-soluble, ring-opened acid form of mevastatin (see Fig. 3.1) produced a more potent and reliable inhibition than did the lactone form in the assays of both sterol synthesis from radiolabeled substrates and HMG-CoA reductase.[9] The inhibition of HMG-CoA reductase by mevastatin was reversible and competitive with respect to HMG-CoA. The K_i value for the ring-opened acid form was $\sim 10^{-9}$ M, while the K_m for HMG-CoA was $\sim 10^{-5}$ M.[9] Thus, the affinity of HMG-CoA reductase for mevastatin was 10 000-fold higher than its affinity for HMG-CoA. The mechanism by which mevastatin inhibited reductase seemed to be ideal for its development as a drug. Kinetic analysis of the reaction catalysed by hepatic HMG-CoA reductase suggested that the lactone portion of the mevastatin molecule bound to the HMG-binding site of the reductase molecule.[44] The structural similarity between the lactone and HMG portions supported this conclusion. Studies of structure–activity relationships indicated that both the 3- and 5-hydroxy groups of the mevastatin molecule (open acid form) played a crucial role in the inhibition of HMG-CoA reductase, as inhibitory activity was abolished by the conversion of either of the hydroxy groups into the methyl ester.[45] The decalin ring was also essential, since HMG, which lacked such structure, was more than 10^6-fold less potent than mevastatin. Further, the α-methylbutyrate ester played a significant role, as analogs that lacked this moiety, ML-236A and ML-236C, had one-tenth or less activity as compared with mevastatin.[9]

Mevastatin strongly inhibited sterol synthesis from [^{14}C]acetate in cultured human skin fibroblasts; inhibition was 50% at 1 nM (0.4 ng/ml) in both normal human cells and cells from patients with familial hypercholesterolaemia (FH). Sterol synthesis from [^{3}H]mevalonate and fatty acid synthesis from [^{14}C]acetate in human cells were not inhibited.[10,46] At higher concentrations, at which sterol synthesis was strongly reduced, mevastatin inhibited cell growth as well. This inhibition was overcome and normal growth was restored by the addition of a small amount of mevalonate, the product of the HMG-CoA reductase reaction.[10,47]

EFFICACY IN ANIMALS

In early 1974, the efficacy of mevastatin was evaluated by feeding rats a diet supplemented with 0.1% mevastatin for seven days.[48] However, no reduction was observed in plasma cholesterol levels. Plasma cholesterol was not lowered even when mevastatin was given at a dose as high as 500 mg/kg for five weeks. Further, mevastatin was ineffective in mice.[48] These findings were unexpected and discouraging. Nevertheless, our previous findings that mevastatin was a reversible, potent, competitive inhibitor of HMG-CoA reductase with very low acute toxicity continued to fascinate us, and led us not to abandon our work but to keep on doing further chemical and biological experiments.

While multiple doses produced no efficacy, a single dose of mevastatin was acutely effective in the rat in both reducing plasma cholesterol levels and inhibiting sterol synthesis *in vivo* in the liver.[10,49] It seemed likely that mevastatin would be more effective in an animal model of FH in which regulation of HMG-CoA reductase was partially or completely lost, resulting in high reductase activity.[50] In the mid-1970s, however, such an animal model was not available. The non-ionic detergent Triton WR-1339 was known to induce hepatic HMG-CoA reductase and thereby elevate plasma cholesterol levels in the rat.[51] Mevastatin was acutely effective in this model, giving a 12–21% reduction of plasma cholesterol at 100 mg/kg.[52] To improve the cholesterol-lowering activity of mevastatin, nearly 80 mevastatin analogs were either derived from mevastatin or synthesized *de novo* and evaluated. However, these new agents were unsuccessful, as none was more efficacious than mevastatin.[45,53]

At the beginning of 1976, we became interested in hens, as they produced one egg every day that contained a large quantity of cholesterol. Preliminary experiments showed that an egg contained about 300 mg of cholesterol, of which two-thirds was derived from the diet and the remainder was supplied by *de novo* synthesis in the body. These findings suggested that cholesterol synthesis in laying hens would be more active than that in cockerels. It was predicted that the activity of hepatic HMG-CoA reductase would be higher in laying hens than in cockerels, and thus it was hoped that mevastatin might lower cholesterol levels of eggs and/or blood. Laying hens were fed with a commercial diet supplemented with 0.1% mevastatin for 30 days. The results showed that after two to four weeks, cholesterol levels in the plasma were reduced by nearly 50%, and those in eggs by 10–15%.[54]

The results obtained with laying hens raised the interesting possibility that mevastatin, which was ineffective in rodents, might be effective in other animal models. Subsequently, we conducted experiments in dogs and then monkeys. In dogs, mevastatin reduced plasma cholesterol by 30% at a daily dose of 20 mg/kg and by 44%

at 50 mg/kg. Plasma LDL levels were markedly reduced by mevastatin, while high-density lipoprotein (HDL) levels were not lowered but rather were increased slightly. In early 1977, we gave mevastatin to cynomolgus monkeys for 11 days. The reduction of plasma cholesterol levels was 21% at 20 mg/kg per day and 36% at 50 mg/kg.[12] Plasma triglyceride levels were not changed significantly in either dogs or monkeys. Faecal excretion of bile acids was slightly elevated in dogs but not significantly changed in monkeys.[11,12] These results strongly suggested that mevastatin would be effective in humans.

CLINICAL EFFICACY

In early 1978, Akira Yamamoto and I gave mevastatin to two patients with homozygous FH. In one of these patients, who was a receptor-negative female, plasma levels of total cholesterol were not reduced detectably at a daily dose of 200 mg for five months, while in another patient, a receptor-defective, three-year-old girl, total cholesterol was lowered by approximately 14% at 150 mg/day for two months.[13] On the other hand, mevastatin was found to be highly effective in other primary hyperlipoproteinaemias. Plasma levels of total cholesterol were reduced by 22–35% (28% on average) at 50–150 mg/day for four to eight weeks in patients with type IIa (apparent FH heterozygotes) and combined hyperlipoproteinaemia; plasma LDL (plus VLDL) was markedly reduced, while HDL was elevated slightly.[13] From mid-1979, clinical trials of mevastatin were carried out by over ten groups in Japan in patients with severe hyperlipoproteinaemia, including types IIa, IIb and III. The results indicated that in these patients, mevastatin lowered plasma levels of total and LDL cholesterol by 20–40% at 15–60 mg/day; no serious side-effects were noticed.[13,55,56] However, in mid-1980, the formal clinical trials of mevastatin were discontinued, and since then its development has never been resumed. A long-term toxicity study in dogs had recently been completed, and it was said that there had been some faults both in designing the study and in judging the experimental results.

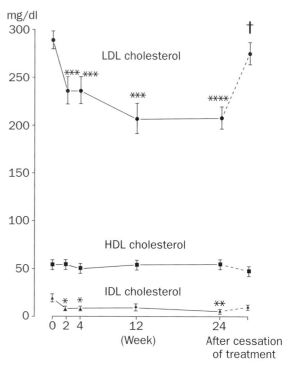

Fig. 3.2 Effects of mevastatin on IDL (intermediary low-density lipoprotein), HDL and LDL cholesterol levels in patients with heterozygous FH. Of seven patients studied, mevastatin was given three times daily for 24 weeks at doses of 60 mg/day in two patients and 30 mg/day in the other five patients. Data are means ± SEM. p-values obtained with Student's paired t-test: before treatment versus after treatment – $*p < 0.05$, $**p < 0.02$, $***p < 0.01$, $****p < 0.001$; after treatment versus after cessation of treatment – $†p < 0.01$.[56] (Reprinted with permission from ref. 56.)

In 1981, Mabuchi et al.[56] reported excellent data obtained with seven patients with heterozygous FH, who received mevastatin at a daily dose of 30 or 60 mg for 24 weeks. LDL cholesterol levels were lowered by 29%, and the decreased levels of LDL cholesterol were sustained during the period of treatment; HDL cholesterol increased slightly (Fig. 3.2). Subsequently, these physicians used a combination of mevastatin and cholestyramine in patients with heterozygous FH. LDL cholesterol was reduced by 50–60% by the combination, without adverse effects (Fig. 3.3).[57] Apparently,

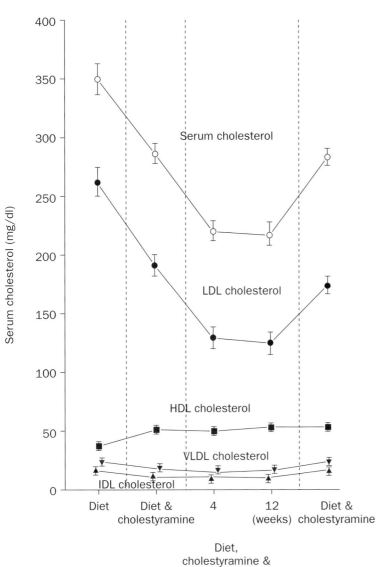

Fig. 3.3 Effects of the three regimens on serum LDL, HDL, VLDL and IDL cholesterol levels. After four to eight weeks of stabilization on an optimal dietary regimen, drug therapy with cholestyramine was started (4 g three times daily). After 2–16 weeks, additional therapy with mevastatin (compactin) was started. Patients were given 30 mg mevastatin three times daily for 12 weeks, after which mevastatin was withdrawn. Data are means ± SEM.[57] (Reprinted with permission from ref. 57.)

these excellent findings of Mabuchi et al. greatly stimulated the development of lovastatin and other statins in the 1980s.

DEVELOPMENT OF LOVASTATIN

In July 1976, in response to a request by Merck, we (Sankyo) concluded a disclosure agreement with Merck in which we would provide information (data on the mechanism of action of mevastatin, and on toxicologic and pharmacologic studies) and samples of mevastatin for the purpose of evaluating such information and the compound itself. Evaluation at Merck continued under our guidance until October 1978. At around that time, investigators at Merck began to search on their own for HMG-CoA reductase inhibitors, and in February 1979 they isolated lovastatin (initially called mevinolin) from *Aspergillus terreus*.[58,59] Lovastatin was independently isolated by us from *Monascus ruber* (and initially called monacolin K).[41,42] The structure of lovastatin is shown in Fig. 3.1. Lovastatin was slightly more potent than mevastatin in both inhibiting HMG-CoA reductase and lowering plasma cholesterol in experimental animals.[41,42,59]

Bilheimer et al.[60] showed that cholesterol lowering by lovastatin was primarily a result of enhanced LDL receptor-mediated catabolism in patients with heterozygous FH. In patients with receptor-negative, homozygous FH who had no capacity to synthesize LDL receptors, treatment with lovastatin at very high doses caused no decrease in LDL cholesterol levels, or an increase in the turnover rate of LDL.[61] These findings strongly supported the view that the principal action of HMG-CoA reductase inhibitors was to increase the number of LDL receptors but not to inhibit the synthesis of lipoproteins. The rates of synthesis of LDL receptors were inversely correlated with the amount of cholesterol in cells.[62] Studies with experimental animals showed that lovastatin increased messenger RNA for LDL receptors in the liver[63] and enhanced the number of LDL receptors expressed on the surface of liver cells.[64] In studies of lipoprotein kinetics in patients with primary moderate hypercholesterolaemia who did not have the clinical characteristics of heterozygous FH, lovastatin lowered the rates of production of LDL but had little effect on its fractional clearance rates.[65]

Clinical trials of lovastatin began in the USA in April 1980 but were halted several months later because of the rumour that the development of mevastatin had been discontinued in Japan because of tumorigenic toxicity in dogs. In 1982, clinical trials of lovastatin were resumed in patients with severe hypercholesterolaemia by physicians in the USA. Lovastatin reduced both total and LDL cholesterol concentrations in patients with heterozygous FH.[66–71] Its effect was potent, sustained and dose-dependent but reached a plateau at high doses. LDL cholesterol levels were reduced by 24–33% at a daily dose of 40 mg and by 38–42% at 80 mg, while HDL cholesterol was increased by up to 11%. Similarly, lovastatin was highly effective in hyperlipoproteinaemias other than FH, including primary moderate and severe hypercholesterolaemia,[65,72,73] type 3 hyperlipoproteinaemia,[74] familial dysbetalipoproteinaemia,[75] diabetic dyslipidaemia[76] and nephrotic hyperlipidaemia.[77]

The combination of lovastatin and a bile acid sequestrant, such as cholestyramine or colestipol, lowered LDL cholesterol levels by 47–56%.[69,70,78–80] This combination enhanced the decrease in LDL levels and permitted the use of smaller doses of both drugs. Large-scale clinical trials of lovastatin started in 1984, and the data on more than 1200 patients with severe hypercholesterolaemia showed that lovastatin was safe and effective.[81] Lovastatin was approved by the US Food and Drug Administration and first marketed in the USA in 1987.

SEMI-SYNTHETIC AND SYNTHETIC STATINS

The experience with mevastatin and lovastatin inspired efforts to chemically modify these natural statins to make even more effective derivatives (semi-synthetic statins). Investigators at Merck synthesized a side-chain ester analogue (called simvastatin) from lovastatin.[82] Simvastatin (Fig. 3.4), which has an additional methyl group on the carbon α to the carboxyl group, was approximately 2.5-fold more active than lovastatin in inhibiting HMG-CoA reductase activity. Many clinical trials showed that while simvastatin was approximately twice as potent on a milligram basis as lovastatin, the effects of these two agents on blood lipid and lipoprotein levels were quantitatively similar if they were administered at equivalent doses.[83–87] Simvastatin has been marketed in many countries. Pravastatin is a mevastatin analogue with a hydroxyl group on the decalin ring (see Fig. 3.4). It was prepared from mevastatin by microbial transformation using *Streptomyces carbophilus*.[88] Pravastatin was comparable to lovastatin in inhibiting HMG-CoA reductase activity and in lowering plasma cholesterol levels in humans.[89–92]

Since lovastatin was first marketed in 1987, mevastatin and lovastatin have frequently been used as models for designing other HMG-CoA reductase inhibitors (synthetic statins). Many synthetic studies worldwide have focused on replacing the highly functionalized decalin ring of the natural statins with a variety of aromatic and heteroaromatic nuclei.[43] Several of these synthetic statins are currently on the market

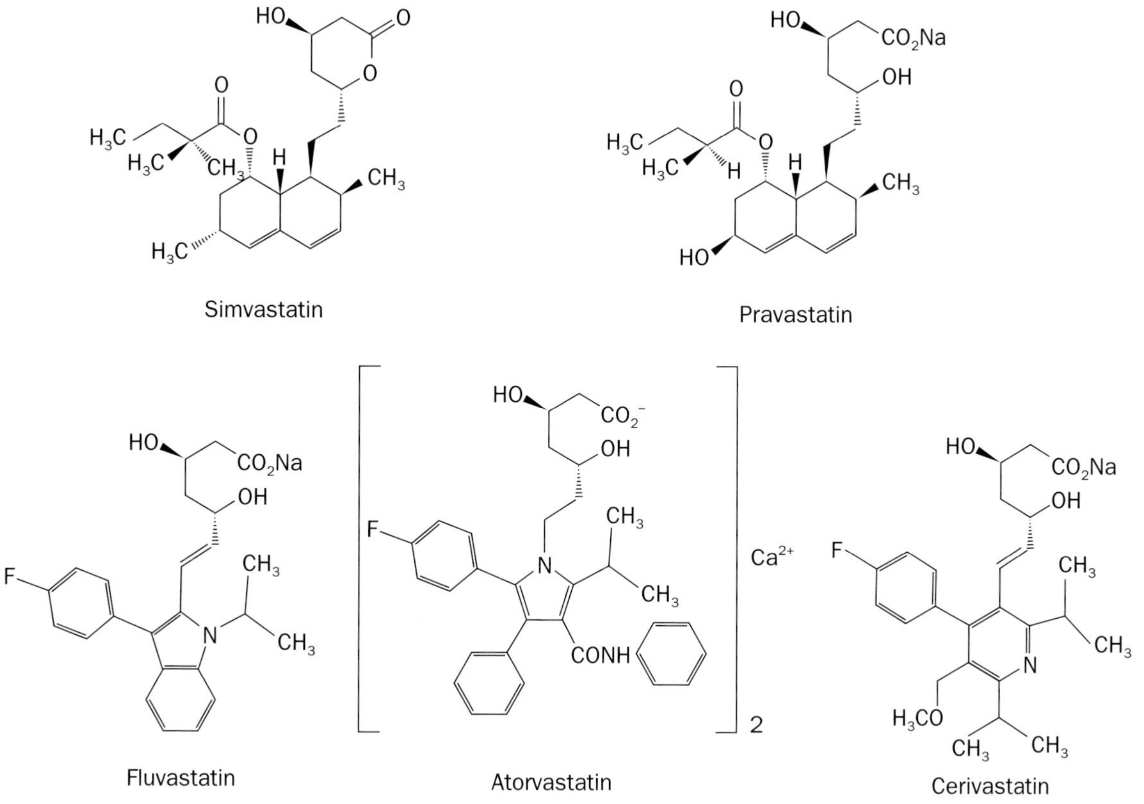

Fig. 3.4 Semi-synthetic and synthetic statins.

(see Fig. 3.4). Fluvastatin, an indolyl derivative, was synthesized by investigators at Sandoz and first marketed in 1993.[93] The 3,5-dihydroxy-carboxylic acid side-chain of fluvastatin corresponds to the lactone portion of mevastatin, whereas the indolyl part is supposed to be a substitute for the complex decalin ring. Fluvastatin was ten times more potent than lovastatin in inhibiting HMG-CoA reductase.[93] However, fluvastatin was less potent than other statins in lowering plasma cholesterol levels in hypercholesterolaemic patients.[94–97] Thus, fluvastatin at 40 and 80 mg/day achieved reductions in total and LDL cholesterol levels equivalent to those achieved by lovastatin and pravastatin at 20 and 40 mg/day, respectively.

Investigators at Warner-Lambert synthesized a substituted H-pyrrole compound, called atorvastatin.[98,99] It was approximately three times more potent than lovastatin in inhibiting rat liver HMG-CoA reductase, and also 4.5 times

more potent than lovastatin in inhibiting cholesterol synthesis in primary rat hepatocytes.[99] Atorvastatin reduced plasma levels of LDL cholesterol by up to 60% in patients with primary hypercholesterolaemia.[100] In patients with homozygous FH, who usually responded poorly to statins, atorvastatin produced a 31% reduction in plasma LDL levels at 80 mg/day.[101] In addition to its cholesterol-lowering activity, atorvastatin reduced plasma levels of triglycerides by over 40%.[102] It was suggested that the greater efficacy of atorvastatin was due to decreased production of hepatic VLDL. This was thought to be caused by prolonged inhibition of *in vivo* cholesterol biosynthesis, as a result of diminished recovery of HMG-CoA reductase activity following drug treatment.[103]

Cerivastatin, an enantiomerically pure derivative of a functionalized pyridine, was synthesized at Bayer. Cerivastatin had a K_i value of

1.3 nM, which was approximately 100-fold lower than the K_i for lovastatin.[104,105] It was effective in lowering serum cholesterol in dogs at a dose of 0.03 mg/kg and was thus at least 200 times more potent than lovastatin. In subjects with primary hypercholesterolaemia, cerivastatin reduced plasma LDL cholesterol concentrations by 30% at a daily dose of 0.2 mg.[104]

Several other statins, including crilvastatin (Pan Medica), HR 780 (Hoechst) and pitavastatin (Nissan-Kowa), have been synthesized and evaluated in both experimental animals and humans. Of these synthetic statins, pitavastatin was, like atorvastatin, effective in reducing plasma levels of both LDL cholesterol and triglycerides.[106] In hyperlipidaemic patients, reductions of LDL cholesterol and triglycerides were 40–50% and 20–30%, respectively, at a dose of 4 mg/day (Y Saito, personal communication). Nisvastatin is currently undergoing large-scale clinical trials and will be marketed within a few years.

REFERENCES

1. Keys A. Coronary heart disease in seven countries. *Circulation* 1970; **41** (Suppl 1): 1–21.
2. Kannel WB, Dawber TR, Kagan A et al. Factors of risk in the development of coronary heart disease – six year follow-up experience: the Framingham Study. *Ann Intern Med* 1961; **55**: 33–50.
3. Leren P. The Oslo diet – heart study: eleven-year report. *Circulation* 1970; **42**: 935–42.
4. A group of physicians of the Newcastle upon Tyne region. Trial of clofibrate in the treatment of ischaemic heart disease. Five year study. *BMJ* 1971; **4**: 767–75.
5. Research Committee of the Scottish Society of Physicians. Ischaemic heart disease: a secondary prevention trial using clofibrate. *BMJ* 1971; **4**: 775–84.
6. Dietschy JM, Wilson JD. Regulation of cholesterol metabolism. *N Engl J Med* 1970; **282**: 1128–38, 1179–83, 1241–9.
7. Siperstein MD. Regulation of cholesterol biosynthesis in normal and malignant tissues. *Curr Top Cell Regul* 1970; **2**: 65–100.
8. Endo A, Kuroda M, Tsujita Y. ML-236A, ML-236B, and ML-236C: new inhibitors of cholesterogenesis produced by *Penicillium citrinum*. *J Antibiot (Japan)* 1976; **29**: 1346–8.
9. Endo A, Kuroda M, Tanzawa K. Competitive inhibition of 3-hydroxy-3-methylglutaryl coenzyme A reductase by ML-236A and ML-2368 fungal metabolites having hypocholesterolemic activity. *FEBS Lett* 1976; **72**: 323–6.
10. Kaneko I, Hazama-Shimada Y, Endo A. Inhibitory effects on lipid metabolism in cultured cells of ML-236B, a potent inhibitor of 3-methylglutaryl coenzyme A reductase. *Eur J Biochem* 1978; **87**: 313–21.
11. Tsujita Y, Kuroda M, Tanzawa K et al. Hypolipidemic effects in dogs of ML-236B, a competitive inhibitor of 3-hydroxy-3-methylglutaryl coenzyme A reductase. *Atherosclerosis* 1979; **32**: 307–13.
12. Kuroda M, Tsujita Y, Tanzawa K, Endo A. Hypolipidemic effects in monkeys of ML-236B, a competitive inhibitor of 3-hydroxy-3-methylglutaryl coenzyme A reductase. *Lipids* 1979; **14**: 585–9.
13. Yamamoto A, Sudo H, Endo A. Therapeutic effects of ML-236B in primary hypercholesterolemia. *Atherosclerosis* 1980; **35**: 259–66.
14. Grundy SM. HMG-CoA reductase inhibitors for treatment of hypercholesterolemia. *N Engl J Med* 1988; **319**: 24–33.
15. Endo A. The discovery and development of HMG-CoA reductase inhibitors. *J Lipid Res* 1992; **33**: 1569–82.
16. Igel M, Sudhop T, von Bergmann K. Pharmacology of 3-hydroxy-3-methylglutaryl-coenzyme A reductase inhibitors (statins), including rosuvastatin and pitavastatin. *J Clin Pharmacol* 2002; **42**: 835–45.
17. Barth JD, Mancini GBJ. An update on lipid-lowering therapy. *Curr Opin Lipidol* 1995; **6**: 32–7.
18. Tikkanen MJ. Statins: within-group comparisons, statin escape and combination therapy, *Curr Opin Lipidol* 1996; **7**: 385–8.
19. Scandinavian Simvastatin Survival Study Group. Randomized trial of cholesterol lowering in 4444 patients with coronary heart disease: the Scandinavian Simvastatin Survival Study. *Lancet* 1994; **344**: 1383–9.
20. Shepherd J, Cobbe SM, Ford I et al. Prevention of coronary heart disease with pravastatin in men with hypercholesterolemia. *N Engl J Med* 1995; **333**: 1301–7.
21. Sever PS, Dahlof B, Poulter NR et al. Prevention of coronary and stroke events with atorvastatin in hypertensive patients who have average or

lower-than-average cholesterol concentrations, in the Anglo-Scandinavian Cardiac Outcomes Trial – Lipid Lowering Arm (ASCOT-LLA): a multicentre randomized controlled trial. *Lancet* 2003; **361**: 1149–58.

22. Altschul R, Hoffer L, Stepher JD. Influence of nicotinic acid on serum cholesterol in man. *Arch Biochem Biophys* 1955; **54**: 558–9.

23. AMA Department of Drugs. *AMA Drugs Evaluations*, 3rd edn. Littleton, Massachusetts: PSG Publishing, 1977: 153–74.

24. Hashin SA, van Itallie TB. Cholestyramine resin therapy for hypercholesterolemia: clinical and metabolic study. *JAMA* 1965; **192**: 289–93.

25. Grundy SM, Ahrens EH Jr, Salen G. Interruption of the enterohepatic circulation of bile acids in man: comparative effects of cholestyramine and ileal exclusion on cholesterol metabolism. *J Lab Clin Med* 1971; **78**: 94–121.

26. Thorp JM, Waring WS. Modification of metabolism and distribution of lipids by ethyl chlorophenoxyisobutyrate. *Nature* 1962; **194**: 948–9.

27. Coronary Drug Project. Clofibrate and niacin in coronary heart disease. *JAMA* 1975; **231**: 360–81.

28. Oliver MF, Heady JA, Morris JN, Cooper MI. A co-operative trial in the primary prevention of ischaemic heart disease using clofibrate. *Br Heart J* 1978; **40**: 1069–118.

29. Pollak OJ. Reduction of blood cholesterol in man. *Circulation* 1953; **7**: 702–6.

30. Taupitz A, Otaguro K. The effects of estrogens on the serum cholesterol of male rats. *Symp Deut Ges Endokrinol* 1959; 430–2.

31. Goldsmith GA, Hamilton JG, Miller ON. Lowering of serum lipid concentrations. Mechanisms used by unsaturated fats, nicotinic acid and neomycin: excretion of sterols and bile acids. *Arch Intern Med* 1960; **105**: 512–17.

32. Hoeg JM, Schaefer EJ, Romano CA et al. Neomycin and plasma lipoproteins in type II hyperlipoproteinemia. *Clin Pharmacol Ther* 1984; **36**: 555–65.

33. Starr P, Roen P, Freibrun JL, Schleissner LA. Reduction of serum cholesterol by sodium D-thyroxine. *AMA Arch Intern Med* 1960; **105**: 830–42.

34. Siperstein MD, Fagan VM. Feedback control of mevalonate synthesis by dietary cholesterol. *J Biol Chem* 1966; **241**: 602–9.

35. Grundy SM. Cholesterol metabolism in man. *West J Med* 1978; **128**: 13–25.

36. Fleming A. History and development of penicillin. In: Fleming A, ed. *Penicillin: Its Practical Application*. London: Butterworth, 1946: 1–33.

37. Florey HW. Penicillin: historical introduction. In: Florey HW, Chain EB, Heatley NG et al., eds. *Antibiotics*. London: Oxford University Press, 1949: 631–71.

38. Waksman SA. *Streptomycin, Nature, and Practical Applications*. Baltimore: Williams & Wilkins, 1949.

39. Gale EF, Cundliffe E, Reynolds PE et al. *The Molecular Basis of Antibiotic Action*. New York: Wiley, 1972.

40. Brown AG, Smale TC, King TJ et al. Crystal and molecular structure of compactin, a new antifungal metabolite from *Penicillium brevicompactum. J Chem Soc Perkin I* 1976; **11**: 1165–70.

41. Endo A, Monacolin K. A new hypocholesterolemic agent produced by a *Monascus* species. *J Antibiot (Japan)* 1979; **32**: 852–4.

42. Endo A, Monacolin K. A new hypocholesterolemic agent that specifically inhibits 3-hydroxy-3-methylglutaryl coenzyme A reductase. *J Antibiot (Japan)* 1980; **33**: 334–6.

43. Endo A, Hasumi K. HMG-CoA reductase inhibitors. *Nat Prod Rep* 1993; **10**: 541–50.

44. Tanzawa K, Endo A. Kinetic analysis of the reaction catalyzed by rat liver 3-hydroxy-3-methylglutaryl coenzyme A reductase using two specific inhibitors. *Eur J Biochem* 1979; **98**: 195–201.

45. Endo A. Compactin (ML-236B) and related compounds as potential cholesterol-lowering agents that inhibit HMG-CoA reductase. *J Med Chem* 1985; **28**: 401–5.

46. Brown MS, Faust JR, Goldstein JL et al. Induction of 3-hydroxy-3-methylglutaryl coenzyme A reductase activity in human fibroblasts incubated with compactin (ML-236B), a competitive inhibitor of the reductase. *J Biol Chem* 1978; **253**: 1121–8.

47. Endo A. Specific non-sterol inhibitors of HMG-CoA reductase. In: Preiss B, ed. *Regulation of HMG-CoA Reductase*. New York: Academic Press, 1985: 49–78.

48. Endo A, Tsujita Y, Kuroda M, Tanzawa K. Effects of ML-236B on cholesterol metabolism in mice and rats: lack of hypocholesterolemic activity in normal animals. *Biochim Biophys Acta* 1979; **575**: 266–76.

49. Endo A, Tsujita Y, Kuroda M, Tanzawa K. Inhibition of cholesterol synthesis *in vitro* and *in vivo* by ML-236A and ML-236B, competitive

inhibitors of 3-hydroxy-3-methylglutaryl co-enzyme A reductase. *Eur J Biochem* 1977; **77**: 31–6.

50. Brown MS, Goldstein JL. Receptor-mediated control of cholesterol metabolism. *Science* 1975; **191**: 150–4.

51. Kandutsch AA, Saucier SE. Prevention of cyclic and Triton-induced increase in hydroxymethyl-glutaryl coenzyme A reductase and sterol synthesis by puromycin. *J Biol Chem* 1969; **244**: 2299–305.

52. Kuroda M, Tanzawa K, Tsujita Y, Endo A. Mechanism for elevation of hepatic cholesterol synthesis and serum cholesterol levels in Triton I WR-1339-induced hyperlipidemia. *Biochim Biophys Acta* 1977; **489**: 119–25.

53. Sato A, Ogiso A, Noguchi R et al. Mevalonolactone derivatives as inhibitors of 3-hydroxy-3-methyl-glutaryl coenzyme A reductase. *Chem Pharm Bull (Japan)* 1980; **28**: 1509–25.

54. Endo A, Kitano N, Fujii S. Effects of ML-236B, a competitive inhibitor of 3-hydroxy-3-methyl-glutaryl coenzyme A reductase, on cholesterol metabolism. *Adv Exp Med Biol* 1978; **109**: 376 (abst).

55. Hata Y, Shigematsu R, Oikawa T et al. Treatment of hypercholesterolemia with an HMG-CoA reductase inhibitor (CS-500). II. Determination of unit weight effect and daily dose by an integration method and observation of safety in initial stage. *Ger Med (Japan)* 1980; **18**: 104–12.

56. Mabuchi H, Haba T, Tatami R et al. Effects of an inhibitor of 3-hydroxy-3-methylglutaryl coenzyme A reductase on serum lipoproteins and ubiquinone-10 levels in patients with familial hypercholesterolemia. *N Engl J Med* 1981; **305**: 478–82.

57. Mabuchi H, Sakai T, Sakai Y et al. Reduction of serum cholesterol in heterozygous patients with familial hypercholesterolemia: additive effects of compactin and cholestyramine. *N Engl J Med* 1983; **308**: 609–13.

58. Alberts AW, Chen J, Curon G et al. Mevinolin: a highly potent competitive inhibitor of hydroxymethylglutaryl-coenzyme A reductase and cholesterol-lowering agent. *Proc Natl Acad Sci USA* 1980; **77**: 3957–61.

59. Vagelos PR. Are prescription drug prices high? *Science* 1991; **252**: 1080–4.

60. Bilheimer DW, Grundy SM, Brown MS, Goldstein IL. Mevinolin and colestipol stimu-late receptor-mediated clearance of low-density lipoprotein from plasma in familial hypercholesterolemia heterozygotes. *Proc Natl Acad Sci USA* 1983; **80**: 4124–8.

61. Uauy R, Vega GL, Grundy SM, Bilheimer DW. Lovastatin therapy in receptor-negative homozygous familial hypercholesterolemia: lack of effect on low-density lipoprotein concentration or turnover. *J Pediatr* 1988; **113**: 383–92.

62. Goldstein IL, Brown MS. The low-density lipoprotein pathway and its relation to athero-sclerosis. *Annu Rev Biochem* 1977; **46**: 897–930.

63. Ma PTS, Gil G, Sudof TC et al. Mevinolin, an inhibitor of cholesterol synthesis, induces mRNA for low-density lipoprotein receptor in livers of hamsters and rabbits. *Proc Natl Acad Sci USA* 1986; **83**: 8370–4.

64. Kovanen PT, Bilheimer DW, Goldstein IL et al. Regulatory role for hepatic low density lipopro-tein receptors *in viva* in the dog. *Proc Natl Acad Sci USA* 1981; **78**: 1194–8.

65. Grundy SM, Vega GL. Influence of mevinolin on metabolism of low-density lipoproteins in primary moderate hypercholesterolemia. *J Lipid Res* 1985; **26**: 1464–75.

66. Illingworth DR, Sexton GI. Hypocholesterolemic effects of mevinolin in patients with hetero-zygous familial hypercholesterolemia. *J Clin Invest* 1984; **74**: 1972–8.

67. Tikkanen MJ, Helve E, Jaatela A et al. Comparison between lovastatin and gemfibrozil in the treatment of primary hyper-cholesterolemia: the Finnish Multicenter Study. *Am J Cardiol* 1988; **62**: J35-J43.

68. Havel R, Hunninghake DB, Illingworth DR et al. Lovastatin (mevinolin) in the treatment of heterozygous familial hypercholesterolemia: a multicenter study. *Ann Intern Med* 1987; **107**: 609–15.

69. Leren TP, Hjermann I, Berg K et al. Effects of lovastatin alone and in combination with cholestyramine on serum lipids and apopro-teins in heterozygotes for familial hyperholes-terolemia. *Atherosclerosis* 1988; **73**: 135–41.

70. Illingworth DR. Mevinolin plus colestipol in therapy for severe heterzygous familial hyper-cholesterolemia. *Ann Intern Med* 1984; **101**: 595–604.

71. Hoeg JM, Maher MB, Zech LA et al. Effectiveness of mevinolin on plasma lipo-protein concentrations in type II hyperlipo-proteinemia. *Am J Cardiol* 1986; **57**: 933–9.

72. The Lovastatin Study Group II. Therapeutic response to lovastatin (mevinolin) in nonfamilial hypercholesterolemia: a multicenter study. *JAMA* 1986; **256**: 2829–34.

73. The Lovastatin Study Group III. A multicenter comparison of lovastatin and cholestyramine therapy for severe primary hypercholesterolemia. *JAMA* 1988; **260**: 359–66.

74. East CA, Grundy SM, Bilheimer DW. Preliminary report. Treatment of type 3 hyperlipoproteinemia with mevinolin. *Metabolism* 1986; **35**: 97–8.

75. Vega GL, East CA, Grundy SM. Lovastatin therapy in familial dysbetalipoproteinemia: effect on kinetics of apoprotein B. *Atherosclerosis* 1988; **70**: 131–43.

76. Garg A, Grundy SM. Lovastatin for lowering cholesterol levels in non-insulin-dependent diabetes mellitus. *N Engl J Med* 1988; **314**: 81–6.

77. Vega GL, Grundy SM. Lovastatin therapy in nephrotic hyperlipidemia: effects on lipoprotein metabolism. *Kidney Int* 1988; **33**: 1160–8.

78. Grundy SM, Vega GL. Influence of combined therapy with mevinolin and interruption of bile acid reabsorption on low-density lipoproteins in heterozygous familial hypercholesterolemia. *Ann Intern Med* 1985; **103**: 339–43.

79. Vega GL, Grundy SM. Treatment of primary moderate hypercholesterolemia with lovastatin (mevinolin) and colestipol. *JAMA* 1987; **257**: 33–8.

80. Vega GL, East C, Grundy SM. Effects of combined therapy with lovastatin and colestipol in heterozygous familial hypercholesterolemia: effects on kinetics of apoprotein B. *Arteriosclerosis* 1989; **9**: 1135–44.

81. Tobert JA. Efficacy and long-term adverse effect pattern of lovastatin. *Am J Cardiol* 1988; **62**: J28–J34.

82. Hoffman WF, Alberts AW, Anderson PS et al. 3-Hydroxy-3-methylglutaryl coenzyme A reductase inhibitors. 4. Side-chain ester derivatives of mevinolin. *J Med Chem* 1986; **29**: 849–52.

83. Pietro DA, Alexander S, Mantell G et al. Effects of simvastatin and probucol in hypercholesterolemia (Simvastatin Multicenter Study Group II). *Am J Cardiol* 1989; **63**: 682–6.

84. Ziegler O, Drouin P and the Simvastatin Study Group. Safety, tolerability, and efficacy of simvastatin and fenofibrate – a multicenter study. *Cardiology* 1990; **77** (Suppl 4): 50–7.

85. Todd PA, Goa KL. Simvastatin – a review of its pharmacological properties and therapeutic potential in hypercholesterolemia. *Drugs* 1990; **40**: 583–607.

86. Boccuzzi SJ, Bocanegra TS, Walker JF et al. Long-term safety and efficacy profile of simvastatin. *Am J Cardiol* 1991; **68**: 1127–31.

87. Molgaard J, Lundh BL, von Schenck H, Olsson AG. Long-term efficacy and safety of simvastatin alone and in combination therapy in treatment of hypercholesterolemia. *Atherosclerosis* 1991; **91**: 21–8.

88. Tsujita Y, Kuroda M, Shimada Y et al. CS-514, a competitive inhibitor of 3-hydroxy-3-methylglutaryl coenzyme A reductase: tissue-selective inhibition of sterol synthesis and hypolipidemic effect on various animal species. *Biochim Biophys Acta* 1986; **877**: 50–60.

89. Mabuchi H, Kamon N, Fujita H et al. Effects of CS-514 on serum lipoprotein lipid and apoprotein levels in patients with familial hypercholesterolemia. *Metabolism* 1987; **36**: 475–9.

90. Hunninghake DB, Knopp RH, Schonfeld G et al. Efficacy and safety of pravastatin, compared to and in combination with bile acid-binding resins, in familial hypercholesterolemia. *J Intern Med* 1990; **228**: 261–6.

91. Vega GL, Krauss RM, Grundy SM. Pravastatin therapy in primary moderate hypercholesterolemia: changes in metabolism of apoprotein B-containing lipoproteins. *J Intern Med* 1990; **227**: 81–94.

92. Betteridge DJ, Bhatnager D, Bing RF et al. Treatment of familial hypercholesterolaemia. United Kingdom Lipid Clinics Study of pravastatin and cholestyramine. *BMJ* 1992; **304**: 1335–8.

93. Kathawala FG. HMG-CoA reductase inhibitors: an exciting development in the treatment of hyperlipoproteinemia. *Med Res Rev* 1991; **11**: 121–46.

94. Leitersdorf E, Eisenberg S, Eliav A et al. Efficacy and safety of high-dose fluvastatin in patients with familial hypercholesterolemia. *Eur J Clin Pharmacol* 1993; **45**: 513–18.

95. Illingworth DR, Tobert JA. A review of clinical trials comparing HMG-CoA reductase inhibitors. *Clin Ther* 1994; **16**: 366–85.

96. Jacotot B, Benghozi R, Pfister P et al. Comparison of fluvastatin versus pravastatin treatment of primary hypercholesterolemia. *Am J Cardiol* 1995; **76** (Suppl): A54–A56.

97. Peters TK, Muratti EN, Mehara M. Fluvastatin in primary hypercholesterolemia: efficacy and safety in patients at high risk. *Am J Med* 1994; **96** (Suppl 6): 79–83.

98. Sliskovic DR, Picard JA, Roark WH et al. Inhibitors of cholesterol biosynthesis. 4. *Trans*-6-y [2-(substituted-quinolinyl)ethenyl/ethyl]tetrahydro-4-hydroxy-2*H*-pyran-2-ones: a novel series of HMG-CoA reductase inhibitors. *J Med Chem* 1991; **34**: 367–72.

99. Shaw MK, Newton RS, Sliskovic DR et al. HepG2 cells and primary rat hepatocytes differ in their response to inhibitors of HMG-CoA reductase. *Biochem Biophys Res Commun* 1990; **170**: 726–34.

100. Nawrocki JW, Weiss SR, Davidson MH et al. Reduction of LDL cholesterol by 25% to 60% in patients with primary hypercholesterolemia by atorvastatin, a new HMG-CoA reductase inhibitor. *Arterioscler Thromb Vasc Biol* 1995; **15**: 678–82.

101. Naoumova RP, Marais AD, Mountney J et al. Atorvastatin augments therapy of homozygous familial hypercholesterolemia by inhibiting upregulation of cholesterol synthesis after apheresis and bile acid sequestrants. *Circulation* 1996; **94**: 1–583.

102. Hakker-Arkema RG, Davidson MH, Goldstein RJ et al. Efficacy and safety of a new HMG-CoA reductase inhibitor, atorvastatin, in patients with hypertriglyceridemia. *JAMA* 1996; **275**: 128–33.

103. Ness GC, Chambers CM, Lopez D. Atorvastatin action involves diminished recovery of hepatic HMG-CoA reductase activity. *J Lipid Res* 1998; **39**: 75–84.

104. Stein E, Sprecher D, Allenby KS et al. Cerivastatin, a new potent synthetic HMG-CoA-reductase inhibitor: effect of 0.2 mg daily in subjects with primary hypercholesterolemia. *J Cardiovasc Pharmacol Ther* 1997; **2**: 7–16.

105. Angerbauer R, Bischoff H, Steinke W et al. BAY 6228: hypolipidemic HMG-CoA reductase inhibitor. *Drugs Future* 1994; **19**: 537–41.

106. Aoki T, Nishimura H, Nakagawa S et al. Pharmacological profile of a novel synthetic inhibitor of 3-hydroxy-3-methylglutaryl-coenzyme A reductase. *Arzneim-ForschDrug Res* 1997; **8**: 904–9.

107. Noji Y, Higashikata T, Inazu A et al. and the NK-104 Study Group. Long-term treatment with pitavastatin (NK-104), a new HMG-CoA reductase inhibitor, of patients with heterozygous familial hypercholesterolemia. *Atherosclerosis* 2002; **163**: 157–64.

4

Comparative chemistry, pharmacology and mechanism of action of the statins

Allan Gaw and Christopher J Packard

INTRODUCTION

With the discovery of the low-density lipoprotein (LDL) receptor by Goldstein and Brown our understanding of the cholesterol economy of the cell took a major step forward.[1] Further breakthroughs by that team and others have now given us the framework to understand in detail the effects of a drug that manipulates and changes that finely balanced economy.[2] The 3-hydroxy-3-methylglutaryl coenzyme A (HMG-CoA) reductase inhibitors or statins are an important group of drugs that have such an effect.

By manipulating intracellular cholesterol concentrations we can achieve the regulation of several key proteins involved in lipid and lipoprotein metabolism. The discovery of the statins is described in Chapter 3, and their widespread use is now testament to their clinical efficacy. It is notable that as a group of drugs they are virtually uniformly effective in changing the plasma lipid profile. Most individuals are responsive to statin therapy irrespective of their baseline phenotype or genotype. This is true even in receptor-negative familial hypercholestrolaemia (FH) homozygotes, where, because of the proposed mechanism of action of the statins, it was believed that they would be ineffective. As described below, the metabolism of lipids and lipoproteins is fundamentally affected by statin therapy, and while changes take place in the clearance rates of various apoB-containing lipoproteins, other important effects have been observed in the synthesis of these lipoproteins.

All statins have structural similarities and from these structures a mechanism of action is immediately apparent: that of competitive inhibition of HMG-CoA reductase through mimicry of this enzyme's substrate. However, there are also important structural differences between the statins that are beginning to be evaluated. What role these differences will play in the final assessment of the clinically beneficial effects of the statins is not yet clear.

This chapter sets forth a review of the basic pharmacology of the statins and examines their comparative pharmacokinetics. Their effect on the elements of plasma lipid profile are discussed in detail. Mechanisms of action beyond lipid regulation, which may have clinical significance, are discussed separately in Chapter 5.

CHEMISTRY AND FUNCTIONAL PROPERTIES

As described in Chapter 3, the statins share a number of common structural features (Fig. 4.1). Firstly, a portion of the molecule comprises the substrate analogue, which is present either in the open-chain form (e.g. in pravastatin) or in the closed-ring lactone form (e.g. in lovastatin). Secondly, a complex hydrophobic ring structure is present to permit tight binding to the reductase enzyme. Thirdly, side-groups on the rings define the solubility properties of the drugs and

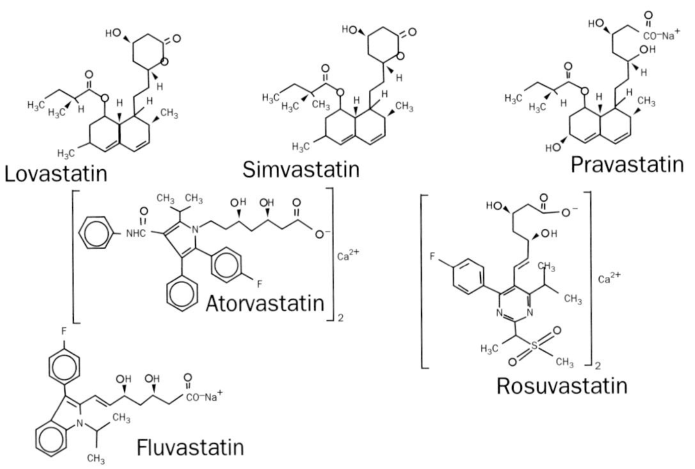

Fig. 4.1 The structures of the marketed statins compared.

Table 4.1 Comparative pharmacokinetics of the statins

Pharmacokinetic parameter	Atorvastatin	Cerivastatin	Fluvastatin	Lovastatin	Pravastatin	Rosuvastatin	Simvastatin
Major metabolic isoenzyme	3A4	3A4, 2C8	2C9	3A4	None	2C9 (small amount)	3A4
Lipophilic	Yes	Yes	Yes	Yes	No	No	Yes
Protein binding (%)	98	>99	>98	>95	~50	90	95–98
Active metabolites	Yes	Yes	No	Yes	No	Few	Yes
Elimination half-life (hours)	14	2–3	1.2	3	1.8	19	2

hence many of their pharmacokinetic properties. Pravastatin, for example, is the most water-soluble, having a hydroxyl group. The next most hydrophilic statin is rosuvastatin, while the remainder are much more hydrophobic (Table 4.1). Lovastatin is a metabolite derived from the fungus *Aspergillus terreus* and is administered unchanged. Simvastatin is prepared by replacing the 2-methylbutyryl side-chain of lovastatin with a 2,2-methylbutyryl group. This increases the potency of the drug substantially. Pravastatin is derived by microbial transformation of the parent compound mevastatin.[3–5] These three 'natural' statins exhibit close structural identity while the other four marketed statins – rosuvastatin, fluvastatin, cerivastatin and atorvastatin – are entirely synthetic and have markedly differing chemical structures.

The clinical importance of the structural variations between statins resides in the differing doses needed to produce a desired reduction in plasma cholesterol and the pleiotropic effects of the drugs. If the latter phenomena turn out to be of significance in preventing coronary heart disease (CHD) then careful attention must be given to discovering which part of the molecule governs the additional beneficial effect, e.g. is the influence of statins on smooth muscle cell proliferation simply a function of their solubility properties?[6]

PHARMACOLOGY AND DRUG INTERACTIONS

Absorption of statins in the gut varies from <30% (pravastatin) to >90% (fluvastatin).[3–5,7–9] Peak plasma levels are attained one to three hours after administration. However, there is extensive first-pass extraction of the drugs in the liver. Since this is the major site of action, the plasma concentrations are not a guide to pharmacodynamic effects. Those compounds that are pro-drugs, i.e. the analogue to HMG-CoA is in the lactone ring formation (lovastatin, simvastatin), undergo ring cleavage and hence activation in the liver. This organ is a major site of cholesterol synthesis and lipoprotein production and catabolism. Thus, it is appropriate that the drugs reach their highest effective concentration at this site. Other tissues are of course exposed to highly variable concentrations of statin in the bloodstream. The consequences of this exposure are a matter of considerable controversy at present. Some statins, i.e. those of a lipophilic nature, will cross the blood–brain barrier and may generate CNS effects. This could arise either from a direct toxic effect of the compound or because of altered cholesterol homeostasis in the brain. Reports have appeared of differential effects of lipophilic (simvastatin) versus hydrophilic (pravastatin) statins on sleep disturbance.[10] The long-term consequences of these potential adverse events are not yet clear. Other cells dependent for their function on cholesterol availability, e.g. adrenal glands or ovaries, could possibly be affected by high systemic levels of statins, but again this theoretical issue has not translated into a chronic clinical problem.[11] Clinical benefit attributed to the pleiotropic effects of statins on, for example, inflammation and smooth muscle cell function will depend on the exposure of these cells to statins and the extent to which the drugs are taken up. The lack of influence of pravastatin on smooth muscle cell replication is likely to be due to low penetration of the cells by the drugs.[6]

Table 4.1 summarizes the major pharmacokinetic properties of marketed statins. A number of features are worthy of comment. Firstly, as rehearsed above, the solubility of the drug will influence its distribution and uptake by non-hepatic tissues with potentially beneficial or detrimental effects; at present these are under active investigation. Secondly, most agents have a short, less than 3 hour, half-life in plasma. Despite this, they cause a chronic stimulation of LDL receptor activity in the liver, presumably secondary to a profound and persistent effect on microsomal membrane cholesterol levels. It is also noteworthy that approximately the same LDL reduction is achieved whether the drugs are given as a single dose at night (when cholesterol synthesis is at the zenith of the diurnal rhythm),[12] in the morning or in divided doses (see, for example, refs 3 and 4). Atorvastatin and rosuvastatin, exceptionally, have long half-lives, as do their active major metabolites. It is this property of these drugs that has been suggested as the source of their greater efficacy in cholesterol lowering. Direct comparison of a single dose of atorvastatin versus simvastatin shows that the initial suppression of HMG-CoA reductase by the two agents is of a similar magnitude but the effect of the former is more persistent, lasting virtually 24 hours, while the enzyme's activity starts to recover within ten hours of administration of the latter.[13] Thirdly, there are differences in the metabolism and excretion of the drugs that have implications for clinical practice, especially in the typical post-myocardial infarction (MI) recipient of a statin, who is likely to be subject to polypharmacy. Lipophilic drugs, in order to be excreted from the body, must first be oxidized or conjugated with polar groups to increase their water solubility. Most compounds are acted on by the cytochrome P450 family of enzymes, which is composed of a large number of isoenzymes. It is the major 3A4 isoform in the liver that metabolizes many drugs and the majority of the statins. Exceptions to this rule are cerivastatin, which is able to interact with 2C8 as well as 3A4,[8] and fluvastatin, which uses 2C9.[14] Pravastatin does not undergo a cytochrome P450-mediated reaction. Its major degradation product is the 3-hydroxy isomer.[4] Rosuvastatin does not undergo any significant metabolism at the 3A4 site but is metabolized to a small extent by the

2C9 isoenzyme system.[15] A large range of pharmaceutical agents and other naturally occurring compounds (e.g. as contained in grapefruit juice) can act as competitive substrates or inhibitors of cytochrome P450 isoforms. If such a compound is co-administered with a statin then the plasma concentration of the latter can increase several-fold. An example is diltiazem, which, when given prior to a single dose of lovastatin, has been shown to cause a three- to fourfold increment in plasma concentration of the latter.[16] Patients' tolerance of statins as a class of drugs is very high and few report serious side-effects. Nevertheless, it is prudent when initiating statin treatment in a patient on medication for hypertension or other disorders to give thought to the potential for drug–drug interactions, which are an increasing medical problem.

SAFETY AND TOLERABILITY

The results of the large-scale outcome trials of statins are remarkable in two ways: the size and consistency of the benefits of treatment and the lack of serious or even moderately serious side-effects. The pathway of cholesterol production which statins inhibit is the route of generation of other molecules critical for cellular processes, including ubiquinone and geranyl and farnesyl derivatives. Ubiquinone (coenzyme Q) is important in electron transport and oxidation phosphorylation, while the geranyl- and farnesyl-related products are key components in cell growth. Early concerns about statin therapy centred on the risk of developing corneal opacities, myopathy and liver damage. Further, the pre-statin trials using fibrates[17] or cholestyramine[18] reported an apparent increase in non-cardiovascular causes of death, including suicide and violence. Increased risk of cancer was also a concern of earlier trials[19] and had to be addressed for statin therapy since such a fundamental cellular pathway was being perturbed.

Experience with the statins in both general use and in clinical trials has been that they provoke few serious adverse events. Side-effects, if they occur, are usually mild: gastrointestinal upsets, headache, fatigue and skin rashes. There are, however, two important, uncommon side-effects that clinicians need to be aware of when prescribing statins. One is an effect on liver enzymes, which is usually not noticed by the patient but may necessitate alanine aminotransferase (ALT) monitoring and sometimes withdrawal of the drug if levels climb to more than three times the upper limit of the laboratory reference range.

The second is that statins can occasionally affect muscle function, causing pain or weakness, and leakage of the muscle enzyme creatine kinase (CK or CPK) into the bloodstream. This is a marker of muscle damage, and if raised by more than ten times the upper limit of the laboratory reference range, the drug should be discontinued.

In its most extreme form this statin-induced myopathy may lead to rhabdomyolysis. This was recently highlighted by the withdrawal from clinical practice of cerivastatin in August 2001. This was the result of a significant increase in the number of cases of fatal rhabdomyolysis in patients receiving this drug. A number of these cases were the result of the co-prescription of cerivastatin and gemfibrozil – a combination that is well known to increase the risk of myopathy. Others could not be attributed to combination therapy but some were linked to the use of a newly introduced higher dose of cerivastatin.

This serves as a reminder that at high doses and in certain combinations, statins can lead to severe and even life-threatening complications, although this has only very rarely been observed with other approved statins. A review of statin safety was recently undertaken by the Committee on Safety of Medicines in the UK and they stated 'Due to pharmacokinetic and lipophilicity differences, the potential for inducing muscle disorders varies with individual drugs.'[20] This committee went on to conclude 'The rare risk of myopathy must be considered in the context of the overwhelmingly beneficial effects of the statins in the prevention of coronary artery disease. These benefits clearly outweigh the potential risks.'

The only other significant side-effect that was suggested early in the life-cycle of the stains, but which has since proved to be unfounded, is the occurrence of lens opacities. This was examined in some detail in the 4S study, and the incidence of opacities of any type was similar in the placebo and simvastatin groups and there appeared to be no cause for concern.[21]

Turning to the clinical trials, it can be seen that pravastatin in WOSCOPS, CARE and LIPID, lovastatin in AFCAPS, and simvastatin in 4S and the HPS caused no discernible increase in risk of non-cardiovascular events.[22–26] Trauma as a cause of death was the same in the treated versus control arms of these studies. The incidence of fatal or non-fatal cancers was, likewise, unaffected by statin treatment and this was also true when event rates were broken down by body system.[22–26] The higher rate of breast cancer seen in women on active treatment in CARE was not confirmed in the larger female cohort in LIPID and is considered a statistical anomaly.[23,24] Similarly, the discrepancy in the total numbers of newly diagnosed cancers between placebo and pravastatin groups in the recently published PROSPER study was thought to be explained by an imbalance in the randomization of patients with early pre-clinical cancer.[27] A meta-analysis of all large-scale pravastatin and non-pravastatin trials shows no effect on cancer rates attributable to statins.[27] Indeed, some workers have proposed that inhibition of HMG-CoA reductase using statin therapy may

be protective against the development of cancer.[28] Tolerability of the drugs used in the trials was very high in that the rates of withdrawal for non-cardiovascular adverse events were similar for patients on placebo and active drug.[22–26] In Scotland, all hospitalizations are recorded in a central registry, and for the WOSCOPS recruits we were able to capture hospitalization rates and discharge diagnosis in addition to the data recorded on case report forms.[29] A reduced number of cardiovascular hospitalizations was seen but no difference in admissions for other causes (Fig. 4.2). With regard to cholesterol lowering causing CNS disturbances (including homicidal tendencies), the relative risk of hospitalization for a psychiatric reason was 0.83 (pravastatin vs placebo; $P = 0.45$). Likewise, trauma and malignancy hospitalizations were equal in the two groups. A significantly lower risk of hepatic/biliary cases of hospitalization was noted in pravastatin-treated WOSCOPS subjects (see Fig. 4.2). This may of course be a spurious finding. However, it is known that statin treatment lowers the lithogenicity of bile[30] and reduced risk of gallstone disease may have been a sequela of active treatment.

A low rate of discontinuations for adverse events was reported in all major statin trials and there was no suggestion of an imbalance in the placebo versus active drug groups (Table 4.2). More specifically, abnormal liver function tests

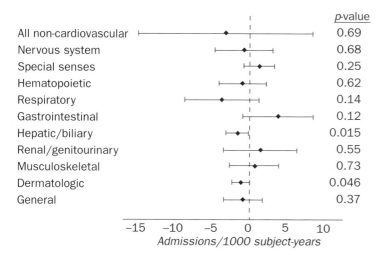

	p-value
All non-cardiovascular	0.69
Nervous system	0.68
Special senses	0.25
Hematopoietic	0.62
Respiratory	0.14
Gastrointestinal	0.12
Hepatic/biliary	0.015
Renal/genitourinary	0.55
Musculoskeletal	0.73
Dermatologic	0.046
General	0.37

−15 −10 −5 0 5 10
Admissions/1000 subject-years

Fig. 4.2 Effect of pravastatin on non-cardiovascular hospital admissions by ICD 8 Body System Code. The point estimate is indicated by a diamond for the difference between placebo and pravastatin groups in the mean number of admissions per 1000 subject-years. Negative values indicate reductions in hospitalization in pravastatin-treated subjects. Approximate 95% confidence intervals with permutation p-value are indicated. (Adapted with permission from ref. 29.)

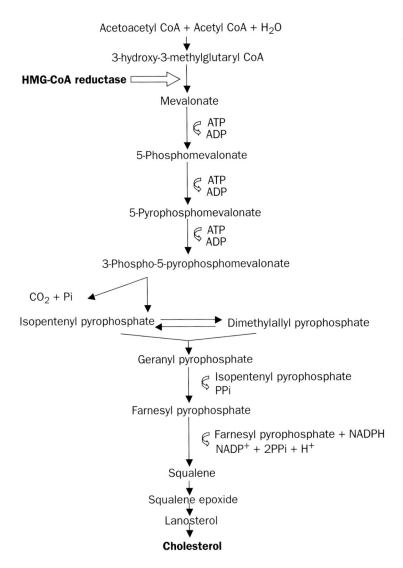

Fig. 4.3 The cholesterol biosynthetic pathway, showing the rate-limiting step catalysed by HMG-CoA reductase.

were not frequent or a feature of treatment, nor was myalgia or myopathy.[22–26] Overall, the lack of an adverse influence on non-cardiovascular death rates by the statins that have been tested means that substantial clinical benefit from CHD prevention can be obtained against a benign background.

Clinically, the major contraindication to the use of statin therapy is active liver disease, although statins should also be avoided in pregnancy and lactation and in women whose contraceptive methods are unreliable. Similarly, care should be taken in patients with renal impairment. None of the statins are licensed for use in

children in the UK but in October 2002 pravastatin was granted a paediatric licence in the USA for use in children aged eight or over with FH.

Statins are available as capsules or tablets to be taken once daily. Many statin manufacturers recommend dosing at night, the rationale for this being that cholesterol synthesis exhibits a diurnal rhythm, the maximum rate occurring at night. Since the statins inhibit cholesterol synthesis by inhibiting the rate-limiting enzyme, the maximum effect should be seen if they are given at the time of peak enzyme activity. In practice, however, if a patient can be encouraged to take their statin therapy at the same

Table 4.2 Adverse events in statin-based outcome trials

	WOSCOPS P/A	*AFCAPS P/A*	*4S P/A*	*CARE P/A*	*LIPID P/A*
Abnormal LFT	20/26	11/18	24/20	73/66	86/95
Discontinuation for adverse event	300/305	445/449	127/126	74/45	122/144
Fatal/non-fatal cancer	106/116	259/252	96/89	161/172	399/379
Death from suicide or violence	6/5	3/1	7/6	4/8	11/6
Total non-cardiovascular deaths	62/56	52/63	49/46	64/68	200/167

P, placebo; A, active drug; LFT, liver function tests.

time each day on a regular basis, this is more important than adhering strictly to evening dosing. And indeed the most recently introduced statin – rosuvastatin – is recommended for dosing at any time of day.

MECHANISMS OF LIPID LOWERING

To understand the mechanisms by which the statins impact upon the plasma cholesterol level we must first explore the regulation of cholesterol homeostasis at a cellular level. The cholesterol economy of the cell is controlled by a family of recently regulatory proteins known as sterol regulatory element-binding proteins (SREBPs).[2] These proteins control the transcription of the LDL receptor and at least six other key enzymatic steps in the cholesterol biosynthetic pathway (see Fig. 4.3).[31] A number of *in vitro* studies have shown that the addition of cholesterol to cells leads to the down-regulation of several key proteins involved in cholesterol homeostasis, including the LDL receptor, HMG-CoA reductase, HMG-CoA synthase and squalene synthase.[2] The SREBP family of proteins are synthesized as 125 kDa precursors that are tethered to the endoplasmic reticulum by two transmembrane domains. A fall in the intracellular cholesterol concentration is thought to lead to the depletion of a regulatory

pool within the membrane of the endoplasmic reticulum. This, in turn, leads to activation of the Site-1 protease that cleaves SREBP. This sterol-regulated cleavage of SREBP is followed by an unregulated second cut catalysed by the recently cloned Site-2 protease.[32] The now mature SREBP consists of a 68 kDa protein containing a basic helix–loop–helix leucine zipper domain. This protein travels to the cell nucleus, where it binds to sterol regulatory elements in the promoter sequences of various genes and activates their transcription.[2,33] When statin therapy is given, the competitive inhibition of the HMG-CoA reductase enzyme leads to a fall in the cholesterol biosynthetic capacity of the cell, and a fall in the intracellular cholesterol concentration. As described above, this sets in motion a train of events that ultimately leads to the enhanced transcription of several proteins involved in cholesterol homeostasis, including, perhaps most importantly, up-regulation of the LDL receptor.

Transcription of HMG-CoA reductase is also up-regulated but this enzyme is not increased enough to overcome the drug effect, i.e. there is more inhibition present than enzyme produced.

The LDL receptor is a single transmembrane glycoprotein with 839 amino acids arranged into five functional domains.[1] The ligand-binding domain is found in the 300-amino-acid

N-terminal segment, which consists of seven 40-amino-acid repeat units, each of which is enriched in aspartate and glutamate residues arranged in a configuration that facilitates electrostatic interaction with complementary arginine and lysine residues found on two apolipoproteins: apoB and apoE.[34] The receptor therefore recognizes and interacts with particles containing these proteins, but with different affinities since apoE binds approximately ten times more effectively than apoB. In theory, the whole spectrum of particles found within the VLDL–LDL interval, which contains one or both of these proteins, could interact with and be degraded by the LDL receptor. Early metabolic studies[35] focused on LDL since it was the lipoprotein recognized to be markedly increased in FH. However, as knowledge developed, it became clearer that the impact of receptor deficiency was felt along the length of the VLDL delipidation cascade, suggesting that the 'LDL' receptor had a wider role in apoB metabolism than its name suggests.

Tracer kinetic analysis following administration of ^{125}I-labeled LDL to humans has shown that approximately 30–40% of the entire LDL mass in the plasma is catabolized each day. Chemical modification of the tracer with agents such as 1,2-cyclohexanedione,[36] glucose[37] or 2-hydroxyacetaldehyde,[38] which interact with arginine or lysine residues on its apolipoprotein moiety, reduces its clearance by 50–70%. Since this treatment blocks binding of the lipoprotein to the receptor, clearly receptor activity must make a major contribution to LDL turnover. The role of the receptor falls by half in those subjects with heterozygous FH and is abolished in homozygous individuals.[36] In consequence, more LDL is directed into alternative catabolic mechanisms which are mediated via the macrophage scavenger receptors.[39]

We know from extensive experiments on cultured cells that the activity of LDL receptors is regulated by variation in the intracellular sterol pool. When the requirement for cholesterol is increased, receptor synthesis is stimulated and LDL uptake promoted. Conversely, in times of surfeit, receptor expression is diminished and LDL assimilation suppressed. Extrapolation of these concepts to man and the recently discovered role of SREBPs has enlightened our understanding of the regulation of LDL metabolism and provided an explanation for the actions of a number of cholesterol-lowering drugs, including the statins.

As indicated earlier, theoretical considerations suggest that we ought to expect the LDL receptor to be implicated in the metabolism of VLDL and IDL. In 1982, Soutar et al. discovered that IDL clearance is retarded in FH.[40] This problem was further examined in detail using cumulative flotation ultracentrifugation to follow the flux of apoB from VLDL through IDL to LDL.[41] FH homozygotes accumulate cholesterol-rich remnants within their VLDL density interval because they lack the capacity to clear them normally. IDL catabolism is also perturbed to such an extent that its pool size increases as much as that of LDL, the level of which rises 3.5-fold in the plasma. Absence of the LDL receptor, therefore, has a profound impact on apoB metabolism in its entirety. But what of its role in normolipaemic subjects? This question may be addressed by following the approach outlined earlier that relies on modification of the ligand to affect its receptor binding. Treatment of large, triglyceride-rich VLDL[42] has no effect on its direct clearance from the plasma or its conversion to IDL. However, subsequent catabolism of apoB-containing particles is significantly retarded. Additional evidence supporting the view that LDL receptors participate in VLDL remnant and IDL clearance comes from clinical observation of patients with dysbetalipoproteinaemia. This condition is accompanied by high circulating levels of both these lipoprotein fractions due to their inability to bind efficiently to hepatic lipoprotein receptors. Up-regulation of the LDL receptor with an HMG-CoA reductase inhibitor lowers the concentration of VLDL remnants and IDL in the plasma of these dysbetalipoproteinaemic patients.[43]

When the detailed mechanism of action of simvastatin was studied in moderately hypercholesterolaemic (non-FH) subjects it was clear that the direct catabolism of lipoproteins throughout the VLDL delipidation cascade was

Table 4.3 Mean percentage change in triglyceride by drug, dose and baseline triglyceride level

	Baseline triglyceride (mg/dl)	Dose (mg)			
		10	20	40	80
Lovastatin	<150	–	+1.3	+4	–9
	150–250	–	–9	–14	–18
	>250	–	–32	–36	–44
Pravastatin	<150	+6	+6	–4	–
	150–250	–11	–11	–15	–
	>250	–22	–25	–35	–
Simvastatin	<150	+0.7	–12	–7	–11
	150–250	–20	–30	–22	–25
	>250	–28	–24	–29	–40

Data from Stein et al.[48]

stimulated.[44] This was a direct consequence of the statin-mediated up-regulation of the LDL receptor. In these subjects the fall in plasma LDL cholesterol concentration as a result of statin therapy was, therefore, not, as expected, due simply to an increase in the clearance of LDL but was also due significantly to a fall in LDL production caused by enhanced clearance of LDL precursors.

Effects on plasma LDL cholesterol

Plasma LDL cholesterol reductions achieved with statin therapy appear to be independent of the baseline lipid phenotype. That said, it must also be appreciated that between statins there are marked differences in cholesterol-lowering effectiveness, and wide inter-individual variation in response to the same dose on one statin. For example, a recent study of simvastatin at 40 mg/day for three months produced anything from a decrement in LDL cholesterol of over 60% to an increment of almost 10%.[45]

There are many small studies defining the biochemical effectiveness of the statins either individually or in comparison with each other. However, any tabular comparison of the cholesterol-lowering effects of the statins inevitably

raises more questions than it answers, as small studies are often included alongside large-scale studies, results achieved in normal practice are compared with the results achieved in a controlled clinical trial setting, and different doses are compared. A fairer comparison may be to highlight the differential potency of the statins, i.e. the LDL cholesterol lowering achieved on a milligram per milligram basis. Using this form of analysis, it is clear that lovastatin is the 'weakest' statin and cerivastatin the 'strongest'. However, even this approach is also misleading as cerivastatin is marketed in microgram doses while the other statins are produced in milligram doses.

What is obvious from studies with all the statins is that the dose-response is not a simple linear one. Doubling the dose of any statin does not double the percentage cholesterol lowering. Indeed, as a rule of thumb, each time the dose is doubled an approximately 6% further reduction is achieved.

While there are clear pharmacological differences between the statins in terms of the cholesterol reductions seen with equivalent doses, it is probably true to say that by adjusting the doses accordingly all statins are capable of producing equivalent reductions in LDL cholesterol. What is not clear from studies completed so far is whether such dose adjustments will be equally free from side-effects for each statin, or whether therapy with all statins, irrespective of their potency in lowering LDL cholesterol, will have the same effect on clinical events.

Effects on plasma triglyceride and HDL

Considering their basic mechanism of action, it was assumed that statins would have no effect on triglyceride levels but this was not the case. Two studies looking at the effects of statins in patients with hypertriglyceridaemia revealed that simvastatin and atorvastatin both reduced plasma triglyceride levels in these subjects in proportion to their effects on LDL cholesterol.[46,47] This prompted a more detailed analysis of the question looking at data from different statins at different doses. Thus, a fixed, non-dose-related triglyceride/LDL cholesterol ratio in subjects on statin therapy with or without baseline hypertriglyceridaemia was discovered.[48] At lower plasma triglyceride levels (<150 mg/dl; 1.7 mmol/l) the percent reduction in triglyceride with statin therapy is modest in comparison with the effects of the drug on LDL. When baseline triglyceride concentration exceeded 250 mg/dl (2.8 mmol/l) the percent triglyceride reduction achieved with any of the statins tested at any dose equaled the corresponding percent reduction in LDL cholesterol. This is shown in Table 4.3. All statins are therefore effective in lowering plasma triglyceride levels, in addition to their effects on plasma LDL cholesterol, but only in baseline hypertriglyceridaemic subjects is this effect comparable to the effects on plasma cholesterol

Two possible mechanisms have been postulated to explain the influence of the statins on triglyceride and, more specifically, VLDL metabolism. In the first, it is proposed that statins inhibit VLDL secretion by limiting the availability of free cholesterol or cholesteryl esters for lipoprotein assembly. There are *in vitro* and animal model studies to support this concept[49–52] and recently atorvastatin has been reported to promote apoB intracellular degradation in HepG2 cells, possibly by so lowering the cholesterol content of nascent lipoprotein

particles that they become unstable.[53] In the second, it is suggested that drug-induced stimulation of LDL receptors promotes the direct catabolism of VLDL, particularly the cholesterol-rich remnants.[44] If the latter mechanism is important then the observation that VLDL (particularly large VLDL1) from hypertriglyceridaemics, by virtue of its surface apoE content, binds to the LDL receptor whereas VLDL from normotriglyceridaemics fails to do so;[54] this provides a possible explanation for the phenotype dependency of plasma triglyceride lowering by statins described above. Recently, clear evidence has emerged from kinetic studies that the principal mechanism whereby statins lower VLDL and plasma triglyceride in hypertriglyceridaemic subjects is by enhanced clearance of VLDL. Production of this lipoprotein was unaffected by therapy.[55,56]

Collectively, what has emerged from these studies is that the initial phenotype of our patients has little bearing on the LDL cholesterol lowering with statin therapy, but when the effects on triglyceride are examined the initial phenotype is paramount. To understand this apparent paradox we must continue our studies of the effects of intracellular lipid availability on lipoprotein assembly and secretion. The more we understand about the latter, the more we will appreciate the putative effects of statins on lipoprotein synthetic mechanisms.

Accompanying the changes in triglyceride there are small increases in HDL cholesterol on statins, usually of the order of 5–10%. The significance of these is not clear, nor is the mechanism for the increase. In WOSCOPS the small rise in HDL could not be linked to any change in the risk of coronary events.[57] HDL of course plays an important role in reverse cholesterol transport and therefore if statins are altering the dynamics of this process without disturbing the steady state concentration of the lipoprotein then further detailed studies will be required to understand what is happening and its impact on atherosclerosis.

The statin-induced rise in HDL has been investigated in detail in the WOSCOPS cohort. Here it was seen that body mass index, alcohol intake and the extent of reduction in plasma triglyceride were important determinants of the size of the increment in HDL cholesterol.[58] It has also been discovered that statins perturb HDL subfraction distribution with treatment generating an increase in apoAI-containing particles and a decrease in apoAI/AII particles.[59]

CONCLUSIONS

Regardless of the lipid phenotype, the individual prescribed statin therapy will achieve clinically significant changes in their lipid profile. The precise nature and extent of these changes will depend in part on the individual's phenotype and in part on the particular statin and dose used.

Most of the statins have been shown to be safe and well tolerated by a very wide range of subjects. Their safety record is remarkable given the early concerns of some clinicians who feared the consequences of inhibiting such a fundamental biochemical pathway in the body. However, as we move from medium- to long-term experience with the original statins and as we see the introduction of new synthetic compounds that hope to emulate the early drugs, we must maintain our vigilance and continually monitor the clinical use of this group of drugs, taking nothing for granted. The withdrawal of cerivastatin from widespread clinical practice because of safety concerns serves as an important reminder of this.

Despite the focus of this chapter on the chemistry and pharmacology of the statins, what remains of paramount importance is their clinical effectiveness. The efficacy of the statins is often discussed in terms of lipid lowering as if this were the real reason why statins are prescribed. In reality, statins are used in an attempt to alter the future of our patients – to reduce the risk of first or subsequent cardiovascular, and more recently cerebrovascular, events. Large controlled clinical trials with lovastatin, simvastatin and pravastatin have proven very conclusively the clinical effectiveness of these statins. Other trials are underway, particularly with atorvastatin and rosuvastatin.

There is no doubt that the statins will continue to have a very prominent place in the cardiovascular formulary. In comparison with many other drugs in common use, this place is appropriate and fully justified.

REFERENCES

1. Brown MS, Goldstein JL. The LDL receptor. In: Gallo LL, ed. *Cardiovascular Disease*. New York: Plenum Press, 1987: 87–91.
2. Brown MS, Goldstein JL. The SREBP pathway: regulation of cholesterol metabolism by proteolysis of a membrane-bound transcription factor. *Cell* 1997; **89**: 331–40.
3. Anon. Lovastatin. In: Dollery C, ed. *Therapeutic Drugs*. Edinburgh: Churchill Livingstone, 1991: L66–L70.
4. Anon. Pravastatin (sodium). In: Dollery C, ed. *Therapeutic Drugs Supplement 2*. Edinburgh: Churchill Livingstone, 1994: 196–200.
5. Anon. Simvastatin. In: Dollery C, ed. *Therapeutic Drugs*. Edinburgh: Churchill Livingstone, 1991: S25–S29.
6. Rosensen RS, Tangney CC. Antiatherothrombotic properties of statins. *JAMA* 1998; **279**: 1643–50.
7. Blum CB. Comparison of the properties of four inhibitors of 3-hydroxy 3-methylglutaryl coenzyme A reductase. *Am J Cardiol* 1994; **73**: 3–11.
8. Muck W. Rationale assessment of the interaction profile of cerivastatin supports its low propensity for drug interactions. *Drugs* 1998; **56** (Suppl 1): 15–23.
9. Lea AP, McTavish D. Atorvastatin 1997: a review of its pharmacology and therapeutic potential in the management of hyperlipidemia. *Drugs* 1997; **53**: 828–47.
10. Eckemas SA, Roos BE, Kvidal P et al. The effects of simvastatin and pravastatin on objective and subjective measures of nocturnal sleep: a comparison of two structurally different HMG-CoA reductase inhibitors in patients with primary moderate hypercholesterolaemia. *Br J Clin Pharmacol* 1993; **35**: 284–9.
11. Travia D, Tosi F, Negri C et al. Sustained therapy with 3-hydroxy-3-methylglutaryl-coenzyme-A reductase inhibitors does not impair steroidogenesis by adrenals and gonads. *J Clin Endocrinol Metab* 1995; **80**: 836–40.
12. Parker TS, McNamara DS, Brown CD et al. Mevalonic acid in human plasma: relationship of concentration and circadian rhythm to cholesterol synthesis rates in man. *Proc Natl Acad Sci USA* 1982; **79**: 3037–41.

13. Naoumova RP, Dunn S, Ralliis L et al. Prolonged inhibition of cholesterol synthesis explains the efficacy of atorvastatin. *J Lipid Res* 1997; **38**: 1496–500.

14. Meadowcroft AM, Williamson KM, Patterson JH et al. The effects of fluvastatin, a CYP2C9 inhibitor, on losartan pharmacokinetics in healthy volunteers. *J Clin Pharmacol* 1999; **39**: 418–24.

15. Martin PD, Mitchell PD, Schneck DW. Disposition of a new HMG-CoA reductase inhibitor ZD4522 following dosing in healthy subjects. *J Clin Pharmacol* 2000; **40**: 1056.

16. Azie NE, Brater DC, Becker PA et al. The interaction of diltiazem with lovastatin and pravastatin. *Clin Pharmacol Ther* 1998; **64**: 369–77.

17. Frick MH, Elo O, Haapa K et al. Helsinki Heart Study: Primary-prevention trial with gemfibrozil in middle-aged men with dyslipidemia. *N Eng J Med* 1987; **317**: 1237–45.

18. Lipid Research Clinics Program. The Lipid Research Clinics Coronary Primary Prevention Trial results. I. Reduction in incidence of coronary heart disease. *JAMA* 1984; **251**: 351–64.

19. Gould AL, Rossouw JE, Santanello NC et al. Cholesterol reduction yields clinical benefit. A new look at old data. *Circulation* 1995; **91**: 2274–82.

20. Committee on the Safety of Medicines. HMG-CoA reductase inhibitors (statins) and myopathy. *Curr Prob Pharmacovigilance* 2002; **28**: 8–9.

21. Pedersen TR, Berg K, Cook TJ et al. Safety and tolerability of cholesterol lowering with simvastatin during 5 years in the Scandinavian Simvastatin Survival Study. *Arch Int Med* 1996; **156**: 2058–92.

22. Shepherd J, Cobbe SM, Ford I et al. Prevention of coronary heart disease with pravastatin in men with hypercholesterolemia. *N Eng J Med* 1995; **333**: 1301–7.

23. Sacks FM, Pfeffer MA, Moye LA et al. The effect of pravastatin on coronary events after myocardial infarction in patients with average cholesterol levels. *N Eng J Med* 1996; **335**: 1001–9.

24. LIPID Study Group. Prevention of cardiovascular events and death with pravastatin in patients with coronary heart disease and a broad range of cholesterol levels. *N Eng J Med* 1998; **339**: 1349–57.

25. Downs JR, Clearfield M, Weis S et al. Primary prevention of acute coronary events with lovastatin in men and women with average cholesterol levels: results of AFCAPS/TEXCAPS Research Group. *JAMA* 1998; **279**: 1615–22.

26. Scandinavian Simvastatin Survival Study Group. Randomised trial of cholesterol lowering in 4444 patients with coronary heart disease: the Scandinavian Simvastatin Survival Study (4S). *Lancet* 1994; **344**: 1383–89.

27. Shepherd J, Blauw GJ, Murphy MB et al. Pravastatin in elderly individuals at risk of vascular disease (PROSPER): a randomised controlled trial. *Lancet* 2002; **360**: 1623–30.

28. Goldstein JL, Brown MS. Regulation of the mevalonate pathway. *Nature* 1990; **343**: 425–30.

29. West of Scotland Coronary Prevention Study Group. The effects of pravastatin on hospital admission in hypercholesterolemic middle-aged men. *J Am Coll Cardiol* 1999; **33**: 909–15.

30. Duane WC. Effects of lovastatin in humans on biliary lipid composition and secretion as a function of dosage and treatment interval. *J Pharmacol Exp Ther* 1994; **270**: 841–5.

31. Horton JD, Shimomura I. Sterol regulatory element-binding proteins: activators of cholesterol and fatty acid biosynthesis. *Curr Opin Lipidol* 1999; **10**: 143–50.

32. Rawson RB, Zelinski NG, Nijhawan D et al. Complementation cloning of S2P, a gene encoding a putative metalloprotease required for intramembrane cleavage of SREBPs. *Mol Cell* 1997; **1**: 47–57.

33. Edwards PA, Ericsson J. Signaling molecules derived from the cholesterol biosynthetic pathway: mechanisms of action and possible roles in human disease. *Curr Opin Lipidol* 1998; **9**: 433–40.

34. Mahley RW, Innerarity TL. Lipoprotein receptors and cholesterol homeostasis. *Biochim Biophys Acta* 1983; **737**: 197–222.

35. Bilheimer DW, Stone NJ, Grundy SM. Metabolic studies in familial hypercholesterolemia. *J Clin Invest* 1979; **64**: 524–33.

36. Shepherd J, Bicker S, Lorimer AR, Packard CJ. Receptor-mediated low density lipoprotein catabolism in man. *J Lipid Res* 1979; **20**: 999–1006.

37. Kesaniemi YA, Witztum JL, Steinbrecher UP. Receptor mediated catabolism of LDL in man. *J Clin Invest* 1983; **71**: 950–9.

38. Slater HR, McKinney L, Packard CJ, Shepherd J. Contribution of the receptor pathway to low-density lipoprotein catabolism in humans. New methods for quantification. *Arteriosclerosis* 1984; **4**: 604–13.

39. Matsumoto A, Naito M, Itakura H et al. Human macrophage scavenger receptors – primary structure, expression and localization in athero-

sclerotic lesions. *Proc Natl Acad Sci USA* 1990; **87**: 9133–7.

40. Soutar AK, Myant NB, Thompson GR. The metabolism of very-low-density and intermediate-density lipoproteins in patients with familial hypercholesterolaemia. *Atherosclerosis* 1982; **43**: 217–31.

41. James RW, Martin B, Pometta D et al. Apolipoprotein B metabolism in homozygous familial hypercholesterolemia. *J Lipid Res* 1989; **30**: 159–69.

42. Packard CJ, Boag DE, Clegg RJ et al. Effects of 1,2-cyclohexanedione modification on the metabolism of VLDL apolipoprotein B. *J Lipid Res* 1985; **26**: 1058–67.

43. Vega GL, East C, Grundy SM. Lovastatin therapy in familial dysbetalipoproteinemia: effects on kinetics of apolipoprotein B. *Atherosclerosis,* 1988; **70**: 131–43.

44. Gaw A, Packard CJ, Murray EF et al. Effects of simvastatin on apoB metabolism and LDL subfraction distribution. *Arterioscler Thromb* 1993; **13**: 170–89.

45. Dujovne CA. New lipid-lowering drugs and new effects of old drugs. *Curr Opin Lipidol* 1997; **8**: 362–8.

46. Stein EA, Davidson MH, Dujovne CA et al. Efficacy and tolerability of low-dose simvastatin and niacin, alone and in combination, in patients with combined hyperlipidemia: a prospective trial. *J Cardiovasc Pharmacol Therapeut* 1996; **1**: 107–16.

47. Bakker-Arkema RG, Davidson MH, Goldstein RJ et al. Efficacy and safety of a new 17 HMG-CoA reductase inhibitor, atorvastatin, in patients with hypertriglyceridemia. *JAMA* 1996; **275**: 128–33.

48. Stein EA, Lane M, Laskarzewski P. Comparison of statins in hypertriglyceridemia. *Am J Cardiol* 1998; **81** (Suppl 4A): B66–B69.

49. Burnett JR, Wilcox LJ, Telford DE et al. Inhibition of HMG-CoA reductase by atorvastatin decreases both VLDL and LDL apolipoprotein B production in miniature pigs. *Arterioscler Thromb Vasc Biol* 1997; **17**: 2589–600.

50. Cianflone K, Yasruel Z, Rodriguez MA et al. Regulation of apoB secretion from HepG2 cells: evidence for a critical role for cholesteryl ester synthesis in the response to a fatty acid challenge. *J Lipid Res* 1990; **31**: 2045–55.

51. Qin W, Infante J, Wang S, Infante R. Regulation of HMG-CoA reductase, apoprotein B and LDL receptor gene expression by the hypocholesterolemic drugs simvastatin and ciprofibrate in HepG2 human and rat hepatocytes. *Biochim Biophys Acta* 1992; **1127**: 57–66.

52. Kasim SE, Elovson J, Khilnani S et al. Effect of lovastatin on the secretion of very low density lipoprotein lipids and apolipoprotein B in the hypertriglyceridemic Zucker obese rat. *Atherosclerosis* 1993; **104**: 147–52.

53. Mohammadi AJ, Macri J, Newton R et al. Effects of atorvastatin on the intracellular stability and secretion of apolipoprotein B in HepG2 cells. *Arterioscler Thromb Vasc Biol* 1998; **18**: 783–93.

54. Gianturco SH, Brown FB, Gotto AM, Bradley WA. Receptor mediated uptake of hypertriglyceridemic very low density lipoproteins by normal human fibroblasts. *J Lipid Res* 1982; **23**: 984–93.

55. Forster LF, Stewart G, Bedford D et al. Influence of atorvastatin and simvastatin on apolipoprotein B metabolism in moderate combined hyperlipidemic subjects with low VLDL and LDL fractional clearance rates. *Atherosclerosis* 2002; **164**: 129–45.

56. Chan DC, Watts GF, Barrett PHR et al. Regulatory effects of HMG-CoA reductase inhibitor and fish oils on apolipoprotein B-100 kinetics in insulin-resistant obese male subjects with dyslipidemia. *Diabetes* 2002; **51**: 2377–86.

57. West of Scotland Coronary Prevention Study Group. Influence of pravastatin and plasma lipids on clinical events in the West of Scotland Coronary Prevention Study (WOSCOPS). *Circulation* 1998; **97**: 1440–5.

58. Streja L, Packard CJ, Shepherd J et al. for the WOSCOPS Group. Factors affecting low-density lipoprotein and high-density lipoprotein cholesterol response to pravastatin in the West of Scotland Coronary Prevention Study (WOSCOPS). *Am J Cardiol* 2002; **90**: 731–6.

59. Asztalos BF, Horvath KV, McNamara JR et al. Comparing the effects of five different statins on the HDL subpopulation profiles of coronary heart disease patients. *Atherosclerosis* 2002; **164**: 361–9.

5

Ancillary benefits of the statins

Brendan M Buckley

INTRODUCTION

HMG-CoA reductase inhibitors (statins) were originally developed to achieve a simple objective: to lower plasma cholesterol concentrations by inhibiting the rate-limiting enzyme in the pathway of cholesterol synthesis in the liver. They do this effectively, decreasing cholesterol synthesis and causing consequent up-regulation of hepatic LDL receptor activity. Their affinity for the active site of HMG-CoA reductase and their elimination half-lives largely determine differences in their efficacy in achieving this. It was anticipated that this would retard the development of atheromatous plaque, which might even regress through lipid loss, rendering plaque less occlusive and less vulnerable to disruption and thrombosis. Over the past decade, however, a number of diverse biological effects of HMG-CoA reductase inhibition by statins have been described in experimental systems, both *in vitro* and *in vivo*, that are difficult to explain on the basis of cholesterol lowering. These ancillary or *pleiotropic* effects (from the Greek πλείων for 'more') have been invoked to explain a number of phenomena that were not expected when statins were first introduced for the treatment of hypercholesterolaemia.

CLINICAL EVIDENCE SUGGESTING THAT STATINS HAVE PLEIOTROPIC ACTIONS

Early onset of clinical benefit with statin therapy

Before statins became available for therapeutic use, bile acid sequestrant resins such as cholestyramine were a mainstay of cholesterol-lowering therapy. These work by interruption of the enterohepatic circulation of bile acids, depleting hepatic cholesterol and inducing expression of LDL receptors. Trials of these agents[1] and of surgical partial ileal bypass,[2] which also decreases sterol enterohepatic circulation, showed that it took more than five years of treatment before significant benefit in reduction of coronary events was observed. This time to benefit was more or less what was anticipated intuitively, as it was believed that plaque lipid deposits would continue to accumulate normally in the untreated group while plaque would grow more slowly or perhaps even become depleted gradually in those on active treatment. While cholestyramine treatment achieved the modest effects of 8.5% lower total cholesterol and 12.6% lower LDL levels than placebo,[1] the effect of partial ileal bypass in the POSCH study[2] was to decrease total cholesterol by 29.2% and LDL by 43.2%, an effect comparable to those of statins. However, when the first landmark statin studies were reported, participants treated with simvastatin in 4S[3] and pravastatin in WOSCOPS[4] and CARE[5] showed benefit as early as six months. This suggested that statins might influence atheroma stability and thrombogenicity by mechanisms of action additional to those influencing LDL deposition in plaque.

Unexpected extent of benefit

Post-hoc multivariate regression analysis of the WOSCOPS trial results[6] showed that the relative risk reduction generated by pravastatin therapy was associated neither with baseline LDL level nor with treatment-induced fall in LDL level. Maximum benefit of an approximately 45% risk reduction was seen in the middle quintile of LDL reduction (mean 24% fall); further mean decrements in LDL (≤ 39%) were not associated with a greater decrease in CHD risk. In the CARE study, comparable analysis also showed that the extent of LDL reduction did not predict CHD event reduction.[7] In WOSCOPS, the Framingham risk equation predicted the observed CHD event rate in the placebo group but the CHD event rate in the pravastatin-treated group was 31% less than predicted.[6] When subjects with the same on-treatment LDL levels were compared, CHD event rates in pravastatin-treated subjects were 36% lower than those on placebo. The authors concluded that LDL reduction alone did not appear to account entirely for the benefits of pravastatin therapy.[6] In the 4S trial,[8] the simvastatin dose was adjusted towards an on-treatment cholesterol target level and it is more difficult to interpret this kind of analysis. However, it was shown that a reduction of the major coronary event rate depended on the extent of LDL lowering on treatment, greater cholesterol reductions giving continuous but progressively smaller decrements in CHD risk. The authors speculated that little would be gained by driving LDL to very low concentrations. In the AFCAPS/TEXCAPS study,[9] on-treatment LDL did not predict a subsequent event rate although apoB did. Similar analyses are awaited for later large outcomes trials. If these analyses are performed, they may demonstrate whether this is a consistent effect of pravastatin and whether it also occurs with other statins.

Effects on transplant survival

A dramatic effect of pravastatin treatment on one-year survival after heart transplantation provided further evidence for the existence of statin effects augmenting those due to LDL lowering.[10] Patients shortly after transplantation, on otherwise usual best care, were randomly assigned to receive either pravastatin (47 patients) or no statin (50 patients). At one year

the pravastatin group had plasma total cholesterol levels 32% lower than the controls, less frequent cardiac rejection accompanied by haemodynamic compromise, better survival and a lower incidence of coronary vasculopathy in the transplant. There was no difference between the two groups in the incidence of mild or moderate episodes of cardiac rejection. There was no correlation between higher cholesterol levels and the development of either cardiac rejection accompanied by haemodynamic compromise or coronary vasculopathy in the transplant (as detected by angiography or at post-mortem). In a subgroup of patients, the cytotoxicity of natural killer cells was lower in the pravastatin group than in the control group (9.8% vs 22.2% specific lysis). This study, with a subsequent analogous study on renal transplant recipients,[11] gave early credence to the concept that statins might have independent immuno-modulatory effects which combine with their primary actions on lipid levels to generate major overall benefit to such patients.

In aggregate, these observations of unexpected speed and extent of benefit of statin therapy in CHD prevention, along with the effect of the drugs in transplant recipients, suggest that factors additional to the lowering of LDL concentrations in plasma may contribute to the overall clinical benefit of treatment. What these factors might be, and the extent to which they contribute to outcomes of statin therapy, have been the subject of considerable recent interest since attention was first drawn to the phenomenon.[12,13]

POTENTIAL MECHANISMS OF STATIN ACTION BEYOND LIPID LOWERING

Effects based on the mevalonate pathway

Mevalonate, the product of HMG-CoA reductase, is a precursor in the synthesis of not only cholesterol but also a range of other important molecules involved in functions as varied as cellular respiration, signal transduction and nitric oxide production. Thus the inhibition of mevalonate synthesis by statins might modify parameters other than LDL that influence

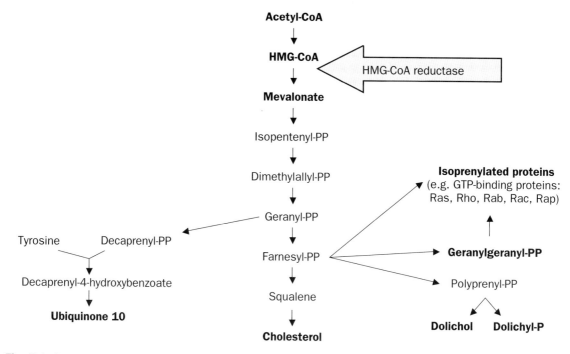

Fig. 5.1 Schematic representation of the mevalonate pathway in human cells.

atherosclerosis and the vascular milieu. Indeed it would be naïve to expect that the pharmaco-dynamic effects of statins do not involve the other pathway products whose synthesis is affected by the drugs. The mevalonate pathway is depicted in Fig. 5.1.

GTP-binding protein isoprenylation

The pathway products that have attracted most attention are the isoprenoids farnesyl pyrophos-phate (FPP) and geranylgeranyl pyrophosphate (GGPP). These molecules are necessary for post-translational modification by isoprenylation of a large number of proteins involved in cytoskeleton integrity and intracellular signal transduction.[14] Consequently, FPP and GGPP production can potentially influence cell sig-nalling, growth, differentiation and motility, as well as gene expression and the intracellular movement of cell structural components. A range of such effects of statins have been described especially on members of the small intracellular GTP-binding protein family such as Ras[15–17] and Rho,[18–26] some of which will be further described below. Table 5.1 shows that

Table 5.1   Potential ancillary mechanisms of action of statins beyond lipid lowering

Effects based on mevalonate pathway inhibition
* Decreased isoprenylation of GTP-binding proteins from farnesyl-PP and geranylgeranyl-PP
* Decreased protein glycosylation from dolichyl-P
* Decreased respiratory chain activity through lower ubiquinone concentrations (unlikely)

Effects independent of the mevalonate pathway
* Direct binding to leukocyte function antigen-1
* Anti-oxidant activity of drug molecule or metabolites within lipoprotein layer

most of the pleiotropic effects described for statins are attributed to decreased isoprenyla-tion of these proteins. Firm evidence for this effect as the mediator of statin action *in vitro* or *ex vivo* is obtained when the observed effect of the statin is reversed by the addition of meval-onate but not of squalene. The identity of the

GTP-binding protein that is the target of the effect may be determined by direct analysis or by further specific inhibitor studies.

There are consistent reports in several model systems *in vitro* that statins down-regulate the activation of the transcription factors NF-κB, AP-1, and hypoxia-inducible factor-1α.[27] This effect is mediated by GTP-binding protein isoprenylation.[28] These factors are important in the regulation of inflammation and of cell differentiation and proliferation.[29]

Dolichol

The term dolichol encompasses a homologous series of α-saturated polyisoprenoid alcohols containing 14–24 isoprene units that are products of a terminal branch of the mevalonate pathway. HMG-CoA reductase inhibition decreases their synthesis. Dolichyl phosphate is a donor of oligosaccharides in glycoprotein synthesis in the endoplasmic reticulum and appears to act as a regulator of cell growth through limiting N-linked glycosylation of the insulin-like growth factor-1 (IGF-1) receptor. In cell cultures, micromolar concentrations of lovastatin inhibited by 95% the N-linked glycosylation of IGF-1 receptors, followed by decreased expression of cell membrane IGF-1 receptors due to inhibition of DNA synthesis[30,31] Ras isoprenylation in the same experiments was inhibited by 50%.[30] It is therefore possible that some of the effects of statins may be exerted through dolichol-mediated changes in cell growth and in other glycosylation-linked membrane receptor functions. This remains to be systematically investigated.

Ubiquinone

Ubiquinone (also known as coenzyme Q), a product of the mevalonate pathway, is an electron carrier in the oxidation–reduction reactions involving complexes I, II and III in the mitochondrial respiratory chain. The assertion is occasionally encountered that ubiquinone depletion may be the basis for some of the cholesterol-independent effects of statins. It is often loosely suggested as a candidate mechanism for the rare cases of myopathy that complicate treatment with the drugs. However, this is not supported by evidence. Whereas ubiquinone concentrations decrease in serum in humans on statin treatment,[32,33] treatment with simvastatin (20 mg/day for six months) did not alter skeletal muscle concentrations of high-energy phosphates and ubiquinone in hypercholesterolaemic patients.[34,35] In rabbits, ubiquinone concentrations in skeletal muscle were decreased after treatment with massive doses of either of two statins (50 mg/kg per day simvastatin and up to 300 mg/kg per day pravastatin) and myopathy occurred in most animals. Nevertheless, mitochondrial activities of respiratory chain enzymes were normal in all groups, indicating that myopathy was not induced by a secondary dysfunction of mitochondrial respiration due to low ubiquinone levels.[36] Ubiquinone is not rate-limiting in mitochondrial respiration and is unlikely to be involved in the ancillary benefits of statins in atherosclerosis–thrombosis.

Effects independent of the mevalonate pathway

The statins are structurally heterogeneous (see Fig. 4.1 in Chapter 4), the HMG-analogous moiety which binds to the active site forming a relatively small part of the drug molecule. Therefore, the relatively large side-chains have potential for pharmacodynamic activity independent of the prime action of the drug.

Direct binding to leukocyte function antigen-1

Some immunomodulatory effects of statins may occur through a mevalonate-independent mechanism. Statins selectively block the β2 integrin leukocyte function antigen-1 (LFA-1), which has an important role in inflammation through mediating T-cell activation, leukocyte migration, adhesion and co-stimulation of lymphocytes. This effect occurs by binding to a novel allosteric site within LFA-1 and appears to be unrelated to inhibition of HMG-CoA reductase.[37] The effect has been shown for lovastatin to be due to the inhibition of the interaction of human LFA-1 with its counter-receptor ICAM-1. Nuclear magnetic resonance spectroscopy and X-ray crystallography have demonstrated that lovastatin binds directly to the highly conserved I-domain of the LFA-1 α-chain.[38]

Antioxidant effects

Plasma LDL from patients chronically treated with either lovastatin or fluvastatin have decreased *ex vivo* susceptibility to copper-induced oxidation.[39,40] If such HMG site-independent effects exist, it could be predicted that they might be shown by metabolites of the parent drug, and this has indeed been shown to be the case. Atorvastatin has no apparent antioxidant effect *in vitro* but pharmacological concentrations of its *o*-hydroxy and *p*-hydroxy metabolites substantially protect LDL, VLDL and HDL from oxidation in a concentration-dependent manner, probably by free-radical scavenging.[41]

INTERPRETATION OF EXPERIMENTAL STUDIES ON ANCILLARY EFFECTS OF STATINS

Before discussing the various suggested pleiotropic effects of statins, it is important to make some cautionary general comments about the interpretation of laboratory studies and their extrapolation to the effects of these drugs in usual therapeutic use in humans.

Atorvastatin, cerivastatin, fluvastatin, lovastatin and simvastatin are lipophilic, with octanol–water partition coefficients (log D at pH 7.4) ranging from about 1.1 to 1.7. Pravastatin and rosuvastatin are hydrophilic, with partition coefficients of –0.84 and –0.33 respectively.[42] This makes interpretation of concentration effects in cell culture difficult as the ratio of free to protein-bound (and presumably inactive) drug cannot be assumed to be the same as in plasma or in interstitial fluid *in vivo*. Comparisons of *in vitro* effects between individual drugs are therefore fraught with difficulty.

Secondly, *in vitro* studies by their very nature are inevitably short term, over hours or days. Thus, it is not possible to extrapolate with any confidence to the long-term biological effects

over years of treatment in clinical practice, since counter-regulatory mechanisms, such as the adaptation of gene expression, may in the longer term cancel out short-term effects.

Lipid concentrations in some species, such as the mouse, are highly resistant to HMG-CoA reductase inhibition. The doses of statins used in many studies in such species are those that have a percentage lipid-lowering effect equivalent to that achieved therapeutically in man and are therefore much higher, up to two orders of magnitude, than those in human therapy. Therefore extrapolation of their results to humans is at best hypothesis generating.

PROPOSED ANCILLARY EFFECTS OF STATINS IN ATHEROSCLEROSIS

Rudolf Virchow (1821–1902) originally proposed that vascular thrombosis was caused by a triad of changes in the constituents of the blood, in the blood vessel wall and in blood flow. The hypotheses to explain the pleiotropic nature of statin pharmacodynamics fit quite neatly into this triad.[10] Clearly the major effects of the drugs are on the lipoprotein constituents of plasma. However, there is strongly suggestive evidence that they modify and stabilize mural arterial plaque, influence blood flow and are antithrombotic. This is summarized in Fig. 5.2 and Table 5.3. Bonetti et al. have comprehensively reviewed the many suggestions for ancillary effects of statins.[43]

Effects on plaque composition and stability

Studies have suggested a possible involvement of statins at virtually every stage in plaque formation and in determining ongoing plaque stability. These stages are outlined in Fig. 5.3, and statins have been shown in experimental systems to influence every step depicted. However, a number of key aspects are worth particular discussion. The overall effect of statins on lipoprotein oxidation, lymphocyte and monocyte recruitment to the intima, and the activation of lymphocytes and macrophages is in essence anti-inflammatory. All observations in experimental systems have shown that

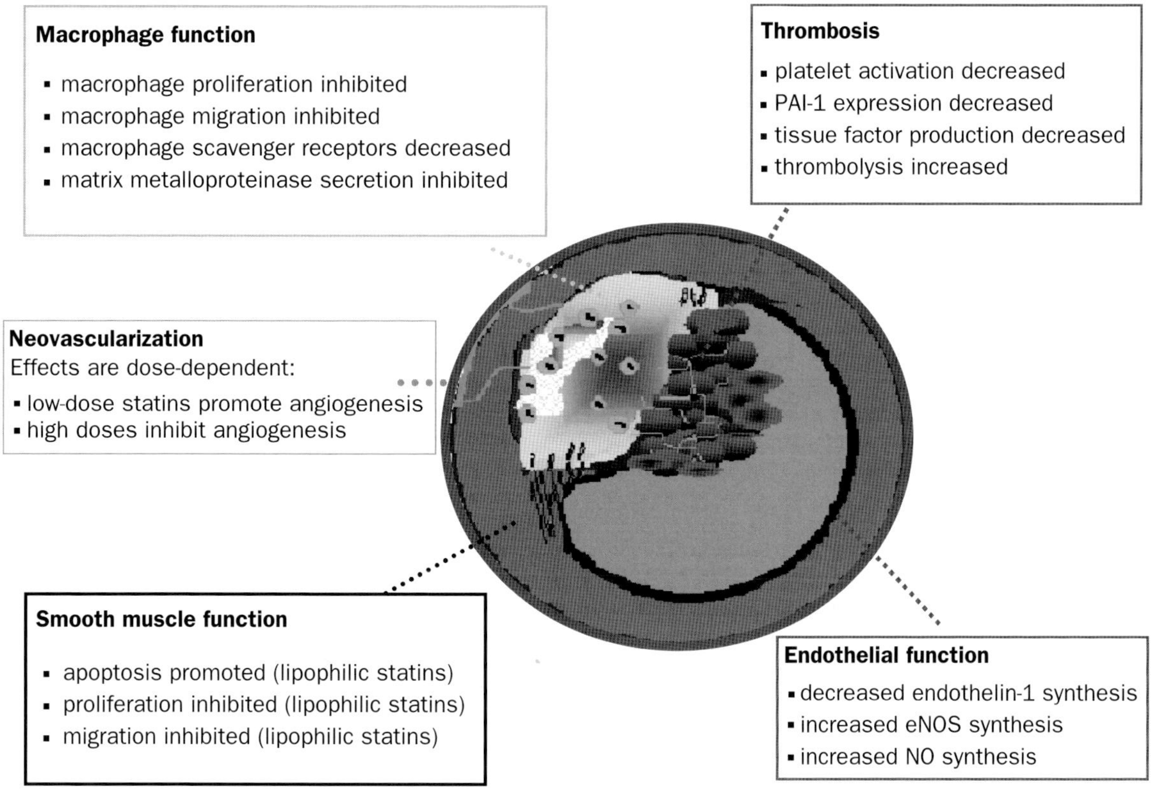

Macrophage function

- macrophage proliferation inhibited
- macrophage migration inhibited
- macrophage scavenger receptors decreased
- matrix metalloproteinase secretion inhibited

Thrombosis

- platelet activation decreased
- PAI-1 expression decreased
- tissue factor production decreased
- thrombolysis increased

Neovascularization

Effects are dose-dependent:

- low-dose statins promote angiogenesis
- high doses inhibit angiogenesis

Smooth muscle function

- apoptosis promoted (lipophilic statins)
- proliferation inhibited (lipophilic statins)
- migration inhibited (lipophilic statins)

Endothelial function

- decreased endothelin-1 synthesis
- increased eNOS synthesis
- increased NO synthesis

Fig. 5.2 Actions of HMG-CoA reductase inhibitors in arteries which appear to be independent of cholesterol lowering. PAI-1, plasminogen activator inhibitor-1; eNOS, endothelial nitric oxide synthase; NO, nitric oxide.

the drugs 'cool down' the cellular response to oxidized lipoprotein, the initial inflammatory stimulus. The likely mechanism, through decreasing the isoprenylation of GTP-binding proteins, is consistent with existing knowledge of mechanisms of inflammation in other fields. It is therefore thought highly plausible that this is a significant contributor to the overall benefit of statin therapy.

The effects of statins on vascular smooth muscle cells (VSMC) are less easily interpreted. There is consistent evidence that lipophilic statins inhibit proliferation and migration of smooth muscle cells and induce apoptosis to an extent that reflects the HMG-CoA reductase-inhibiting potency and the dose of the drug.[44] The hydrophilic pravastatin has minimal effect, possibly because of limitation to its ability to enter the cells. The lipophilic statins decrease isoprenylation of the GTP-binding protein Rho,

which is required for smooth muscle proliferation.[45] However, these findings from cell culture studies may not reflect the situation *in vivo*. When simvastatin and pravastatin were compared in a 12-month study in monkeys in which all plasma lipoprotein classes were held at the same level in all treatment groups, both pravastatin and simvastatin increased smooth muscle content of plaque lesions compared with controls.[46]

It is difficult to decide whether or not the effect of lipophilic statins on smooth muscle is desirable. Smooth muscle cells are important in the repair of damage inflicted on the arterial wall by inflammation in plaque, when, stimulated by growth factors released by plaque components, they proliferate, migrate to the sites of inflammation and secrete matrix proteins such as collagen to repair defects left by matrix metalloproteinase activity.[47] It has on the

Table 5.2   Proposed mechanisms of action of HMG-CoA reductase inhibitors which appear to be independent of cholesterol synthesis occurring in arteries

Function	Mediator proposed	In vitro	In vivo	In clinical use
Improved endothelial function				
Increased eNOS activity	Rho isoprenylation	+	+	
Increased NO production	Increased eNOS	+	+	+
Decreased endothelin-1 synthesis	Rho isoprenylation; increased NO	+		
Decreased LDL and HDL oxidation				
Decreased O_2^- from NADH oxidase	Rac isoprenylation	+		
Increased catalase activity	Isoprenylation	+	+	
Antioxidant effect of drug bound to lipoprotein	Drug molecule direct effect	+		+
Inhibition of LDL oxidation by macrophages	Isoprenylation	+		+
Diminished inflammatory cell recruitment				
Expression of ICAM-1 and P-selectin decreased	Rho isoprenylation	+	+	+
Release of pro-inflammatory cytokines decreased	Rho isoprenylation	+	+	+
MHC-II expression decreased	Isoprenylation (likely)	+		
Effects on atheromatous plaque				
VSMC apoptosis promoted (lipophilic statins)	Rho isoprenylation	+		
VSMC proliferation inhibited (lipophilic statins)	Ras, Rho isoprenylation	+		
VSMC migration inhibited (lipophilic statins)	Isoprenylation	+		
Macrophage proliferation inhibited	Isoprenylation	+		
Macrophage migration inhibited	Isoprenylation	+		
Macrophage scavenger receptors decreased	Isoprenylation	+		
Matrix metalloproteinase secretion inhibited	Isoprenylation	+		
Reversal of calcification of plaque	Not known			+
Effects on thrombogenesis				
Platelet activation decreased	Rho isoprenylation; effects of NO	+	+	+
Tissue factor expression in plaque decreased	Rho isoprenylation	+	+	+
PAI-1 expression decreased	Rho isoprenylation	+	+	
Endothelial tissue plasminogen activator increased	Rho isoprenylation	+	+	+
Effects on fibrinogen unclear: may depend on drug	Unclear			+

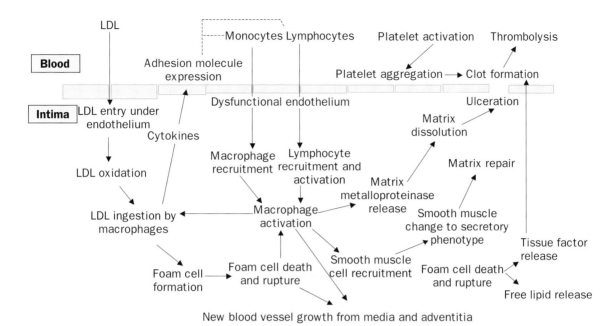

Fig. 5.3 Steps in the pathway of atherogenesis and thrombosis in arteries which are modified by HMG-CoA reductase inhibitors independently of cholesterol lowering.

other hand been claimed to be an advantage that inhibition of these activities and apoptosis of cells should prevent stenosis.[48] Whichever point of view is correct, the fact remains that both lipophilic and hydrophilic statins are about equally effective in clinical trials in preventing coronary occlusion, suggesting that *in vitro* studies on smooth muscle can be overextrapolated to the clinical situation and that the large differences seen between drugs in cell culture experiments may not have any clinical significance.

The clearest evidence that statins stabilize plaque by ancillary mechanisms independent of lipid lowering comes from an elegant experiment[49] in which male cynomolgus monkeys fed for two years on an atherogenic diet were randomized to receive pravastatin ($n = 14$) or to control ($n = 18$). Their lipid levels were manipulated to ensure that plasma LDL, VLDL and HDL concentrations were kept the same in both groups for a further two years. At the end of this period, post-mortem studies revealed significant decreases in the pravastatin group in carotid artery macrophage content, and while 17 out of 18 controls had calcified vessels none

of the statin group manifested this. In the control group 11 out of 18 had neovascularization in the carotid arteries, while none of the statin group showed this. The pravastatin group had a vasodilator response to acetylcholine stimulation, while the controls had a constrictor response. These significantly beneficial effects occurred without question by mechanisms independent of plasma lipid concentrations.[49] Similar results were obtained in an analogous study by the same group comparing pravastatin with simvastatin and control.[46]

Effects on blood flow

Hypercholesterolaemia impairs endothelial-mediated vasoreactivity. Lowering plasma LDL concentrations, for instance by LDL apheresis, immediately improves flow in coronary and peripheral arteries.[50] Statin therapy augments this by mechanisms in which increased nitric oxide synthesis and decreased endothelin expression are central.[43] This is clear from studies *in vitro* using isolated artery preparations. In clinical studies, improved peripheral arterial flow was seen in normolipidaemic volunteers after 24 hours of treatment with high-dose atorvastatin 80 mg/day, some 24 hours before the drug altered their plasma lipid concentrations. Withdrawal of the drug caused an acute impairment of arterial flow, well before plasma lipid concentrations responded.[51] Cerivastatin had similar effects on brachial artery flow in diabetic patients, also manifest before plasma lipid concentrations changed, and there was evidence that the effect was due to increased nitric oxide levels.[52] The very rapid onset of improvement of arterial flow due to direct effects of statins on vasoreactivity, augmented and sustained by lipid lowering, is probably a prime reason for the early onset of benefit seen in statin outcome studies, and is justification for the acute initiation of statin therapy in acute coronary syndrome.[53]

Effects on clotting

Lowering LDL concentrations, by any means, decreases platelet aggregation by decreasing LDL-mediated ADP-induced fibrinogen binding to platelets. Statins have been shown to decrease platelet aggregation in clinical use[54–56] and *ex vivo* experiments suggest that this is in part due to stimulation of endothelial nitric oxide generation.[57] Hypercholesterolaemia is associated with increased platelet-dependent thrombin generation. Pravastatin, simvastatin and cerivastatin normalize the generation of thrombin.[58,59] In addition of course, the action of statins in stabilizing plaque inevitably diminishes the local stimuli to platelet aggregation in the vicinity.

Tissue factor is a powerful stimulus trigger of the intrinsic clotting cascade. Its secretion by macrophages is inhibited in culture by statins through diminished GGPP-mediated isoprenylation and consequent NF-κB activation.[60]

The literature is quite contradictory on the effects of individual statins on plasma fibrinogen concentrations, with different studies in human volunteers suggesting increased, unchanged or decreased levels resulting from treatment with the same drug. This is likely to be due to methodological difficulties and possibly to the different responses in the cohorts studied.

Small thrombi probably form from time to time in older peoples' coronary arteries, with effective spontaneous thrombolytic activity preventing disaster. Statins probably help to encourage this protection by inhibiting the expression of the anti-fibrinolytic factor plasminogen activator inhibitor-1 (PAI-1) in endothelium and smooth muscle, by inhibiting Rho isoprenylation.[25,61,62]

THE CONTRIBUTION OF THE ANCILLARY ACTIONS OF STATINS TO THEIR CLINICAL EFFECTS

The large clinical trials that have shed so much light on the clinical application of statin therapy tell us little about how the drugs work. We intuitively attribute their benefits to their effects on lipoproteins. The trials hint that there may be additional mechanisms at work. However, the pharmacodynamic effects of the drugs, whatever they are, are inextricably intertwined. It is not possible to manipulate study cohorts so that, for instance, plasma lipids are maintained identical between statin and placebo groups. There is a prospect, however, that it may be possible to disentangle cholesterol-dependent from non-cholesterol-dependent mechanisms in future studies in which newer non-statin drugs, for instance those that interfere with intestinal sterol absorption, may be compared with statins of comparable cholesterol-lowering efficacy. Until then, we have to rely on acute studies that observe effects such as blood flow that change before lipid concentrations are altered and on extrapolation from the few long-term studies in animals in which lipid levels were manipulated to equate those in the statin-treated groups with those in controls.

THE FUTURE: STATIN EFFECTS OUTSIDE OF THE ARTERY

The description of the pleiotropic effects of statins in vascular disease has led to interest in their use in other therapeutic areas, although this is still poorly explored in clinical trials. The three main areas of interest are in inflammatory disease, osteoporosis and cancer.

Inflammatory diseases

Simvastatin in a Th1-driven model of mouse inflammatory arthritis markedly inhibited developing and clinically evident collagen-induced arthritis in doses that were unable to significantly alter cholesterol concentrations *in vivo*. Treatment caused significant suppression of collagen-specific Th1 humoral and cellular immune responses and reduced anti-CD3/anti-CD28 proliferation and IFN-γ release from mononuclear cells from peripheral blood and synovial fluid. Pro-inflammatory cytokine production by T-cell contact-activated macrophages was suppressed *in vitro* by simvastatin.[63]

There is increasing interest in the potential use of statins in multiple sclerosis (MS), particularly since there is evidence that the drugs have a significant ameliorating effect on the animal model of the disease, experimental allergic encephalomyelitis.[64–66] There is a clear need for a large outcomes trial of statin treatment in MS, given the many unsatisfactory aspects of existing treatments for this condition.

The extent of the anti-inflammatory effect of statins in animals is quite significant; simvastatin had a comparable potency to indomethacin in preventing carrageenan-induced foot-pad oedema in mice, the effect being manifest within four hours, long before any effect was seen in lipid levels.[67]

Osteoporosis

Considerable interest was aroused by the report that simvastatin and lovastatin enhanced new bone formation when injected subcutaneously over the calvaria of mice and increased cancellous bone volume when orally administered to rats. This effect was associated with increased expression of the bone morphogenetic protein-2 (BMP-2) gene in bone cells.[68] Simvastatin significantly improves fracture healing in mice.[69] Subsequent retrospective case-control studies reported that statin users seemed to have fewer osteoporotic fractures than non-users.[70–73] although *post-hoc* analysis of the LIPID trial participants showed no difference in fracture rates between treated and placebo groups.[74] The pro-

posed effect of statins on bone formation is biologically plausible, as protein geranylgeranylation but not farnesylation (e.g. Ras) is important for osteoclast-mediated bone resorption and nitrogen-containing bisphosphonates exert their anti-resorptive action by affecting enzymes of the mevalonate pathway involved in the generation of GGPP.[75,76] Here again, however, the issue of clinical relevance will only be resolved by a randomized controlled trial.

Cancer

There are many reports of inhibition of cancer growth and induction of apoptosis by statins in human and animal cell lines *in vitro* and also *in vivo* in animals.[77–83] These are usually attributed to effects on GTP-binding proteins, especially Rho, in the tumour cells themselves.[81,84–86] In addition, atorvastatin and cerivastatin have lipid-independent biphasic dose-dependent effects on angiogenesis. This is associated with alterations in endothelial apoptosis and vascular endothelial growth factor (VEGF) signalling. Statins have pro-angiogenic effects at low therapeutic concentrations but angiostatic effects at high concentrations (including in a mouse Lewis lung tumour model) that are reversed by GGPP.[87,88] The effect is Rho-mediated.[86]

There is no evidence, however, for a consistent effect of statin therapy on cancer incidence in the many participants in large outcomes trials. This may be due to the relatively short duration of the studies in relation to the long period over which cancers are thought to develop. It may also be the case that the doses used in clinical practice cannot deliver the degree of exposure to the drug required to produce effects in cell culture studies *in vitro*. It is clear in this area of cancer treatment, as in all other areas in medicine, that we cannot assess whether a biological effect seen in the laboratory is of any clinical use until the drug is put to the test in a properly designed controlled clinical trial.

CONCLUSION

It is a fortunate chance that the ancillary effects of statins have turned out to be beneficial, with a very low incidence of adverse effects. The drugs designed to do the single task of lowering plasma lipid concentrations have yielded an unexpected bonus. How important a relative contribution this makes in the overall sum of clinical utility of the drugs remains to be determined. This is not just a matter of academic curiosity, as it is very relevant to our expectation of efficacy of the newer classes of lipid-lowering medicines in the pipeline, such as ACAT inhibitors, absorption inhibitors, etc. Time may reveal the answer to this. In the meantime, statins continue to show new actions and their potential for therapeutic use in other diseases remains to be investigated in trials.

The relative importance of lipid-dependent and non-lipid mechanisms of action cannot yet be determined with confidence for any individual statin and it may differ from one drug to another in the group. It is not appropriate to compare drugs on the basis of lipid-lowering effects alone when making selection for therapy. The therapeutic goal is the prevention of vascular mortality and morbidity, not some biochemical surrogate clinical outcomes. The purpose of end-point trials is to provide a clinical evidence base for therapy – comparisons between individual statins must be based on these.

REFERENCES

1. The Lipid Research Clinics Coronary Primary Prevention Trial results. I. Reduction in incidence of coronary heart disease. *JAMA* 1984; **251**: 351–64.
2. Buchwald H, Varco RL, Matts JP et al. Effect of partial ileal bypass surgery on mortality and morbidity from coronary heart disease in patients with hypercholesterolemia. Report of the Program on the Surgical Control of the Hyperlipidemias (POSCH). *N Engl J Med* 1990; **323**: 946–55.
3. The Scandinavian Simvastatin Survival Study (4S). Randomised trial of cholesterol lowering in 4444 patients with coronary heart disease. *Lancet* 1994; **344**: 1383–9.
4. Shepherd J, Cobbe SM, Ford I et al. Prevention of coronary heart disease with pravastatin in men with hypercholesterolemia. West of Scotland Coronary Prevention Study Group. *N Engl J Med* 1995; **333**: 1301–7.
5. Sacks FM, Pfeffer MA, Moye LA et al. The effect of pravastatin on coronary events after myocardial infarction in patients with average cholesterol levels. Cholesterol and Recurrent Events Trial Investigators. *N Engl J Med* 1996; **335**: 1001–9.
6. Influence of pravastatin and plasma lipids on clinical events in the West of Scotland Coronary Prevention Study (WOSCOPS). *Circulation* 1998; **97**: 1440–5.
7. Sacks FM, Moye LA, Davis BR et al. Relationship between plasma LDL concentrations during treatment with pravastatin and recurrent coronary events in the Cholesterol and Recurrent Events Trial. *Circulation* 1998; **97**: 1446–52.
8. Pedersen TR, Olsson AG, Faergeman O et al. Lipoprotein changes and reduction in the incidence of major coronary heart disease events in the Scandinavian Simvastatin Survival Study (4S). *Circulation* 1998; **97**: 1453–60.
9. Gotto AM Jr, Whitney E, Stein EA et al. Relation between baseline and on-treatment lipid parameters and first acute major coronary events in the Air Force/Texas Coronary Atherosclerosis Prevention Study (AFCAPS/TexCAPS). *Circulation* 2000; **101**: 477–84.
10. Kobashigawa JA, Katznelson S, Laks H et al. Effect of pravastatin on outcomes after cardiac transplantation. *N Engl J Med* 1995; **333**: 621–7.
11. Katznelson S, Kobashigawa JA. Dual roles of HMG-CoA reductase inhibitors in solid organ transplantation: lipid lowering and immunosuppression. *Kidney Int Suppl* 1995; **52**: S112–S115.
12. Vaughan CJ, Murphy MB, Buckley BM. Statins do more than just lower cholesterol. *Lancet* 1996; **348**: 1079–82.
13. Rosenson RS, Tangney CC. Antiatherothrombotic properties of statins: implications for cardiovascular event reduction. *JAMA* 1998; **279**: 1643–50.
14. Edwards PA, Ericsson J. Sterols and isoprenoids: signaling molecules derived from the cholesterol biosynthetic pathway. *Annu Rev Biochem* 1999; **68**: 157–85.
15. Bouterfa HL, Sattelmeyer V, Czub S et al. Inhibition of Ras farnesylation by lovastatin leads to downregulation of proliferation and migration in primary cultured human glioblastoma cells. *Anticancer Res* 2000; **20**: 2761–71.

16. Bassa BV, Roh DD, Vaziri ND et al. Effect of inhibition of cholesterol synthetic pathway on the activation of Ras and MAP kinase in mesangial cells. *Biochim Biophys Acta* 1999; **1449**: 137–49.

17. Cuthbert JA, Lipsky PE. Regulation of proliferation and Ras localization in transformed cells by products of mevalonate metabolism. *Cancer Res* 1997; **57**: 3498–505.

18. Yamamoto T, Takeda K, Harada S et al. HMG-CoA reductase inhibitor enhances inducible nitric oxide synthase expression in rat vascular smooth muscle cells: involvement of the Rho/Rho kinase pathway. *Atherosclerosis* 2003; **166**: 213–22.

19. Nagata K, Ishibashi T, Sakamoto T et al. Rho/Rho-kinase is involved in the synthesis of tissue factor in human monocytes. *Atherosclerosis* 2002; **163**: 39–47.

20. Kaneider NC, Egger P, Dunzendorfer S, Wiedermann CJ. Rho-GTPase-dependent platelet–neutrophil interaction affected by HMG-CoA reductase inhibition with altered adenosine nucleotide release and function. *Arterioscler Thromb Vasc Biol* 2002; **22**: 1029–35.

21. Eto M, Kozai T, Cosentino F et al. Statin prevents tissue factor expression in human endothelial cells: role of Rho/Rho-kinase and Akt pathways. *Circulation* 2002; **105**: 1756–9.

22. Blanco-Colio LM, Villa A, Ortego M et al. 3-Hydroxy-3-methyl-glutaryl coenzyme A reductase inhibitors, atorvastatin and simvastatin, induce apoptosis of vascular smooth muscle cells by downregulation of Bcl-2 expression and Rho A prenylation. *Atherosclerosis* 2002; **16**: 17–26.

23. Eberlein M, Heusinger-Ribeiro J, Goppelt-Struebe M. Rho-dependent inhibition of the induction of connective tissue growth factor (CTGF) by HMG-CoA reductase inhibitors (statins). *Br J Pharmacol* 2001; **133**: 1172–80.

24. Takeuchi S, Kawashima S, Rikitake Y et al. Cerivastatin suppresses lipopolysaccharide-induced ICAM-1 expression through inhibition of Rho GTPase in BAEC. *Biochem Biophys Res Commun* 2000; **269**: 97–102.

25. Essig M, Vrtovsnik F, Nguyen G et al. Lovastatin modulates in vivo and in vitro the plasminogen activator/plasmin system of rat proximal tubular cells: role of geranylgeranylation and Rho proteins. *J Am Soc Nephrol* 1998; **9**: 1377–88.

26. Koch G, Benz C, Schmidt G et al. Role of Rho protein in lovastatin-induced breakdown of

actin cytoskeleton. *J Pharmacol Exp Ther* 1997; **283**: 901–9.

27. Dichtl W, Dulak J, Frick M et al. HMG-CoA Reductase inhibitors regulate inflammatory transcription factors in human endothelial and vascular smooth muscle cells. *Arterioscler Thromb Vasc Biol* 2003; **23**: 58–63.

28. Ortego M, Bustos C, Hernandez-Presa MA et al. Atorvastatin reduces NF-kappaB activation and chemokine expression in vascular smooth muscle cells and mononuclear cells. *Atherosclerosis* 1999; **147**: 253–61.

29. De Martin R, Hoeth M., Hoeffer-Warbinek R et al. The transcription factor NF-kappaB and the regulation of vascular cell function. *Arterioscler Thromb Vasc Biol* 2000; **20**: E83–E88.

30. Dricu A, Wang M, Hjertman M et al. Mevalonate-regulated mechanisms in cell growth control: role of dolichyl phosphate in expression of the insulin-like growth factor-1 receptor (IGF-1R) in comparison to Ras prenylation and expression of c-myc. *Glycobiology* 1997; **7**: 625–33.

31. Carlberg M, Dricu A, Blegen H et al. Mevalonic acid is limiting for N-linked glycosylation and translocation of the insulin-like growth factor-1 receptor to the cell surface. Evidence for a new link between 3-hydroxy-3-methyl glutaryl coenzyme A reductase and cell growth. *J Biol Chem* 1996; **271**: 17453–62.

32. Laaksonen R, Ojala JP, Tikkanen MJ, Himberg JJ. Serum ubiquinone concentrations after short- and long-term treatment with HMG-CoA reductase inhibitors. *Eur J Clin Pharmacol* 1994; **46**: 313–17.

33. Ghirlanda G, Oradei A, Manto A et al. Evidence of plasma CoQ10-lowering effect by HMG-CoA reductase inhibitors: a double-blind, placebo-controlled study. *J Clin Pharmacol* 1993; **33**: 226–9.

34. Laaksonen R, Jokelainen K, Sahi T et al. Decreases in serum ubiquinone concentrations do not result in reduced levels in muscle tissue during short-term simvastatin treatment in humans. *Clin Pharmacol Ther* 1995; **57**: 62–6.

35. Laaksonen R, Jokelainen K, Laakso J et al. The effect of simvastatin treatment on natural antioxidants in low-density lipoproteins and high-energy phosphates and ubiquinone in skeletal muscle. *Am J Cardiol* 1996; **77**: 851–4.

36. Nakahara K, Kuriyama M, Sonoda Y et al. Myopathy induced by HMG-CoA reductase inhibitors in rabbits: a pathological, electrophysio-

logical, and biochemical study. *Toxicol Appl Pharmacol* 1998; **152**: 99–106.

37. Weitz-Schmidt G, Welzenbach K, Brinkmann V et al. Statins selectively inhibit leukocyte function antigen-1 by binding to a novel regulatory integrin site. *Nat Med* 2001; **7**: 687–92.

38. Kallen J, Welzenbach K, Ramage P et al. Structural basis for LFA-1 inhibition upon lovastatin binding to the CD11a I domain. *J Mol Biol* 1999; **292**: 1–9.

39. Hussein O, Schlezinger S, Rosenblat M et al. Reduced susceptibility of low-density lipoprotein (LDL) to lipid peroxidation after fluvastatin therapy is associated with the hypocholesterolemic effect of the drug and its binding to the LDL. *Atherosclerosis* 1997; **128**: 11–18.

40. Aviram M, Hussein O, Rosenblat M et al. Interactions of platelets, macrophages, and lipoproteins in hypercholesterolemia: antiatherogenic effects of HMG-CoA reductase inhibitor therapy. *J Cardiovasc Pharmacol* 1998; **31**: 39–45.

41. Aviram M, Rosenblat M, Bisgaier CL, Newton RS. Atorvastatin and gemfibrozil metabolites, but not the parent drugs, are potent antioxidants against lipoprotein oxidation. *Atherosclerosis* 1998; **138**: 271–80.

42. Matsuyama K, Nakagawa K, Nakai A et al. Evaluation of myopathy risk for HMG-CoA reductase inhibitors by urethane infusion method. *Biol Pharm Bull* 2002; **25**: 346–50.

43. Bonetti PO, Lerman LO, Napoli C, Lerman A. Statin effects beyond lipid lowering – are they clinically relevant? *Eur Heart J* 2003; **24**: 225–48.

44. Negre-Aminou P, van Vliet AK, van Erck M et al. Inhibition of proliferation of human smooth muscle cells by various HMG-CoA reductase inhibitors: comparison with other human cell types. *Biochim Biophys Acta* 1997; **1345**: 259–68.

45. Negre-Aminou P, van Erck M, van Leeuwen RE et al. Differential effect of simvastatin on various signal transduction intermediates in cultured human smooth muscle cells. *Biochem Pharmacol* 2001; **61**: 991–8.

46. Sukhova GK, Williams JK, Libby P. Statins reduce inflammation in atheroma of nonhuman primates independent of effects on serum cholesterol. *Arterioscler Thromb Vasc Biol* 2002; **22**: 1452–8.

47. Weissberg PL, Clesham GJ, Bennett MR. Is vascular smooth muscle cell proliferation beneficial? *Lancet* 1996; **347**: 305–7.

48. Corsini A, Bernini F, Quarato P et al. Non-lipid-related effects of 3-hydroxy-3-methyl glutaryl coenzyme A reductase inhibitors. *Cardiology* 1996; **8**: 458–68.

49. Williams JK, Sukhova GK, Herrington DM, Libby P. Pravastatin has cholesterol-lowering independent effects on the artery wall of atherosclerotic monkeys. *J Am Coll Cardiol* 1998; **31**: 684–91.

50. Kroon AA, van Asten WN, Stalenhoef AF. Effect of apheresis of low-density lipoprotein on peripheral vascular disease in hypercholesterolemic patients with coronary artery disease. *Ann Intern Med* 1996; **125**: 945–54.

51. Laufs U, Wassmann S, Hilgers S et al. Rapid effects on vascular function after initiation and withdrawal of atorvastatin in healthy, normocholesterolemic men. *Am J Cardiol* 2001; **88**: 1306–7.

52. Tsunekawa T, Hayashi T, Kano H et al. Cerivastatin, a hydroxymethylglutaryl coenzyme a reductase inhibitor, improves endothelial function in elderly diabetic patients within 3 days. *Circulation* 2001; **104**: 376–9.

53. Schwartz GG, Olsson AG, Ezekowitz MD et al. Effects of atorvastatin on early recurrent ischemic events in acute coronary syndromes: the MIRACL study: a randomized controlled trial. *JAMA* 2001; **285**: 1711–18.

54. Thompson PD, Moyna NM, White CM et al. The effects of hydroxy-methyl-glutaryl co-enzyme A reductase inhibitors on platelet thrombus formation. *Atherosclerosis* 2002; **161**: 301–6.

55. Osamah H, Mira R, Sorina S et al. Reduced platelet aggregation after fluvastatin therapy is associated with altered platelet lipid composition and drug binding to the platelets. *Br J Clin Pharmacol* 1997; **44**: 77–83.

56. Tsakiris DA, Keller U, Zulewski H et al. Simvastatin reduces activation of normal platelets by LDL isolated from patients with familial hypercholesterolaemia and familial defective apolipoprotein B [Letter]. *Eur J Clin Pharmacol* 1997; **53**: 277–9.

57. Tannous M, Cheung R, Vignini A, Mutus B. Atorvastatin increases ecNOS levels in human platelets of hyperlipidemic subjects. *Thromb Haemost* 1999; **82**: 1390–4.

58. Kaneider NC, Egger P, Dunzendorfer S et al. Reversal of thrombin-induced deactivation of CD39/ATPDase in endothelial cells by HMG-CoA reductase inhibition: effects on Rho-GTPase and adenosine nucleotide metabolism. *Arterioscler Thromb Vasc Biol* 2002; **22**: 894–900.

59. Aoki I, Aoki N, Kawano K et al. Platelet-dependent thrombin generation in patients

with hyperlipidemia. *J Am Coll Cardiol* 1997; **30**: 91–6.

60. Colli S, Eligini S, Lalli M et al. Vastatins inhibit tissue factor in cultured human macrophages. A novel mechanism of protection against atherothrombosis. *Arterioscler Thromb Vasc Biol* 1997; **17**: 265–72.

61. Essig M, Nguyen G, Prie D et al. 3-Hydroxy-3-methyl glutaryl coenzyme A reductase inhibitors increase fibrinolytic activity in rat aortic endothelial cells. Role of geranylgeranylation and Rho proteins. *Circ Res* 1998; **83**: 683–90.

62. Bourcier T, Libby P. HMG-CoA reductase inhibitors reduce plasminogen activator inhibitor-1 expression by human vascular smooth muscle and endothelial cells. *Arterioscler Thromb Vasc Biol* 2000; **20**: 556–62.

63. Leung BP, Sattar N, Crilly A et al. A novel anti-inflammatory role for simvastatin in inflammatory arthritis. *J Immunol* 2003; **170**: 1524–30.

64. Stanislaus R, Singh AK, Singh I. Lovastatin treatment decreases mononuclear cell infiltration into the CNS of Lewis rats with experimental allergic encephalomyelitis. *J Neurosci Res* 2001; **66**: 155–62.

65. Stanislaus R, Pahan K, Singh AK, Singh I. Amelioration of experimental allergic encephalomyelitis in Lewis rats by lovastatin. *Neurosci Lett* 1999; **269**: 71–4.

66. Youssef S, Stuve O, Patarroyo JC et al. The HMG-CoA reductase inhibitor, atorvastatin, promotes a Th2 bias and reverses paralysis in central nervous system autoimmune disease. *Nature* 2002; **420**: 78–84.

67. Sparrow CP, Burton CA, Hernandez M et al. Simvastatin has anti-inflammatory and antiatherosclerotic activities independent of plasma cholesterol lowering. *Arterioscler Thromb Vasc Biol* 2001; **21**: 115–21.

68. Mundy G, Garrett R, Harris S et al. Stimulation of bone formation in vitro and in rodents by statins. *Science* 1999; **286**: 1946–9.

69. Skoglund B, Forslund C, Aspenberg P. Simvastatin improves fracture healing in mice. *J Bone Miner Res* 2002; **17**: 2004–8.

70. Edwards CJ, Hart DJ, Spector TD. Oral statins and increased bone-mineral density in postmenopausal women [Letter]. *Lancet* 2000; **355**: 2218–19.

71. Pasco JA, Kotowicz MA, Henry MJ et al. Statin use, bone mineral density, and fracture risk: Geelong Osteoporosis Study. *Arch Intern Med* 2002; **162**: 537–40.

72. Wang PS, Solomon DH, Mogun H, Avorn J. HMG-CoA reductase inhibitors and the risk of hip fractures in elderly patients *JAMA* 2000; **283**: 3211–16.

73. Meier CR, Schlienger RG, Kraenzlin ME et al. HMG-CoA reductase inhibitors and the risk of fractures. *JAMA* 2000; **283**: 3205–10.

74. Reid IR, Hague W, Emberson J et al. Effect of pravastatin on frequency of fracture in the LIPID study: secondary analysis of a randomised controlled trial. Long-term Intervention with Pravastatin in Ischaemic Disease. *Lancet* 2001; **357**: 509–12.

75. Fisher JE, Rogers MJ, Halasy JM et al. Alendronate mechanism of action: geranylgeraniol, an intermediate in the mevalonate pathway, prevents inhibition of osteoclast formation, bone resorption, and kinase activation in vitro. *Proc Natl Acad Sci USA* 1999; **96**: 133–8.

76. Luckman SP, Hughes DE, Coxon FP et al. Nitrogen-containing bisphosphonates inhibit the mevalonate pathway and prevent post-translational prenylation of GTP-binding proteins, including Ras. *J Bone Miner Res* 1998; **13**: 581–9.

77. Seeger H, Wallwiener D, Mueck AO. Statins can inhibit proliferation of human breast cancer cells in vitro. *Exp Clin Endocrinol Diabetes* 2003; **111**: 47–8.

78. Wong WW, Dimitroulakos J, Minden MD, Penn LZ. HMG-CoA reductase inhibitors and the malignant cell: the statin family of drugs as triggers of tumor-specific apoptosis. *Leukemia* 2002; **16**: 508–19.

79. Wang W, Collie-Duguid E, Cassidy J. Cerivastatin enhances the cytotoxicity of 5-fluorouracil on chemosensitive and resistant colorectal cancer cell lines. *FEBS Lett* 2002; **531**: 415–20.

80. Denoyelle C, Albanese P, Uzan G et al. Molecular mechanism of the anti-cancer activity of cerivastatin, an inhibitor of HMG-CoA reductase, on aggressive human breast cancer cells. *Cell Signal* 2003; **15**: 327–38.

81. Kusama T, Mukai M, Iwasaki T et al. 3-Hydroxy-3-methyl glutaryl coenzyme A reductase inhibitors reduce human pancreatic cancer cell invasion and metastasis. *Gastroenterology* 2002; **122**: 308–17.

82. Schmidt F, Groscurth P, Kermer M et al. Lovastatin and phenylacetate induce apoptosis, but not differentiation, in human malignant glioma cells. *Acta Neuropathol (Berl)* 2001; **101**: 217–24.

83. Agarwal B, Bhendwal S, Halmos B et al. Lovastatin augments apoptosis induced by chemotherapeutic agents in colon cancer cells. *Clin Cancer Res* 1999; **5**: 2223–9.

84. Kusama T, Mukai M, Iwasaki T et al. Inhibition of epidermal growth factor-induced RhoA translocation and invasion of human pancreatic cancer cells by 3-hydroxy-3-methyl glutaryl coenzyme A reductase inhibitors. *Cancer Res* 2001; **61**: 4885–91.

85. Denoyelle C, Vasse M, Korner M et al. Cerivastatin, an inhibitor of HMG-CoA reductase, inhibits the signaling pathways involved in the invasiveness and metastatic properties of highly invasive breast cancer cell lines: an in vitro study. *Carcinogenesis* 2001; **22**: 1139–48.

86. Park HJ, Kong D, Iruela-Arispe L et al. 3-Hydroxy-3-methyl glutaryl coenzyme A reductase inhibitors interfere with angiogenesis by inhibiting the geranylgeranylation of RhoA. *Circ Res* 2002; **91**: 143–50.

87. Weis M, Heeschen C, Glassford AJ, Cooke JP. Statins have biphasic effects on angiogenesis. *Circulation* 2002; **105**: 739–45.

88. Urbich C, Dernbach E, Zeiher AM, Dimmeler S. Double-edged role of statins in angiogenesis signaling. *Circ Res* 2002; **90**: 737–44.

6

Angiographic and IVUS techniques evaluating progression and regression of coronary atherosclerosis: statin intervention trials in perspective

Philippine Kiès, Albert VG Bruschke and J Wouter Jukema

INTRODUCTION

For many years, trials evaluating the effect of interventions to improve the prognosis of patients with coronary atherosclerosis could be divided into two categories:

- Trials evaluating the effect of the intervention by counting clinical events, the so-called 'clinical event trials'.
- Trials evaluating the effect of the intervention by measuring angiographic changes of the coronary arteries over time, the so-called 'angiographic trials'.

Since coronary atherosclerosis is essentially a chronic progressive disease and, in patients with coronary atherosclerosis, progression of the disease is one of the major factors which determine clinical prognosis,[1–3] angiographic coronary atherosclerosis trials thus provide valid (surrogate) endpoints. The purpose of this chapter is to discuss what we have learned from these trials and the additional insights we obtained from newer techniques, such as intravascular ultrasound (IVUS), on which some trials have recently started.

Clinical events occurring during angiographic or US trials may give additional information to morphological changes, so the outcomes of clinical event trials and angiographic trials show some overlap. Clinical trials as well as angiographic trials have advantages and disadvantages. The advantages of clinical event trials are:

- The results are clinically most relevant.
- The study costs per subject are generally low.
- No invasive examination is needed.

The disadvantages of clinical event trials are:

- A large number of patients must be followed over a relatively long period of time in order to obtain a sufficient number of clinical events.
- To be certain that all subjects have coronary atherosclerosis, only patients with unequivocal evidence of coronary artery disease – frequently a history of myocardial infarction (MI) – are included. This induces a selection bias towards patients with advanced coronary artery disease making the results only valid for a limited group of patients.
- Hardly any information is obtained about the anatomical substrate.

The advantages of angiographic trials are:

- They provide an accurate diagnosis, which allows inclusion of patients with mild or moderate coronary artery disease.

- The study's duration can often be significantly shorter than for clinical event trials.
- A smaller number of patients than for clinical event trials is generally sufficient to demonstrate a treatment effect.
- Angiographic trials provide information about the morphological substrate of a treatment effect.

However, angiographic trials also have disadvantages:

- They are rather expensive.
- There is always some risk related to the invasive examination.
- The fact that an invasive procedure is needed may also induce a selection bias.
- The clinical relevance of the angiographic outcome was sometimes unclear.

However, more recently a good correlation has been shown to exist between progression of coronary atherosclerosis and the occurrence of clinical events.[1–3] Thus angiographic as well as clinical event trials provide unique and mutually complementary information.

This chapter discusses the most important angiographic trials performed to date, focusing on the trials with HMG-CoA reductase inhibitors (statins). At the end of the chapter we shall discuss new (non-)invasive techniques to characterize the atherosclerotic plaque. One of these is IVUS, which is considered to be the new gold standard in conjunction with coronary angiography, in studying the process of progression and/or regression of atherosclerosis.

ANGIOGRAPHIC STUDIES

General considerations

To study the anatomical changes caused by the progression of coronary atherosclerosis, and factors which may influence this process, repeated coronary arteriographic examinations in patients with coronary artery disease are required. Ideally, studies should comprise patients in whom repetitive arteriographic examinations are performed at regular intervals, e.g. every one or two years. However,

such studies are neither feasible nor ethical and therefore in practice all progression studies are limited to patients who underwent coronary arteriography twice.[4] This makes such studies liable to several biases. In the first place, the interval between the two angiographic studies may influence the findings in that during short intervals disease progression, although present, may not be marked enough to be detectable by angiography, whereas during long intervals an increasing mortality and morbidity among patients with marked progression may lead to a selection of patients in favour of those with little progression, thus causing an underestimation of the true rate of progression.[5] In the second place, progression of coronary atherosclerosis is a non-linear process (as discussed below) and progression over a certain period of time may not automatically be extrapolated to longer intervals. This may be of importance in studies designed to demonstrate the influence of interventions on progression or regression of coronary artery disease because such studies generally use a fixed and relatively short time interval.

In spite of these and other limitations, the results of most studies on progression are fairly consistent, which allows us to draw some general conclusions. Reviewing some of the most important progression studies, we will divide these studies into observational and intervention studies (and emphasize methodological aspects, which, in reviews on this subject, often receive little attention).

Observational studies

Observational studies may be defined as studies based on observations in regular patient populations. Typically, the patients have not been subjected to a specific intervention and the studies are basically retrospective. Sometimes the term 'natural history' is used, which is only appropriate if this is defined as the evolution of the disease under usual treatment, in the case of coronary disease excluding mechanical interventions (bypass surgery and catheter interventions). Strictly speaking it is not possible to study the true natural history of coronary artery

Table 6.1   Observational studies comprising 100 or more patients

First author	No. of patients	Mean interval (months)	% progression	Correlation with time	Correlation with other risk factors
Kramer[9,125,126]	317	30	49	+	None
Bruschke[5]	286	39	56	+	None
Moise[10]	313	39	44	+	Young age
Visser[14]	300	30	56	+	None
Ishikawa[11]	227	36	32	–	Not reported
Sainsous[127]	122	34	57	+	None
Vanhaecke[12]	100	35	60	+	Diabetes mellitus

disease (or any other disease) because 'it is the function of the physician to make the history as desirably unnatural as possible'.[6] Table 6.1 presents an overview of observational studies that include at least 100 patients. Most of these studies are relatively old, which is mainly due to the increasing number of mechanical interventions and perhaps also to the large number of ongoing intervention trials, which include a significant proportion of patients on medical therapy. All studies include a wide range of intervals between the two angiographic examinations, which allows evaluation of the time factor. It appears that time is the most consistent and, in several studies, most powerful determinant of progression. However, even after very long intervals some patients do not show progression. This is in agreement with survival studies, which also demonstrated that a small proportion of patients with severe coronary artery disease survive uneventfully periods of 15 years or longer.[7] Apparently in some cases the disease process is 'burnt out' but unfortunately it has not been possible to identify these patients on the basis of a single clinical and arteriographic evaluation.

Correlations between the commonly recognized (non-angiographic) risk factors and progression were absent or of little consequence in most studies. However, this finding should be interpreted cautiously. In the first place, in the majority of the observational studies, no attempt was made to reduce risk factors drastically as may be necessary to influence progres-

sion. In the second place, these studies do not fulfil the requirements currently accepted for angiographic intervention studies,[8] and thus small changes in obstructions may have escaped recognition.

There is some controversy as to the type of lesions most likely to progress. Some investigations found that there is a positive correlation between severity of narrowing and change of progression,[5,9] whereas others found no such correlation.[10–12] Using the Coronary Artery Surgery Study (CASS) data, Ellis et al. analysed the morphology of lesions in the left anterior descending artery and tried to determine their prognostic significance. Lesions with rough borders and involving long segments frequently led to myocardial infarction, which may suggest a high progression rate, but angiographic follow-up data were not available.[13] The situation is even more complex if, rather than separate lesions, patients are considered. As was demonstrated in several studies, in most patients the presence of a relatively large number of slight or moderate narrowings (with a low change of progression) and a small number of severe narrowings (with a high change of progression) makes the prediction of progression in individual cases very uncertain.[5,14,15] Progression, if present, involved only significant lesions in about one-third of the cases. In all other cases progression followed an unexpected pattern.

Many angiographers intuitively feel that progression itself is of predictive significance. If, for

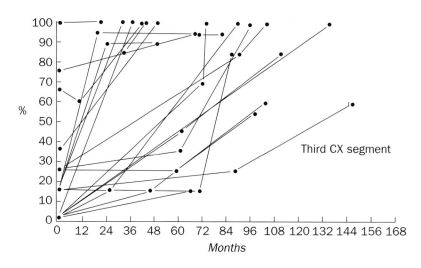

Fig. 6.1 Progression in one coronary segment in a study on patients who underwent two follow-up coronary angiographies.[15] Progression is clearly a non-linear process.

example, in two years an obstruction progresses from 25% to 60% diameter narrowing, it is often assumed that in the near future this will result in a critical stenosis and frequently this is interpreted as an indication for mechanical intervention. However, in a study on patients who had more than one follow-up angiogram it was frequently found that progression of individual lesions did not continue, at least not in a more or less linear fashion.[15] Conversely, if a lesion showed no progression over a certain period of time, this did not mean that the lesion had become inactive, because occasionally significant progression was noted afterwards (Fig. 6.1).

These inconsistencies were not only present in individual lesions but were found if groups of patients were considered: patients who showed progression during the first interval (from angiogram 1 to angiogram 2) often had no progression during the second interval (from angiogram 2 to angiogram 3) and vice versa. These findings indicate that the progression of coronary atherosclerosis occurs in bouts rather than as a continuous process, which makes accurate prediction in individual cases practically impossible.

Regression
Regression of coronary atherosclerosis has been observed in practically all studies, occurring in 2–6% of patients. This includes a large proportion of cases showing recanalization of occluded

arteries; regression is often associated with progression elsewhere in the coronary system. A high incidence of regression (13.4% if recanalizations are not counted) was found by Roskamm et al. in young patients at an average of 3.8 years after acute MI.[16] Apart from this possible correlation with MI (e.g. further clearance of remnants of thrombi), regression seems to be as unpredictable as progression.

Intervention studies

Mechanical interventions
Since mechanical interventions such as percutaneous transluminal coronary angioplasty (PTCA) and coronary artery bypass graft surgery (CABG) influence the evolution of coronary obstructions in a specific manner, which is different from the naturally occurring process of coronary atherosclerosis, we will focus on the natural process of atherosclerosis by reviewing non-mechanical interventions.

Methodological considerations concerning non-mechanical intervention studies
Most intervention studies have been designed as prospective (placebo-controlled) studies, which makes it possible to define in advance strict criteria for quality assurance; this is of particular importance for the angiographic part. If these criteria are fulfilled then automated quantitative analysis of the coronary angiograms is war-

ranted. Quality assurance involves two aspects of major importance, namely that the projections in which the coronary arteries are visualized at baseline and follow-up should be absolutely identical and the influence of vasomotor tone must be reduced to a minimum,[17] and because quantitative analysis uses not only relative (percentage) but also absolute measures, a reliable calibration object must be present. All aspects of quality assurance, as well as the importance of endpoint selection in quantitative coronary arteriography studies, are discussed in detail elsewhere.[8,18,19] The IVUS technique uses direct planimetry performed on a cross-sectional image for measurement of lumen and atheroma areas. This is independent of the projection angle. Since the technique relies on an internal electronic distance scale overlaid on the image, IVUS does not require any special calibration methods. Other (methodological) aspects of the implementation of the IVUS technique in research activities are discussed at the end of this chapter.

Examples of intervention studies

Types of interventions used to reduce the progression of coronary atherosclerosis or to stimulate regression and the placebo-controlled trials in these specific fields are listed in Table 6.2. For the lipid-lowering intervention trials, the number of included patients, study duration and intervention medication are listed in Table 6.3 and the inclusion criteria as well as the entry serum lipids in Table 6.4. The interventions consisted of lipid lowering with drugs, lifestyle risk factor modifications, ileal bypass and low-density lipoprotein (LDL) cholesterol aphereses. The tables show that although all studies are placebo-controlled intervention trials, large differences in design exist, resulting in different clinical implications of their outcomes. Over a period of 15 years a large number of intervention studies have been published. Here we will discuss only the (in our opinion) most important placebo-controlled drug lipid-lowering trials, focusing on the statin trials. A comprehensive overview of the results with regard to influencing progression of coronary atherosclerosis by risk factor modification, changes in lifestyle, ileal bypass

Table 6.2 Lipid intervention trials – placebo-controlled angiographic trials with year of publication

Drug intervention

+ NHLB I–II[128]	1984
+ CLAS I[22]	1987
+ CLAS II[7]	1990
* SCOR[26]	1990
* FATS[25]	1990
* STARS[27]	1992
* MARS[129]	1993
* CCAIT[130]	1994
* MAAS[131]	1994
* HARP[32]	1994
* REGRESS[30]	1995
* PLAC I[40]	1995
* BECAIT[28]	1996
* CIS[132]	1997
* CARS[133]	1997
* LCAS[134]	1997
* PostCABG[135]	1997
* LOCAT[136]	1997
* LIPS[41]	2002

Risk factor modification

* Lifestyle Heart[137]	1990
* Heidelberg[138]	1992
* SCRIP[139]	1994
* Estrogen Replacement and Atherosclerosis Trial[29]	2000

Ileal bypass

# POSCH[140]	1990

Low-density lipoprotein cholesterol apheresis

* FHRS[141]	1995
* LAARS[20]	1996

+ partly analysed by quantitative coronary analysis;
* designed for quantitative coronary analysis;
# angiographic analysis not primary end-point.

surgery, LDL-apheresis and calcium channel blocker therapy can be found elsewhere.[20]

Drug lipid intervention trials

Following the Leiden Intervention Trial,[21] which was lacking a control group, the CLAS (Cholesterol Lowering Atherosclerosis Study),

Table 6.3   Drug lipid-lowering intervention trials – number of included patients, study duration and intervention medication

Trial	No. of patients (finished)	Study duration in months (extension)	Study medication
NHBL I–II	143 (116)	60	Cholestyramine
CLAS I	188 (162)	24 (48)	Colestipol + niacin
SCOR	97 (72)	26	Colestipol + niacin/lovastatin
FATS	146 (120)	30	Lovastatin/colestipol/niacin
STARS	90 (74)	39	Diet/diet + cholestyramine
MARS	270 (246)	26	Lovastatin
CCAIT	331 (299)	24	Lovastatin
MAAS	381 (345)	24 (48)	Simvastatin
HARP	91 (79)	29	Pravastatin/niacin/cholestyramine/gemfibrozil
REGRESS	885 (778)	24	Pravastatin
PLAC I	408 (320)	36	Pravastatin
BECAIT	92 (81)	24 (60)	Bezafibrate
CIS	254 (203)	28	Simvastatin
CARS	90 (80)	24	Pravastatin
LCAS	429 (340)	30	Fluvastatin (cholestyramine)
PostCABG	1351 (1192)	51	Lovastatin (cholestyramine; warfarin)
LOCAT	395 (372)	32	Gemfibrozil
LIPS	1677 (1640)	47	Fluvastatin

For trial references see Table 6.2.

initiated by Blankenhorn et al., is one of the first well-designed placebo-controlled studies that was published.[22] For this study 162 non-smoking men were selected who had previously undergone CABG surgery. The patients were randomized to diet plus placebo or diet plus combined therapy of colestipol and nicotinic acid. The patients were pre-selected to ensure tolerance to both therapeutics. Two years of treatment with a combination of colestipol and niacin resulted in a 26% reduction of serum cholesterol and a 37% elevation in high-density lipoprotein (HDL) cholesterol. Progression was somewhat less in the treated group but, more remarkably, regression was present in 16.2% of the drug treated versus 3.6% in the placebo group. Initially no quantitative analysis was performed; however, the investigators used a sophisticated method of panel assessments. This may be an appropriate way to evaluate changes in patients with previous

bypass surgery,[23] although it makes comparison with other studies, analysed by quantitative coronary analysis, difficult. Furthermore, the final angiographic classification contains a significant degree of subjectivity, especially in those patients who showed a combination of progression and regression. A subgroup of the patients included in CLAS later underwent a third coronary arteriography. The results of the latter study appeared to corroborate the initial findings and indicated that therapy had a beneficial effect for at least four years.[24]

FATS (Familial Atherosclerosis Treatment Study) showed that in patients with a high apolipoprotein B level (≥125 mg/dl) and a family history of vascular disease, treatment with lovastatin and colestipol, or niacin and colestipol, reduced the frequency of progression and increased the frequency of regression of coronary lesions compared with placebo and colestipol.[25] Clinical events (death, MI or revas-

Table 6.4   Drug lipid-lowering intervention trials – inclusion criteria and entry serum lipids

Trial	Inclusion criteria	Entry serum lipids
NHBL I–II	Type II hypercholesterolaemia	LDL chol >95 percentile
CLAS I	Previous coronary bypass surgery	Total chol 4.8–9.1 mmol/l
SCOR	Heterozygous familial hypercholesterolaemia	LDL chol >5.17 mmol/l
FATS	Family history of vascular disease	Apolipoprotein B >125 mg/dl
STARS	Coronary artery disease	Total chol 6.0–10.0 mmol/l
MARS	Coronary artery disease	Total chol 4.9–7.6 mmol/l
CCAIT	Coronary artery disease	Total chol 5.7–7.6 mmol/l
MAAS	Coronary artery disease	Total chol 5.5–8.0 mmol/l
HARP	Coronary artery disease	Total chol 4.6–6.4 mmol/l
REGRESS	Coronary artery disease	Total chol 4.0–8.0 mmol/l
PLAC I	Coronary artery disease	LDL chol 3.4–4.9 mmol/l
BECAIT	Myocardial infarction survivors <45 years	Total chol ≥5.2 mmol/l and TG ≤1.6 mmol/l
CIS	Coronary artery disease	Total chol 5.4–9.0 mmol/l
CARS	Coronary artery disease	Total chol 4.1–5.7 mmol/l
LCAS	Coronary artery disease	LDL chol 3.0–4.9 mmol/l
PostCABG	Previous coronary bypass surgery	LDL chol 3.4–4.5 mmol/l
LOCAT	Previous coronary bypass surgery	LDL chol ≤4.5 mmol/l and HDL chol ≤1.1 mmol/l
LIPS	Previous percutaneous coronary intervention (first time)	Tot chol 3.5–7.0 mmol/l

For trial references see Table 6.2.
Note that the definition of coronary artery disease differs between studies, ranging from vessels (only minimally) visibly involved with atherosclerosis to at least one segment with ≥50% diameter stenosis
LDL, low-density lipoprotein; chol, cholesterol; HDL, high-density lipoprotein; TG, triglycerides.

cularization for worsening symptoms) occurred significantly less in the treatment groups than in the placebo group. Concerning the analysis of the coronary angiograms, it must be noted that the quantitative assessment or edge detection algorithm was not fully automated.

The SCOR (Specialized Center of Research) Intervention Trial randomized 97 patients with heterozygous familial hypercholesterolaemia (FH) to test whether reducing plasma low-density lipoprotein levels by diet and combined drug regimens (see Table 6.3) could reduce progression of coronary lesions.[26] For the analysis of the coronary angiograms, the investigators used in part the same (semi-)quantitative analysis method as was used in FATS.[25] The mean change in percent area stenosis among controls was +0.80, indicating progression, while the mean change for the treatment group was –1.53,

indicating regression. Of note was the fact that regression among women, analysed separately, was also significant, which had not been convincingly demonstrated before.

STARS (St Thomas' Atherosclerosis Regression Study) randomized 90 men with coronary artery disease to receive usual care (controls), dietary intervention or diet plus cholestyramine.[27] Angiography was performed at baseline and after a mean of 39 months. The investigators used change of mean absolute width of segments (MAWS) as the principal angiographic endpoint. For each patient an overall MAWS change, averaged from all changes of measurable segments, was calculated. MAWS decreased by 0.201 mm in controls, increased by 0.003 mm in the dietary group and increased by 0.103 mm in the diet- plus drug-treated group. Although only a relatively small number of segments were analysed, the results of this study appear to warrant intensive lipid-lowering therapy as part of secondary prevention. It should be noted, however, that a minimum plasma cholesterol concentration of 6.0 mmol/l was an inclusion criterion and the mean plasma cholesterol was 7.23 mmol/l, and that vasomotor tone was not standardized, as is nowadays considered state of the art,[16] because lipid lowering itself may reduce vasomotor tone, mimicking regression.

BECAIT (Bezafibrate Coronary Atherosclerosis Intervention Trial) studied the effect of lipid-modifying and fibrinogen-lowering therapy with bezafibrate in young (<45 years) survivors of an acute MI.[28] For 39 placebo patients and 42 bezafibrate patients quantitative coronary angiography was available at baseline and after two and five years. Diffuse as well as focal atherosclerosis progression was retarded in the treatment group. The amount of treatment effect was comparable to that found in the 'statin' trials. Furthermore, 11 out of 45 placebo patients and 3 out of 47 bezafibrate patients suffered a clinical event.

The Estrogen Replacement and Atherosclerosis Trial[29] is a randomized, double-blind, placebo-controlled clinical trial that examined the effects of hormone replacement therapy on the progression of coronary atherosclerosis in women. A total of 309 post-menopausal women who had angiographically verified coronary artery disease at baseline were randomly assigned to receive unopposed oestrogen, estrogen plus medroxyprogesterone acetate, or placebo, and were scheduled for coronary angiography about three years after randomization. Although oestrogen and oestrogen plus medroxyprogesterone acetate produced significant reductions in LDL cholesterol levels and significant increase in HDL cholesterol levels, the progression of coronary atherosclerosis was not affected by any of the three groups.

The 'angiographic statin monotherapy' trials
In the late 1980s a new powerful class of lipid-lowering drugs became available, with only few side-effects, the 3-hydroxy-3-methylglutaryl coenzyme A (HMG-CoA) reductase inhibitors, the so-called 'statins'. This led to a number of large well-designed angiographic trials with statins as monotherapy (see Table 6.2). The results of these trials gave rise to a large upswing in the number of patients with coronary atherosclerosis treated with lipid-lowering therapy, especially with these statins.

In spite of the diversity in number and type of patients included, the medication used and the angiographic techniques and end-points, there is a remarkable consistency in the outcome of the described statin trials: MARS, CCAIT, MAAS, REGRESS, PLAC 1, CIS, CARS, LCAS, PostCABG and LIPS. Therefore we do not describe the results of all these trials undertaken in specific patient groups but describe, as an example, results of the large Regression Growth Evaluation Statin Study (REGRESS). Before the REGRESS results became available a beneficial effect of lipid lowering by HMG-CoA reductase inhibitors had been fairly well demonstrated in patients with various forms of hypercholesterolaemia and other specific groups of patients, e.g. patients with a history of CABG surgery. However, little was known about the potential benefit of lipid lowering in a broader range of patients, including patients with normal to moderately elevated serum cholesterol levels. In other words, it was uncertain if the beneficial effect demonstrated in selected groups of patients could be extrapolated to the average patient most frequently seen in clinical practice. REGRESS specifically addressed this large group of patients. The design and main outcome of the study are described in detail elsewhere.[30] Here we will briefly review this trial and the insights derived from it, and we will relate the results of REGRESS to the results of the other statin trials.

REGRESS was designed as a double-blind, placebo-controlled, multi-centre study to assess the effect of the HMG-CoA reductase inhibitor pravastatin on progression of angiographically documented coronary atherosclerosis in male patients with a baseline serum cholesterol between 4 and 8 mmol/l (155 and 310 mg/dl). Coronary angiography was performed at base-

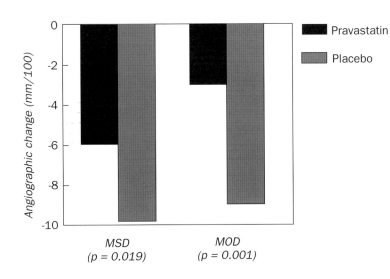

Fig. 6.2 Change of mean (mean segment diameter: MSD) and median (minimum obstruction diameter: MOD) in mm/100 for the pravastatin versus placebo group during the study. A highly significant treatment effect as assessed by these primary end-points is present.

line and after two years of follow-up. Eleven hospitals in the Netherlands participated in the study. All male patients who were scheduled to undergo coronary angiography at one of the participating centres were considered for entry in the study. In both the placebo and the pravastatin groups there was a decrease of the mean segment diameter (MSD) and of the minimum obstruction diameter (MOD), representing progression of coronary atherosclerosis in a diffuse way and a focal way, respectively. In the placebo group mean MSD decreased 0.10 mm whereas in the pravastatin group mean MSD decreased 0.06 mm ($p = 0.019$). In the placebo group median MOD decreased 0.09 mm whereas in the pravastatin group median MOD decreased 0.03 mm ($p = 0.001$). Thus, there was a highly significant treatment effect as assessed by the two primary endpoints of the study (see Fig. 6.2). Furthermore, a significant 41% reduction in clinical events was observed, within the two years of study follow-up.

Overall angiographic results
The other angiographic statin trials showed results that were in general remarkably consistent with those of the REGRESS trial described above, in spite of the described diversity in number and type of patients included in the studies.[31] Practically all the listed studies have shown that lipid lowering significantly retards

progression of coronary atherosclerosis. In only one study, the Harvard Atherosclerosis Reversibility Project (HARP), was there no beneficial treatment effect.[32] However, HARP included only 79 normocholestrolaemic men who finished the study. Of these, 31 had a history of CABG surgery, which makes the interpretation of the angiographic findings cumbersome.

On average, in the statin groups progression is not abolished and there is no regression. However, if a categorical classification is used, most studies show that in both the placebo and the treatment groups there are individual patients who show regression (without progression elsewhere in the coronary tree) while the number of regressors is highest, up to 20%, in the statin treatment group. Thus a significant and non-negligible portion of treated patients may actually show regression of coronary atherosclerosis within two years induced by statin therapy.

Angiographic treatment effect related to baseline lipid profiles: possibilities for risk stratification
The average treatment effect on serum lipids in the trials with statin monotherapy, approximately, was a reduction in total cholesterol of 22%, in LDL cholesterol of 30% and in triglycerides of 13%, and an increase in HDL cholesterol of 6%.

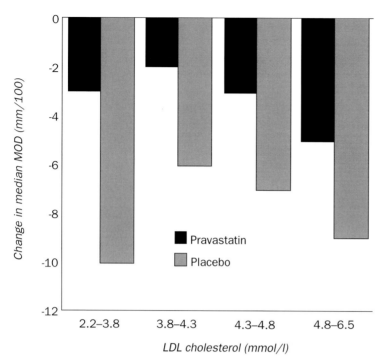

Fig. 6.3 Change of median (minimum obstruction diameter: MOD) in mm/100 related to baseline low-density lipoprotein (LDL) cholesterol level (patient quartiles) for the pravastatin versus placebo group during the study. Treatment effect is independent of baseline LDL cholesterol level.

An important finding is the absence of a correlation between baseline lipid levels and treatment effect. This aspect was extensively analysed in REGRESS and FATS,[30,33] and is illustrated in Fig. 6.3. In practice this means that baseline lipid levels should not be regarded as the only (and perhaps not even an important) criterion upon which a decision to treat patients with HMG-CoA reductase inhibitors should be based. Of course this is only true for patients with proven coronary artery disease. If the disease had developed in the presence of normal or only mildly elevated serum lipid levels, we surmise that in these patients the vascular wall is more susceptible to atherosclerosis-causing agents, including lipids, than is normally the case, which may explain the beneficial effect of lipid lowering. It may also be an indication that HMG-CoA reductase inhibitors have an effect beyond lipid lowering by a direct influence on atherosclerotic plaques, as discussed in the subsection below on ancillary mechanisms. Thus baseline cholesterol is not a good discriminator for those who are at a high risk for progression of coronary artherosclerosis. However, identifying patients at increased risk

for (premature) coronary atherosclerosis and increased progression rate of coronary atherosclerosis is important because these patients might benefit from (early) lipid-lowering treatment. As indicated, it has been proven to be difficult to identify patients at increased risk for progression of coronary atherosclerosis when lipoprotein disturbances were only moderate. REGRESS has provided data on how to treat the individual patient optimally, based on a combination of lipid parameters such as Lp(a) and co-medication with calcium channel blockers and various genetic patient characteristics, as well as a mutation in the gene coding for lipoprotein lipase, and polymorphisms in the gene coding for Apo E and the cholesteryl ester transfer protein.[34–38] This kind of approach will lead us in the future from a population-based therapy strategy to individualized therapy, based on patient characteristics.

Treatment effect on clinical outcome
Angiographic trials are not designed to determine the impact of treatment on clinical events and therefore usually lack sufficient statistical

power to demonstrate a reduction in clinical event rate in the intervention group. However, since coronary atherosclerosis is essentially a chronic progressive disease and, in patients with coronary atherosclerosis, progression of the disease is one of the major factors which determine clinical prognosis, regression of angiographic coronary atherosclerosis may be expected to show a trend to improved clinical outcome, even though the follow-up time is relatively short.[1-3]

Indeed, despite the fact that the angiographic trials were not designed to study clinical events *per se*, most statin studies showed some reduction of cardiac events; however, as may be expected, this did reach statistical significance only in a minority of the trials, e.g. in a study on lovastatin by Andrews et al.[39] and the PLAC I, REGRESS and LIPS trials.[30,40,41]

Mega-trials and meta-analyses
As noted above, the statistical power of individual studies was limited by study size. A few mega-trials have specifically been designed to overcome this problem. The Scandinavian Simvastatin Survival Study (4S) evaluated 4444 patients with CHD (angina or previous MI). The patients were treated with placebo or simvastatin. The treatment group experienced significantly less major cardiac events, cardiac deaths and cerebrovascular events. There was no difference between both groups in non-cardiovascular deaths. The long-standing concern, based on an unexpected outcome of early primary prevention trials (WHO Cooperative Trial and the Helsinki Heart Study), regarding the safety of cholesterol-lowering therapy, particularly in a relatively low-risk population, has been shown to be incorrect.[42-44]

The LIPID study was terminated prematurely (mean follow-up of 60 months) because pravastatin was associated with significant risk reductions in the same categories as the 4S trial.[45-49] The CARE (Cholesterol and Recurrent Events) trial established the same benefit even with pravastatin therapy among patients without markedly elevated lipid levels.[27,50-54] The Heart Protection Study established a 25% reduction in rates of MI, stroke and revascularization for a wide range of high-risk patients, irrespective of their initial cholesterol concentrations.[55]

In meta-analyses by Byngton et al., describing a pooled analysis of the pravastatin atherosclerosis intervention programme,[56] and Vos, describing all monostatin trials until 1996,[31] a significant decrease in all cardiac events, i.e. mortality, non-fatal MI, CABG and PTCA, was observed, corroborating the validity of the concept of angiographic trials and the results of statin therapy. The analysis of the pravastatin atherosclerosis intervention programme also provided evidence for a reduced stroke/TIA rate (which was no prior hypothesis) in the pravastatin group compared with the placebo group.[56] These findings were compatible with several other meta-analyses involving an average of 20 000 patients. The risk reduction appeared to be approximately similar for men and women, elderly and middle-aged, and for various types of risk factors for coronary heart disease.[57-62]

A deeper understanding

Ancillary mechanisms of statin therapy
Statins inhibit the rate-limiting enzyme of cholesterol synthesis in the liver, decreasing the hepatic production of LDL and upgrading the expression of hepatic LDL receptors, consequently lowering concentrations of circulating LDL. Lower plasma LDL concentrations should retard or even regress plaque development due to lipid loss.[63] However, the clinical benefit of statins is manifest within six months after initiation of therapy, which is before plaque regression can occur. The suggestion that statins may have effects beyond lipid lowering is supported by the observation of Byington et al. that in the pravastatin trials the treatment group effect was still statistically significant after adjustment for LDL cholesterol reduction.[56]

Statins may influence plaque stability by preventing macrophage activation, reducing the uptake and endogenous synthesis of cholesterol (reducing plaque size), tissue factor (which promotes thrombus formation) and the production of metalloproteinases (MMP), which weakens the fibrous cap, particularly at the 'vulnerable' shoulder region.[63-66]

Normal endothelial function involves the regulation of vasomotor tone, inhibition of platelet activity, thromboresistance and the promotion of fibrinolysis. Regulation of these processes is partly dependent on nitric oxide (NO), which is produced by the endothelium itself. Statins improve endothelial function by the activation of NO release, partly due to a reduction in serum-oxidized LDL and the concurrent inactivation of endothelin-1, improving overall vasodilator capacity and myocardial blood flow reserve.[63,67-71] That this may indeed be of clinical importance is shown by the fact that in the REGRESS trial a significant reduction of transient myocardial ischaemia could be demonstrated in the pravastatin group with 48-hour ambulatory ECGs (AECG) with continuous ST-segment analysis.[72] In addition to this, statins improve endothelial integrity, reducing its permeability to LDL cholesterol.[73] Most recently Walter et al.[74] have established that statins stimulate mobilization and the incorporation of bone marrow-derived endothelial progenitor cells. This leads to an accelerated re-endothelization of balloon-injured arterial segments. Statins also have anti-inflammatory properties, consisting of the inhibition of leukocyte–endothelium interactions and the reduction of inflammatory cell numbers within the plaque.[75] Statins reduce the expression of adhesion molecules (e.g. ICAM-1), which are involved in the recruitment of circulating monocytes. A reduced monocyte expression of pro-inflammatory cytokines might reduce the serum concentration of C-reactive protein (CRP).[63,75] The potential importance of statin-induced reduction in serum markers of inflammation was illustrated by an analysis from the CARE trial. Patients with the highest serum levels of CRP and amyloid had a relative risk which was 75% higher than those with the lowest levels of the study patient population.[71,76]

Circulating platelets are associated with mural thrombus formation at the site of the plaque rupture, and statin therapy has a variety of effects that may reduce thrombus formation, reduce expression of tissue factor (in endothelial cells and by macrophages), decrease prothrombin activation and thrombin generation and improve fibrinolytic profile.[77,78]

Early use of statins after an acute myocardial infarction

The role of statin therapy initiated three or more months after an acute MI has been extensively established. However, statins may decrease cardiovascular events by a number of mechanisms that can be important directly after a MI. This has led to the investigation of immediate initiation of statin therapy (within the first 24 hours of an acute MI).[79]

The MIRACL (Myocardial Ischemia Reduction with Aggressive Cholesterol Lowering) trial looked specifically at the short-term benefits (16 weeks' follow-up) and established a 16% relative reduction in its combined primary endpoint (death, recurrent non-fatal infarction, resuscitated cardiac arrest and recurrent symptomatic ischaemia requiring hospitalization).[80] The Florida (Fluvastatin on Risk Diminishing After Acute Myocardial Infarction) trial proved neither benefit nor harm. The L-CAD trial (Lipid–Coronary Artery Disease) found fewer major cardiac events in the aggressive lipid-lowering group after two years of follow-up.[81,82] Stenestrand and Wellentin found a reduced one-year mortality in patients who received statin therapy at discharge, compared with those who did not (3.7% vs 5%).[83] In a subgroup analysis of the PRISM (Platelet Receptor Inhibition in Ischemic Syndrome Management) trial Heeschen et al. showed an improved clinical outcome in patients with an acute coronary syndrome who were pre-treated with statins. However, the discontinuation of statins after the onset of symptoms completely abrogated this beneficial effect, despite a lack of change in the cholesterol levels during the first 72 hours. This is consistent with the hypothesis that statins increase the release of endothelial NO independently of cholesterol levels and with animal studies demonstrating a profound rebound phenomenon with impaired NO bioavalability after the withdrawal of statin therapy.[64,84] At the time of writing we are awaiting the results of two randomized controlled trials which address this issue. These are the A-to-Z (Aggrastat and Zocor) and the PROVE IT (Pravastatin or Atorvastatin Evaluation and Infection Therapy) trials.[81] Princess (Prevention of Re-infarction with Cerivastatin Study) and PACT (Pravastatin Acute Coronary Trial) have been interrupted, respectively due to the withdrawal of cerivastatin before conclusions could be reached and due to very slow recruitment (Table 6.5).

Other techniques characterizing the coronary atherosclerotic plaque

Based on tremendous research efforts, we now know that an acute coronary syndrome is caused by plaque vulnerability. Consequently, we have tried to find ways to assess the vulnerability of the plaque by its main features:

- thickness of the fibrous cap
- size and composition of the lipid core
- vessel function
- inflammation.

There is a relatively weak relationship between plaque size and subsequent risk for acute coronary syndromes, since coronary arteries remodel in the presence of developing plaque. This emphasizes the limitation of contrast angiography for the detection of the (vulnerable) plaque.

It is this vulnerable plaque that is partly dealt with by statins. We call this 'pleiotropic effects' (see the subsection above on ancillary mechanisms of statin therapy). In the quest to find a way to be able to predict which plaque is rupture-prone, many new invasive techniques have been developed.

Intravascular ultrasound

IVUS is the only invasive technique mentioned here that has gained substantial clinical importance. It is a catheter-based imaging technique that provides visualization of the full vessel wall, as opposed to the two-dimensional projection of the lumen provided by angiography. The IVUS probe emits high US (20–50 MHz)

and the signal reflected from the arterial wall structures is used to generate an image.[85] Changes in acoustic impedance between adjacent tissue layers produce a strong reflection, resulting in an apparent boundary in the image. Particularly, the interface between the blood-filled lumen and the endothelium (intima) and the interface between the media and the external elastic lamina are acoustically strong. *In vitro* and *in vivo* studies have demonstrated the accuracy and reproducibility to assess quantatively lumen area, plaque area and vessel area as well as some morphological features such as fibromuscular tissue versus fibrous tissue versus calcifications (Fig. 6.4).[86–88] In studies comparing results of US and angiography studies, IVUS appeared to detect atherosclerosis at angiographically (almost) normal sites.[86,88–91] This is understood through a number of important limitations of contrast angiography.

Apart from limited resolution and motion blur, angulations (foreshortening) and irregularities of the luminal shape misrepresent the true extent of luminal narrowing.[92] Due to the fact that atherosclerosis is often a diffuse process, which can affect the full length of a vessel, there is no uninvolved reference segment, resulting in an angiographic appearance of a small artery, with minimal stenosis.[93] Angiography often misses the presence of atherosclerotic disease due to the process of 'remodelling'. Remodelling is the response of the artery (in an early stage) to the atherosclerotic process. An increase in arterial size in order to compensate for the plaque burden is positive remodelling. Negative remodelling consists of a decrease in arterial size.[94] Due to this, a vessel can contain extensive atherosclerosis within the wall but show little or no evidence of luminal obstruction. All these features do not cause a problem for the US technique, although this technique also has limitations. 'Ring-down artefact' impairs the ability to image structures adjacent to the transducer. In small coronary arteries lesional morphology and quantitative measurements can be distorted by the physical size of the catheter (currently approx. 1.0 mm). Geometric distortion can result from imaging in

Table 6.5   Overview of trials on early use of statins after an acute myocardial infarction

Trial	Patient characteristic	Drug	Initiation of statin	Randomization period	Switch to open label Tx	Primary end-points	Sample size	Duration of study
A-to-Z	ACS	Simvastatin (40 mg/d for 30 d then 80 mg/d vs usual care for 120 d)	120 h after hosp	120 h to 120 d	Simvastatin 80 mg/d vs 20 mg/d	CV death, reinfarction, hosp for ACS, stroke	About 4500	FU until 970 primary events occur
PROVE IT	ACS	Atorvastatin 80 mg/d vs pravastatin 40 mg/d for 2 y	≤10 d after hosp	2 y	No switch	Death, hosp for MI or UA, CABG or PCI, stroke	About 4000	2 y

ACS, acute coronary syndrome (MI or UA); CABG, coronary artery bypass grafting; CV, cardiovascular; FU, follow-up; hosp, hospitalization; MI, myocardial infarction; PCI, percutaneous coronary intervention; Tx, treatment; UA, unstable angina.
Adapted with permission from ref. 81.

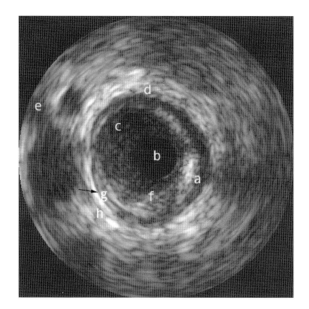

Fig. 6.4 Intravascular ultrasound (IVUS) image is established with a 20 MHz Avanar catheter (JOMED). (a) Calcified plaque with its acoustic echo. (b) Catheter. (c) Vessel lumen. (d) External elastic membrane border. (e) Collateral artery. (f) Intimal thickening (fibrous tissue). (g) Media. (h) Adventitia.

an oblique plane instead of perpendicular to the long axis of the vessel. Inherent to this technique, IVUS only supplies images of the site in the coronary tree in which the catheter is situated. This means that this technique is incapable of visualizing the whole coronary tree, unlike coronary angiography. Since the process of progression and regression of coronary atherosclerosis is a dynamic one, as shown in, for example, the REGRESS trial, this is a major limitation. Additionally, if the operator wants to see another epicardial vessel, he has to replace the coronary guide wire in advance of replacing the catheter, which is an extra manipulation in the (diseased) coronary vessel.

IVUS has greatly improved our understanding of atherosclerosis. IVUS studies have demonstrated that lesions, which cause acute coronary syndromes or MI, are angiographically barely visible due to extensive positive remodelling.[95] IVUS will be a valuable tool in the ongoing research activities of assessing the (vulnerable) plaque, as well as assessing the

effects of risk-factor reduction and statin therapy on the atherosclerotic process. An international expert panel has standardized IVUS measurements and nomenclature, which is very important for the quality of future IVUS-based longitudinal studies on coronary artery disease.[96] Usual protocols of IVUS regression studies consist of a motorized pullback with the selection of every 60th frame, starting from a site located just distally to the intended point, usually a side branch. After a follow-up period of 12–24 months the procedure is repeated according to the exact same methodology. Comparison of the atheroma area of comparable slices then generates the primary end-point and the percent change in atheroma volume. It is expected that this procedure will prove to be very sensitive in detecting drug-induced changes in atherosclerosis. IVUS is expected to become the new gold standard in conjunction with coronary arteriography in (statin) intervention trials. Consequently a number of statin trials have been started, which are either entirely IVUS-based or at least underpowered for angiographic analysis.

Takagi et al.[97] assigned 36 patients with an acute coronary syndrome to either conventional risk-factor modification or additional treatment with pravastatin 10 mg/day. After three years there were no angiographic changes between the two groups, but with IVUS they found a 10% increase versus a 9% decrease in lumen area in the pravastatin group. In the SARIS trial (effects of Statin on Atherosclerosis and vascular Remodeling assessed with Intravascular Sonography) patients are randomized to one-year treatment with either 10 mg or 80 mg atorvastatin. IVUS is the only available technique to measure the effect of atorvastatin on both intimal hyperplasia and vascular remodelling in this trial.[98] In the REVERSAL trial (Reversal of Atherosclerosis with Lipitor) patients are randomly assigned to two different intensities of lipid-lowering therapy: 80 mg atorvastatin versus 40 mg pravastatin daily. All patients undergo IVUS at baseline and at 18 months' follow-up in order to assess the primary end-point: the percentage change in atheroma volume. Apart from other secondary end-points the hypothesis that US will be able to detect changes while angiography will not will be tested. The study has nearly completed enrolment.[99] As mentioned above, several more invasive as well as non-invasive new techniques have been developed. Many of these techniques are still in the process of being validated in order to become a true diagnostic tool.

Other invasive imaging techniques
IVUS elastography demarcates regions within the plaque by their strain; increased strain is lipid-rich while low strain represents fibrous plaque. The information is obtained by processing several US images in a complex mathematical model.[100,101]

Angioscopy generates a full-colour three-dimensional image, which is obtained by observing the intra-coronary lumen directly by means of optical fibres. It can discriminate between stable (white) and unstable (yellow) plaque. Due to the fact that the blood has to be washed from the vessel wall, this technique is already obsolete.[102–104]

Optical coherence tomography (OCT) is an optical analogue of US imaging because it measures the amplitude of backscattered light (optical echoes).[87,105] It measures the thickness of the separate layers of the vessel wall and characterizes the plaque: lipid versus calcium versus fibrous tissue. OCT is a promising imaging modality for plaque characterization due to its high resolution and the fact that it can be easily incorporated into a thin catheter.

Raman spectroscopy assesses the chemical composition ('fingerprint') of the plaque (cholesterol vs calcium).[106,107]

Thermometry uses intracoronary thermistor devices to measure the temperature of the plaque. A 'hot' plaque is associated with inflammation.[108] These techniques are more extensively discussed in detail elsewhere.[109,110]

Non-invasive imaging techniques
B-mode US imaging of carotid and femoral artery walls allows recognition of the early stages of atherosclerosis. Through the separation of the lumen–intima interface from the

media–adventitia interface the intima–media thickness (IMT) is obtained. An increase in IMT is regarded as an early sign of atherogenesis. This is a very patient-friendly technique. However, the correlation between peripheral wall thickness and coronary lumen measurements is low,[111] which makes this technique unsuitable for predicting coronary lumen stenosis on an individual patient basis.

A promising non-invasive tool for studying the progression and regression of atherosclerosis is magnetic resonance imaging (MRI). MRI discriminates luminal boundaries by visualizing the blood flow. It allows discrimination of the lipid core, fibrosis, calcification and thrombus deposits.[112,113] Corti et al.[114] used MRI to study the effect of statin therapy in asymptomatic, untreated, hypercholesterolaemic patients with carotid and aortic atherosclerosis. The effect of simvastatin was measured in terms of changes in lumen area, vessel wall thickness and vessel wall area. At six weeks total cholesterol and LDL cholesterol were significantly reduced, and at 12 months there were significant reductions in vessel wall thickness and vessel wall area, without any changes in lumen area. According to this study, MRI can confidently be used to detect a change in plaque burden of approximately 5% in the aorta or carotid arteries.

Electron beam computed tomography (EBCT) allows direct visualization of the coronary arteries and detects coronary calcium within a plaque. EBCT has been compared with IVUS[115,116] and resulted in the same capacity in detecting calcium. EBCT has also been compared with coronary angiography.[117–121] This generated no results since angiography visualized the lumen and EBCT the vessel wall. However, further development of the technique, such as multislice computed tomography (MSCT), has lead to the possibility of discriminating the wall from the lumen and calcified from non-calcified lesions when contrast is injected.[122] Most recently, Nieman et al.[123,124] were able to reliably perform non-invasive coronary angiographies of the major coronary artery branches in patients with low heart rates by means of MSCT.

CONCLUSION

Observational and intervention studies, in combination with new sources of information, especially IVUS studies, have supplied additional information on vessel wall, plaque area and composition and the principle of remodelling. This is slowly bringing us to a deeper understanding of the processes which take place underlying the progression and regression of atherosclerosis. Intervention by means of statins has proven to be beneficial on progression and induction of regression of coronary atherosclerosis as well as on clinical events. This is probably due to the cholesterol-lowering quality of statins but may also be partly due to their pleiotropic aspects. Whether the underlying mechanisms of these aspects also have a beneficial influence on the occurrence of (in-stent) restenosis remains a subject of further investigation. IVUS will play an important role in this, since this technique is expected to become the new gold standard in statin intervention trials in addition to coronary angiography.

REFERENCES

1. Buchwald H, Matts JP, Fitch LL et al. Changes in sequential coronary arteriograms and subsequent coronary events. Surgical Control of the Hyperlipidemias (POSCH) Group. *JAMA* 1992; **268**: 1429–33.
2. Waters D, Craven TE, Lesperance J. Prognostic significance of progression of coronary atherosclerosis. *Circulation* 1993; **87**: 1067–75.
3. Azen SP, Mack WJ, Cashin-Hemphill L et al. Progression of coronary artery disease predicts clinical coronary events. Long-term follow-up from the Cholesterol Lowering Atherosclerosis Study. *Circulation* 1996; **93**: 34–41.
4. Bruschke AV. Progression of coronary artery disease. *Curr Opin Cardiol* 1987; **2**: 996–1001.
5. Bruschke AV, Wijers TS, Kolsters W, Landmann J. The anatomic evolution of coronary artery disease demonstrated by coronary arteriography in 256 nonoperated patients. *Circulation* 1981; **63**: 527–36.
6. Proudfit WL, Bruschke AV, Sones FM Jr. Natural history of obstructive coronary artery disease: ten-year study of 601 nonsurgical cases. *Prog Cardiovasc Dis* 1978; **21**: 53–78.

7. Proudfit WJ, Bruschke AV, MacMillan JP et al. Fifteen-year survival study of patients with obstructive coronary artery disease. *Circulation* 1983; **68**: 986–97.
8. Reiber JHC, Jukema JW, Koning G, Bruschke AVG. *Quality Control in Quantitative Coronary Arteriography.* Lancaster: Kluwer Academic Publishers, 1986: 45–63.
9. Kramer JR, Kitazume H, Proudfit WL et al. Segmental analysis of the rate of progression in patients with progressive coronary atherosclerosis. *Am Heart J* 1983; **106**: 1427–31.
10. Moise A, Theroux P, Taeymans Y et al. Clinical and angiographic factors associated with progression of coronary artery disease. *J Am Coll Cardiol* 1984; **3**: 659–67.
11. Ishikawa H, Uwatoko M, Watabe S et al. Analysis of the evolution of coronary artery disease – evaluation of 227 cases by restudy of coronary arteriography. *Jpn Circ J* 1986; **50**: 575–86.
12. Vanhaecke J, Piessens J, van de Werf F et al. Angiographic evolution of coronary atherosclerosis in non-operated patients. *Eur Heart J* 1983; **4**: 547–56.
13. Ellis S, Alderman EL, Cain K et al. Morphology of left anterior descending coronary territory lesions as a predictor of anterior myocardial infarction: a CASS Registry Study. *J Am Coll Cardiol* 1989; **13**: 1481–91.
14. Visser RF, van der Werf T, Ascoop CA, Bruschke AV. The influence of anatomic evolution of coronary artery disease on left ventricular contraction: an angiographic follow-up study of 300 nonoperated patients. *Am Heart J* 1986; **112**: 963–72.
15. Bruschke AV, Kramer JR Jr, Bal ET et al. The dynamics of progression of coronary atherosclerosis studied in 168 medically treated patients who underwent coronary arteriography three times. *Am Heart J* 1989; **117**: 296–305.
16. Roskamm H, Gohlke H, Sturzenhofecker P et al. Myocardial infarction at a young age (under 40 years). *Int J Sports Med* 1984; **5**: 1–10.
17. Jost S, Rafflenbeul W, Reil GH et al. Reproducible uniform coronary vasomotor tone with nitrocompounds: prerequisite of quantitative coronary angiographic trials. *Cathet Cardiovasc Diagn* 1990; **20**: 168–73.
18. Jukema JW, van Boven AJ, Zinderman AH et al. The influence of angiographic endpoints on the outcome of lipid intervention studies. A proposal

for standardization. REGRESS Study Group. *Angiology* 1996; **47**: 633–42.

19. Bruschke AVG, Jukema JW, van Boven AJ et al. *Angiographic Endpoints in Progression Trials. Lipid-lowering Therapy and Progression of Coronary Atherosclerosis.* Lancaster: Kluwer Academic Publishers, 1996: 71–7.

20. Kroon AA, Aengevaeren WR, van der Werf T et al. LDL-Apheresis Atherosclerosis Regression Study (LAARS). Effect of aggressive versus conventional lipid-lowering treatment on coronary atherosclerosis. *Circulation* 1996; **93**: 1826–35.

21. Arntzenius AC, Kromhout D, Barth JD et al. Diet, lipoproteins, and the progression of coronary atherosclerosis. The Leiden Intervention Trial. *N Engl J Med* 1985; **312**: 805–11.

22. Blankenhorn DH, Nessim SA, Johnson RL et al. Beneficial effects of combined colestipol–niacin therapy on coronary atherosclerosis and coronary venous bypass grafts. *JAMA* 1987; **257**: 3233–40.

23. Azen SP, Cashin-Hemphill L, Pogoda J et al. Evaluation of human panelists in assessing coronary atherosclerosis. *Arterioscler Thromb* 1991; **11**: 385–94.

24. Cashin-Hemphill L, Mack WJ, Pogoda JM et al. Beneficial effects of colestipol–niacin on coronary atherosclerosis. A 4-year follow-up. *JAMA* 1990; **264**: 3013–17.

25. Brown G, Albers JJ, Fisher LD et al. Regression of coronary artery disease as a result of intensive lipid-lowering therapy in men with high levels of apolipoprotein B. *N Engl J Med* 1990; **323**: 1289–98.

26. Kane JP, Malloy MJ, Ports TA et al. Regression of coronary atherosclerosis during treatment of familial hypercholesterolemia with combined drug regimens. *JAMA* 1990; **264**: 3007–12.

27. Watts GF, Lewis B, Brunt JN et al. Effects on coronary artery disease of lipid-lowering diet, or diet plus cholestyramine, in the St Thomas' Atherosclerosis Regression Study (STARS). *Lancet* 1992; **339**: 563–9.

28. Ericsson CG, Hamsten A, Nilsson J et al. Angiographic assessment of effects of bezafibrate on progression of coronary artery disease in young male postinfarction patients. *Lancet* 1996; **347**: 849–53.

29. Herrington DM, Reboussin DM, Brosnihan KB et al. Effects of estrogen replacement on the progression of coronary artery atherosclerosis. *N Engl J Med* 2000; **343**: 522–9.

30. Jukema JW, Bruschke AV, van Boven AJ et al. Effects of lipid lowering by pravastatin on progression and regression of coronary artery disease in symptomatic men with normal to moderately elevated serum cholesterol levels. The Regression Growth Evaluation Statin Study (REGRESS). *Circulation* 1995; **91**: 2528–40.

31. Vos J. *Retardation of Progression of Coronary Atherosclerosis* (Thesis). Rotterdam: Erasmus University, 1997.

32. Sacks FM, Pasternak RC, Gibson CM et al. Effect on coronary atherosclerosis of decrease in plasma cholesterol concentrations in normocholesterolaemic patients. Harvard Atherosclerosis Reversibility Project (HARP) Group. *Lancet* 1994; **344**: 1182–6.

33. Stewart BF, Brown BG, Zhao XQ et al. Benefits of lipid-lowering therapy in men with elevated apolipoprotein B are not confined to those with very high low-density lipoprotein cholesterol. *J Am Coll Cardiol* 1994; **23**: 899–906.

34. Jukema JW, Zwinderman AH, van Boven AJ et al. Evidence for a synergistic effect of calcium channel blockers with lipid-lowering therapy in retarding progression of coronary atherosclerosis in symptomatic patients with normal to moderately raised cholesterol levels. The REGRESS Study Group. *Arterioscler Thromb Vasc Biol* 1996; **16**: 425–30.

35. Groenemeijer BE, Hallman MD, Reymer PW et al. Genetic variant showing a positive interaction with beta-blocking agents with a beneficial influence on lipoprotein lipase activity, HDL cholesterol, and triglyceride levels in coronary artery disease patients. The Ser447-stop substitution in the lipoprotein lipase gene. REGRESS Study Group. *Circulation* 1997; **95**: 2628–35.

36. Jukema JW, van Boven AJ, Groenemeijer B et al. The Asp9 Asn mutation in the lipoprotein lipase gene is associated with increased progression of coronary atherosclerosis. REGRESS Study Group, Interuniversity Cardiology Institute, Utrecht, The Netherlands. Regression Growth Evaluation Statin Study. *Circulation* 1996; **94**: 1913–18.

37. Kuivenhoven JA, Jukema JW, Zwinderman AH et al. The role of a common variant of the cholesteryl ester transfer protein gene in the progression of coronary atherosclerosis. The Regression Growth Evaluation Statin Study Group. *N Engl J Med* 1998; **338**: 86–93.

38. Cobbaert C, Jukema JW, Zwinderman AH et al. Modulation of lipoprotein(a) atherogenicity by

high-density lipoprotein cholesterol levels in middle-aged men with symptomatic coronary artery disease and normal to moderately elevated serum cholesterol. Regression Growth Evaluation Statin Study (REGRESS) Study Group. *J Am Coll Cardiol* 1997; **30**: 1491–9.

39. Andrews TC, Raby K, Barry J et al. Effect of cholesterol reduction on myocardial ischemia in patients with coronary disease. *Circulation* 1997; **95**: 324–8.

40. Pitt B, Mancini GB, Ellis SG et al. Pravastatin limitation of atherosclerosis in the coronary arteries (PLAC I): reduction in atherosclerosis progression and clinical events. PLAC I Investigation. *J Am Coll Cardiol* 1995; **26**: 1133–9.

41. Serruys PW, de Feyter P, Macaya C et al. Fluvastatin for prevention of cardiac events following successful first percutaneous coronary intervention: a randomized controlled trial. *JAMA* 2002; **287**: 3215–22.

42. Report from the Committee of Principal Investigators. A co-operative trial in the primary prevention of ischaemic heart disease using clofibrate. *Br Heart J* 1978; **40**: 1069–118.

43. World Health Organization. WHO cooperative trial on primary prevention of ischaemic heart disease using clofibrate to lower serum cholesterol: mortality follow-up. Report of the Committee of Principal Investigators. *Lancet* 1980; **ii**: 379–85.

44. Frick MH, Elo O, Haapa K et al. Helsinki Heart Study: primary prevention trial with gemfibrozil in middle-aged men with dyslipidemia. Safety of treatment, changes in risk factors, and incidence of coronary heart disease. *N Engl J Med* 1987; **317**: 1237–45.

45. The Long-Term Intervention with Pravastatin in Ischemic Disease (LIPID) Study Group. Prevention of cardiovascular events and death with pravastatin in patients with coronary heart disease and a broad range of initial cholesterol levels. *N Engl J Med* 1998; **339**: 1349–57.

46. Simes RJ, Marschner IC, Hunt D et al. Relationship between lipid levels and clinical outcomes in the Long-term Intervention with Pravastatin in Ischemic Disease (LIPID) Trial: to what extent is the reduction in coronary events with pravastatin explained by on-study lipid levels? *Circulation* 2002; **105**: 1162–9.

47. Tonkin AM, Colquhoun D, Emberson J et al. Effects of pravastatin in 3260 patients with unstable angina: results from the LIPID study. *Lancet* 2000; **356**: 1871–5.

48. Marschner IC, Colquhoun D, Simes RJ et al. Long-term risk stratification for survivors of acute coronary syndromes. Results from the Long-term Intervention with Pravastatin in Ischemic Disease (LIPID) Study. LIPID Study Investigators. *J Am Coll Cardiol* 2001; **38**: 56–63.

49. Secondary prevention by raising HDL cholesterol and reducing triglycerides in patients with coronary artery disease: the Bezafibrate Infarction Prevention (BIP) study. *Circulation* 2000; **102**: 21–7.

50. Rosengren A, Hagman M, Wedel H, Wilhelmsen L. Serum cholesterol and long-term prognosis in middle-aged men with myocardial infarction and angina pectoris. A 16-year follow-up of the Primary Prevention Study in Goteborg, Sweden. *Eur Heart J* 1997; **18**: 754–61.

51. Executive Summary of the Third Report of the National Cholesterol Education Program (NCEP) Expert Panel on Detection, Evaluation, and Treatment of High Blood Cholesterol in Adults (Adult Treatment Panel III). *JAMA* 2001; **285**: 2486–97.

52. Rosenson RS, Frauenheim WA, Tangney CC. Dyslipidemias and the secondary prevention of coronary heart disease. *Dis Mon* 1994; **40**: 369–464.

53. De Lorgeril M, Renaud S, Mamelle N et al. Mediterranean alpha-linolenic acid-rich diet in secondary prevention of coronary heart disease. *Lancet* 1994; **343**: 1454–9.

54. Arntzenius AC, Kromhout D, Barth JD et al. Diet, lipoproteins, and the progression of coronary atherosclerosis. The Leiden Intervention Trial. *N Engl J Med* 1985; **312**: 805–11.

55. MRC/BHF Heart Protection Study of cholesterol lowering with simvastatin in 20,536 high-risk individuals: a randomised placebo-controlled trial. *Lancet* 2002; **360**: 7–22.

56. Byington RP, Jukema JW, Salonen JT et al. Reduction in cardiovascular events during pravastatin therapy. Pooled analysis of clinical events of the Pravastatin Atherosclerosis Intervention Program. *Circulation* 1995; **92**: 2419–25.

57. Hebert PR, Gaziano JM, Chan KS, Hennekens CH. Cholesterol lowering with statin drugs, risk of stroke, and total mortality. An overview of randomized trials. *JAMA* 1997; **278**: 313–21.

58. Marchioli R, Marfisi RM, Carinci F, Tognoni G. Meta-analysis, clinical trials, and transferability of research results into practice. The case of

cholesterol-lowering interventions in the secondary prevention of coronary heart disease. *Arch Intern Med* 1996; **156**: 1158–72.

59. LaRosa JC, He J, Vupputuri S. Effect of statins on risk of coronary disease: a meta-analysis of randomized controlled trials. *JAMA* 1999; **282**: 2340–6.

60. Sacks FM, Tonkin AM, Craven T et al. Coronary heart disease in patients with low LDL-cholesterol: benefit of pravastatin in diabetics and enhanced role for HDL-cholesterol and triglycerides as risk factors. *Circulation* 2002; **105**: 1424–8.

61. Simes J, Furberg CD, Braunwald E et al. Effects of pravastatin on mortality in patients with and without coronary heart disease across a broad range of cholesterol levels. The Prospective Pravastatin Pooling Project. *Eur Heart J* 2002; **23**: 207–15.

62. LaRosa JC. Prevention and treatment of coronary heart disease: who benefits? *Circulation* 2001; **104**: 1688–92.

63. Liao J. Beyond lipid lowering: the role of statins in vascular protection. *Int J Cardiol* 2002; **86**: 5.

64. Heeschen C, Hamm CW, Laufs U et al. Withdrawal of statins increases event rates in patients with acute coronary syndromes. *Circulation* 2002; **105**: 1446–52.

65. Ambrose JA, Martinez EE. A new paradigm for plaque stabilization. *Circulation* 2002; **105**: 2000–4.

66. Crisby M, Nordin-Fredriksson G, Shah PK et al. Pravastatin treatment increases collagen content and decreases lipid content, inflammation, metalloproteinases, and cell death in human carotid plaques: implications for plaque stabilization. *Circulation* 2001; **103**: 926–33.

67. John S, Schlaich M, Langenfeld M et al. Increased bioavailability of nitric oxide after lipid-lowering therapy in hypercholesterolemic patients: a randomized, placebo-controlled, double-blind study. *Circulation* 1998; **98**: 211–16.

68. Kalinowski L, Dobrucki LW, Brovkovych V, Malinski T. Increased nitric oxide bioavailability in endothelial cells contributes to the pleiotropic effect of cerivastatin. *Circulation* 2002; **105**: 933–8.

69. Hernandez-Perera O, Perez-Sala D, Navarro-Antolin J et al. Effects of the 3-hydroxy-3-methylglutaryl-CoA reductase inhibitors, atorvastatin and simvastatin, on the expression of endothelin–1 and endothelial nitric oxide synthase in vascular endothelial cells. *J Clin Invest* 1998; **101**: 2711–19.

70. Laufs U, La F, V, Plutzky J, Liao JK. Upregulation of endothelial nitric oxide synthase by HMG-CoA reductase inhibitors. *Circulation* 1998; **97**: 1129–35.

71. Kaesemeyer WH, Caldwell RB, Huang J, Caldwell RW. Pravastatin sodium activates endothelial nitric oxide synthase independent of its cholesterol-lowering actions. *J Am Coll Cardiol* 1999; **33**: 234–41.

72. Van Boven AJ, Jukema JW, Zwinderman AH et al. Reduction of transient myocardial ischemia with pravastatin in addition to the conventional treatment in patients with angina pectoris. REGRESS Study Group. *Circulation* 1996; **94**: 1503–5.

73. Nieuw Amerongen GP, Vermeer MA, Negre-Aminou P et al. Simvastatin improves disturbed endothelial barrier function. *Circulation* 2000; **102**: 2803–9.

74. Walter DH, Rittig K, Bahlmann FH et al. Statin therapy accelerates re-endothelialization: a novel effect involving mobilization and incorporation of bone marrow-derived endothelial progenitor cells. *Circulation* 2002; **105**: 3017–24.

75. Vaughan CJ, Murphy MB, Buckley BM. Statins do more than just lower cholesterol. *Lancet* 1996; **348**: 1079–82.

76. Ridker PM, Rifai N, Pfeffer MA et al. Inflammation, pravastatin, and the risk of coronary events after myocardial infarction in patients with average cholesterol levels. Cholesterol and Recurrent Events (CARE) Investigators. *Circulation* 1998; **98**: 839–44.

77. Eto M, Kozai T, Cosentino F et al. Statin prevents tissue factor expression in human endothelial cells: role of Rho/Rho-kinase and Akt pathways. *Circulation* 2002; **105**: 1756–9.

78. Undas A, Brummel KE, Musial J et al. Simvastatin depresses blood clotting by inhibiting activation of prothrombin, factor V, and factor XIII and by enhancing factor Va inactivation. *Circulation* 2001; **103**: 2248–53.

79. Bybee KA, Wright RS, Williams BA et al. Effect of concomitant or very early statin administration on in-hospital mortality and reinfarction in patients with acute myocardial infarction. *Am J Cardiol* 2001; **87**: 771–4.

80. Schwartz GG, Olsson AG, Ezekowitz MD et al. Effects of atorvastatin on early recurrent ischemic events in acute coronary syndromes. The MIRACL Study: a randomized controlled trial. *JAMA* 2001; **285**: 1711–18.

81. Wright RS, Murphy JG, Bybee KA et al. Statin lipid-lowering therapy for acute myocardial infarction and unstable angina: efficacy and mechanism of benefit. *Mayo Clin Proc* 2002; **77**: 1085–92.

82. Arntz HR, Agrawal R, Wunderlich W et al. Beneficial effects of pravastatin (+/– colestyramine/niacin) initiated immediately after a coronary event (the randomized Lipid-Coronary Artery Disease [L-CAD] Study). *Am J Cardiol* 2000; **86**: 1293–8.

83. Stenestrand U, Wallentin L. Early statin treatment following acute myocardial infarction and 1-year survival. *JAMA* 2001; **285**: 430–6.

84. Laufs U, Endres M, Custodis F et al. Suppression of endothelial nitric oxide production after withdrawal of statin treatment is mediated by negative feedback regulation of rho GTPase gene transcription. *Circulation* 2000; **102**: 3104–10.

85. Schoenhagen P, Nissen S. Understanding coronary artery disease: tomographic imaging with intravascular ultrasound. *Heart* 2002; **88**: 91–6.

86. Erbel R, Ge J, Bockisch A et al. Value of intracoronary ultrasound and Doppler in the differentiation of angiographically normal coronary arteries: a prospective study in patients with angina pectoris. *Eur Heart J* 1996; **17**: 880–9.

87. Pasterkamp G, Falk E, Woutman H, Borst C. Techniques characterizing the coronary atherosclerotic plaque: influence on clinical decision making? *J Am Coll Cardiol* 2000; **36**: 13–21.

88. Topol EJ, Nissen SE. Our preoccupation with coronary luminology. The dissociation between clinical and angiographic findings in ischemic heart disease. *Circulation* 1995; **92**: 2333–42.

89. Tuzcu EM, Berkalp B, De Franco AC et al. The dilemma of diagnosing coronary calcification: angiography versus intravascular ultrasound. *J Am Coll Cardiol* 1996; **27**: 832–8.

90. Nissen SE, Gurley JC, Grines CL et al. Intravascular ultrasound assessment of lumen size and wall morphology in normal subjects and patients with coronary artery disease. *Circulation* 1991; **84**: 1087–99.

91. Mintz GS, Painter JA, Pichard AD et al. Atherosclerosis in angiographically 'normal' coronary artery reference segments: an intravascular ultrasound study with clinical correlations. *J Am Coll Cardiol* 1995; **25**: 1479–85.

92. De Franco A. Understanding the pathophysiology of the arterial wall: which method should we choose? Intravascular ultrasound. *Eur Heart J* 2002; **4** (Suppl F): F29–F40.

93. Nissen SE. Application of intravascular ultrasound to characterize coronary artery disease and assess the progression or regression of atherosclerosis. *Am J Cardiol* 2002; **89**: 24B–31B.

94. Glagov S, Weisenberg E, Zarins CK et al. Compensatory enlargement of human atherosclerotic coronary arteries. *N Engl J Med* 1987; **316**: 1371–5.

95. Schoenhagen P, Ziada KM, Kapadia SR et al. Extent and direction of arterial remodeling in stable versus unstable coronary syndromes: an intravascular ultrasound study. *Circulation* 2000; **101**: 598–603.

96. Mintz GS, Nissen SE, Anderson WD et al. American College of Cardiology clinical expert consensus document on standards for acquisition, measurement and reporting of intravascular ultrasound studies (IVUS). A report of the American College of Cardiology Task Force on Clinical Expert Consensus Documents. *J Am Coll Cardiol* 2001; **37**: 1478–92.

97. Takagi T, Yoshida K, Akasaka T et al. Intravascular ultrasound analysis of reduction in progression of coronary narrowing by treatment with pravastatin. *Am J Cardiol* 1997; **79**: 1673–6.

98. Hagenaars T, Gussenhoven EJ, Poldermans D et al. Rationale and design for the SARIS trial; effect of statin on atherosclerosis and vascular remodeling assessed with intravascular sonography. Effect of statin on atherosclerosis and vascular remodeling assessed with intravascular sonography. *Cardiovasc Drugs Ther* 2001; **15**: 339–43.

99. Nissen S. Assessing the effects of statins on atherosclerosis progression using intravascular ultrasound: rationale and design of the REVERSAL Study. *Atherosclerosis* 2001; **2**(Suppl 2): 51–2.

100. De Korte CL, Pasterkamp G, van der Steen AF et al. Characterization of plaque components with intravascular ultrasound elastography in human femoral and coronary arteries in vitro. *Circulation* 2000; **102**: 617–23.

101. De Korte CL, Carlier SG, Mastik F et al. Morphological and mechanical information of coronary arteries obtained with intravascular elastography; feasibility study in vivo. *Eur Heart J* 2002; **23**: 405–13.

102. Mizuno K, Arakawa K, Isojima K et al. Angioscopy, coronary thrombi and acute coronary syndromes. *Biomed Pharmacother* 1993; **47**: 187–91.

103. Bauters C, LaBlanche JM, Renaud N et al. Morphological changes after percutaneous transluminal coronary angioplasty of unstable plaques. Insights from serial angioscopic follow-up. *Eur Heart J* 1996; **17**: 1554–9.

104. Hoher M, Hombach V, Wohrle J. Angioscopic predictors of restenosis following coronary angioplasty – the impact of yellow smooth plaques. *Z Kardiol* 2001; **90**: 111–19.

105. Jang IK, Bouma BE, Kang DH et al. Visualization of coronary atherosclerotic plaques in patients using optical coherence tomography: comparison with intravascular ultrasound. *J Am Coll Cardiol* 2002; **39**: 604–9.

106. Brennan JF III, Romer TJ, Lees RS et al. Determination of human coronary artery composition by Raman spectroscopy. *Circulation* 1997; **96**: 99–105.

107. Buschman HP, Marple ET, Wach ML et al. In vivo determination of the molecular composition of artery wall by intravascular Raman spectroscopy. *Anal Chem* 2000; **72**: 3771–5.

108. Casscells W, Hathorn B, David M et al. Thermal detection of cellular infiltrates in living atherosclerotic plaques: possible implications for plaque rupture and thrombosis. *Lancet* 1996; **347**: 1447–51.

109. Jukema JW, Visseren FLJ. Plaque stabilisation and lipid lowering in clinical practice. In: Gaw A, Shepherd J, eds. *Lipids and Atherosclerosis Annual*. London: Martin Dunitz, 2001: 95–130.

110. Pasterkamp G, Falk E, Woutman H, Borst C. Techniques characterizing the coronary atherosclerotic plaque: influence on clinical decision making? *J Am Coll Cardiol* 2000; **36**: 13–21.

111. De Groot E, Jukema JW, Montauban van Swijndregt AD et al. B-mode ultrasound assessment of pravastatin treatment effect on carotid and femoral artery walls and its correlations with coronary arteriographic findings: a report of the Regression Growth Evaluation Statin Study (REGRESS). *J Am Coll Cardiol* 1998; **31**: 1561–7.

112. Fayad ZA, Fuster V. Characterization of atherosclerotic plaques by magnetic resonance imaging. *Ann NY Acad Sci* 2000; **902**: 173–86.

113. Fayad ZA, Fuster V. Clinical imaging of the high-risk or vulnerable atherosclerotic plaque. *Circ Res* 2001; **89**: 305–16.

114. Corti R, Fayad ZA, Fuster V et al. Effects of lipid lowering by simvastatin on human atherosclerotic lesions: a longitudinal study by high-resolution, noninvasive magnetic resonance imaging. *Circulation* 2001; **104**: 249–52.

115. Schmermund A, Baumgart D, Adamzik M et al. Comparison of electron-beam computed tomography and intracoronary ultrasound in detecting calcified and noncalcified plaques in patients with acute coronary syndromes and no or minimal to moderate angiographic coronary artery disease. *Am J Cardiol* 1998; **81**: 141–6.

116. Baumgart D, Schmermund A, Goerge G et al. Comparison of electron beam computed tomography with intracoronary ultrasound and coronary angiography for detection of coronary atherosclerosis. *J Am Coll Cardiol* 1997; **30**: 57–64.

117. Kajinami K, Seki H, Takekoshi N, Mabuchi H. Coronary calcification and coronary atherosclerosis: site by site comparative morphologic study of electron beam computed tomography and coronary angiography. *J Am Coll Cardiol* 1997; **29**: 1549–56.

118. Tanenbaum SR, Kondos GT, Veselik KE et al. Detection of calcific deposits in coronary arteries by ultrafast computed tomography and correlation with angiography. *Am J Cardiol* 1989; **63**: 870–2.

119. Rumberger JA, Sheedy PF III, Breen JF, Schwartz RS. Coronary calcium, as determined by electron beam computed tomography, and coronary disease on arteriogram. Effect of patient's sex on diagnosis. *Circulation* 1995; **91**: 1363–7.

120. Kaufmann RB, Peyser PA, Sheedy PF et al. Quantification of coronary artery calcium by electron beam computed tomography for determination of severity of angiographic coronary artery disease in younger patients. *J Am Coll Cardiol* 1995; **25**: 626–32.

121. Budoff MJ, Georgiou D, Brody A et al. Ultrafast computed tomography as a diagnostic modality in the detection of coronary artery disease: a multicenter study. *Circulation* 1996; **93**: 898–904.

122. Schroeder S, Kopp AF, Baumbach A et al. Noninvasive detection and evaluation of atherosclerotic coronary plaques with multislice computed tomography. *J Am Coll Cardiol* 2001; **37**: 1430–5.

123. Nieman K, Cademartiri F, Lemos PA et al. Reliable noninvasive coronary angiography with fast submillimeter multislice spiral computed tomography. *Circulation* 2002; **106**: 2051–4.

124. Nieman K, Rensing BJ, van Geuns RJ et al. Non-invasive coronary angiography with multislice spiral computed tomography: impact of heart rate. *Heart* 2002; **88**: 470–4.

125. Kramer JR, Kitazume H, Proudfit WL et al. Progression and regression of coronary atherosclerosis: relation to risk factors. *Am Heart J* 1983; **105**: 134–44.

126. Kramer JR, Matsuda Y, Mulligan JC et al. Progression of coronary atherosclerosis. *Circulation* 1981; **63**: 519–26.

127. Sainsous J, Baragan P, Benichou M et al. Repeated coronarographies in 122 medically treated patients. *Arch Mal Coeur Vaiss* 1985; **78**: 184–90. (In French.)

128. Brensike JF, Levy RI, Kelsey SF et al. Effects of therapy with cholestyramine on progression of coronary arteriosclerosis: results of the NHLBI Type II Coronary Intervention Study. *Circulation* 1984; **69**: 313–24.

129. Blankenhorn DH, Azen SP, Kramsch DM et al. Coronary angiographic changes with lovastatin therapy. The Monitored Atherosclerosis Regression Study (MARS). The MARS Research Group. *Ann Intern Med* 1993; **119**: 969–76.

130. Waters D, Higginson L, Gladstone P et al. Effects of monotherapy with an HMG-CoA reductase inhibitor on the progression of coronary atherosclerosis as assessed by serial quantitative arteriography. The Canadian Coronary Atherosclerosis Intervention Trial. *Circulation* 1994; **89**: 959–68.

131. Effect of simvastatin on coronary atheroma: the Multicentre Anti-Atheroma Study (MAAS). *Lancet* 1994; **344**: 633–8.

132. Bestehorn HP, Rensing UF, Roskamm H et al. The effect of simvastatin on progression of coronary artery disease. The Multicenter Coronary Intervention Study (CIS). *Eur Heart J* 1997; **18**: 226–34.

133. Tamura A, Mikuriya Y, Nasu M. Effect of pravastatin (10 mg/day) on progression of coronary atherosclerosis in patients with serum total cholesterol levels from 160 to 220 mg/dl and angiographically documented coronary artery disease. Coronary Artery Regression Study (CARS) Group. *Am J Cardiol* 1997; **79**: 893–6.

134. Herd JA, Ballantyne CM, Farmer JA et al. Effects of fluvastatin on coronary atherosclerosis in patients with mild to moderate cholesterol elevations. Lipoprotein and Coronary Atherosclerosis Study (LCAS). *Am J Cardiol* 1997; **80**: 278–86.

135. The Post Coronary Artery Bypass Graft Trial Investigators. The effect of aggressive lowering of low-density lipoprotein cholesterol levels and low-dose anticoagulation on obstructive changes in saphenous vein coronary-artery bypass grafts. *N Engl J Med* 1997; **336**: 153–62.

136. Frick MH, Syvanne M, Nieminen MS et al. Prevention of the angiographic progression of coronary and vein-graft atherosclerosis by gemfibrozil after coronary bypass surgery in men with low levels of HDL cholesterol. Lopid Coronary Angiography Trial (LOCAT) Study Group. *Circulation* 1997; **96**: 2137–43.

137. Ornish D, Brown SE, Scherwitz LW et al. Can lifestyle changes reverse coronary heart disease? The Lifestyle Heart Trial. *Lancet* 1990; **336**: 129–33.

138. Schuler G, Hambrecht R, Schlierf G et al. Regular physical exercise and low-fat diet. Effects on progression of coronary artery disease. *Circulation* 1992; **86**: 1–11.

139. Haskell WL, Alderman EL, Fair JM et al. Effects of intensive multiple risk factor reduction on coronary atherosclerosis and clinical cardiac events in men and women with coronary artery disease. The Stanford Coronary Risk Intervention Project (SCRIP). *Circulation* 1994; **89**: 975–90.

140. Buchwald H, Varco RL, Matts JP et al. Effect of partial ileal bypass surgery on mortality and morbidity from coronary heart disease in patients with hypercholesterolemia. Report of the Program on the Surgical Control of the Hyperlipidemias (POSCH). *N Engl J Med* 1990; **323**: 946–55.

141. Thompson GR, Maher VM, Matthews S et al. Familial Hypercholesterolaemia Regression Study: a randomised trial of low-density lipoprotein apheresis. *Lancet* 1995; **345**: 811–16.

7

The Scandinavian Simvastatin Survival Study (4S)

Ole Faergeman

INTRODUCTION

The interest of some readers of this book will have been kindled by the current competition between manufacturers of statins for shares of a big market. Several interesting scientific issues are discussed in this context in other chapters but they are trivial compared with the central question answered by the statin trials. That question was whether coronary heart disease (CHD) could be effectively and safely prevented by lowering plasma cholesterol. It had not been satisfactorily answered in the mid-1980s and, unanswered, it kept most physicians from doing anything about hypercholesterolaemia.

There were reasons for questioning the safety of cholesterol reduction. The WHO trial of clofibrate, especially, had left a legacy of concern about the safety of reducing plasma cholesterol. That trial, designed and executed two decades before the large statin trials were begun, showed that non-fatal CHD could be prevented with clofibrate, but also that treatment was inexplicably associated with deaths due to a wide variety of causes.[1] The chief investigator of the trial, Michael F Oliver, wrote much later that 'lowering cholesterol does not reduce total mortality'.[2] This statement was based on an appraisal of the literature since the WHO trial and it was largely true, even though a few small trials had in fact demonstrated reduction of total mortality by reduction of cholesterol.[3] The statement was echoed by many others, and it greatly affected medical policy.

The concern about total mortality was directed selectively at the cholesterol issue. No one bothered to ask whether cessation of smoking or treatment of high blood pressure or treatment of diabetes had been shown to decrease total mortality. Smoking, high blood pressure and diabetes are, of course, the other commonly occurring conditions that clearly increase the risk of CHD. Since then the treatment of high blood pressure has been shown to reduce total mortality in the aged,[4] whereas the hope that deaths can be postponed by stopping smoking and treating hyperglycaemia is still not supported by trial evidence.[5,6] It is one of the peculiarities of the age of clinical science that scientists and clinicians in closely related fields of medicine accept fundamentally different standards of evidence on which to base therapy and prevention.

With the advent of the statins it became easier to test the cholesterol question, because statins were more effective than earlier drugs, including the fibrates such as clofibrate. The methology of the randomized clinical trial had also been substantially improved since the WHO trial was designed. Terje Pedersen, a Norwegian cardiologist, had performed the timolol trial in collaboration with Merck, Sharpe & Dohme,[7] and in 1987, after discussions with the company, he proposed that it should sponsor a trial of cholesterol reduction with simvastatin to test whether treatment would delay death. The structure of the Scandinavian Simvastatin Survival Study (4S), including a steering committee and programmes for data management, was in place later that year, and the first patient was randomized in May 1988.[8] When the trial's Data Monitoring and Safety Committee had completed the third and final interim analysis in May 1994, it advised the steering committee that the trial should be stopped as soon as possible. 1 August was selected as the cut-off date, at which time it was anticipated that the protocol-specified target of 440 deaths would have been reached.

MAIN RESULTS

Entry requirements included CHD, age from 35 to 70 years, serum cholesterol between 5.5 and 8.0 mmol/l (213–309 mg/dl) and triglycerides less than 2.5 mmol/l (<221 mg/dl). CHD was a history of myocardial infarction (MI), angina pectoris or both. Of 7027 patients recruited for the pre-trial diet period, 4444 fulfilled entry criteria and were randomized to treatment with placebo (*n* = 2223) or 20 mg per day of simvastatin (*n* = 2221). In 37% of the latter patients, cholesterol exceeded the target range of 3.0–5.2 mmol/l (116–200 mg/dl) during the first six months of the study, and the dose of active drug was increased to 40 mg per day in a manner maintaining the double-blind nature of the study. Over the whole course of the study, total cholesterol was reduced by 25%, low-density lipoprotein (LDL) cholesterol by 35% and triglycerides by 10%; high-density lipoprotein (HDL) cholesterol was increased by 8%. Corresponding changes in the placebo group were + 1%, + 1%, + 7% and + 1%, respectively. Rates of withdrawal from study medication were low in both groups: 10% in the simvastatin group and 13% in the placebo group. No patient was lost to follow-up and analysis of results was according to the intention-to-treat principle.[9]

The 4S trial was the first and is still the only major trial to have used total mortality as the primary end-point. After a median 5.4 years of follow-up, 8.2% of the patients treated with simvastatin had died (*n* = 182), compared with 11.5% of placebo patients (*n* = 256). In absolute terms, risk of dying was therefore reduced by 3.3%, and in relative terms it was reduced by 30% (*p* = 0.0003). This result was entirely due to a 42% relative reduction in coronary deaths and it changed the way in which clinicians thought about cholesterol and the prevention of CHD.

The secondary end-point, analysed by the time of first events, was major coronary events. They comprised coronary death, definite or probable hospital-verified non-fatal acute MI, resuscitated cardiac arrest and definite silent MI verified electrocardiographically. One or more major coronary events occurred in 431 simvastatin patients (19%) and in 622 placebo patients (28%). In relative terms, treatment reduced the risk of a major coronary event by 34%.

TERTIARY END-POINTS AND HEALTH ECONOMICS

Tertiary end-points included any CHD-related event, other atherosclerosis-related events, hospitalizations for angina pectoris, coronary bypass surgery and balloon angioplasty, and costs. Earlier studies of the health economics of preventing CHD with statin drugs had been based on extrapolations from epidemiological data.[10–12] Since the study had demonstrated a significant reduction in total deaths, the measure of effectiveness was life-years saved. [Costs per life-year saved = (cost of drug – cost savings)/life-years saved.]

In the first report,[10] only direct cost savings were used. They were the costs of hospitalizations, coronary bypass surgery and percutaneous transluminal coronary angioplasty (PTCA) avoided due to treatment. Calculated in this manner, costs per life-year saved were £5502 (approx. US$9100).

Another report also included indirect cost savings.[12] They were the difference between labour production per patient-year before and after a coronary event estimated from patients in the placebo group who sustained non-fatal events. Calculated in this manner, costs per life-year saved varied from savings in those aged 35 years to US$13 300 (approx. £8000) in women aged 70 years with the lowest concentrations of plasma cholesterol.

The authors calculated the sensitivity of the results to varying assumptions concerning the magnitude of reductions in risk, of risk of dying after a coronary event, of morbidity-associated costs, of intervention costs and of discounting rates, as well as adjustments for quality of life with CHD. This sensitivity analysis showed that direct plus indirect costs could vary from savings to a cost of US$9300 (£5600) per year of life gained in men and from US$100 (£60) to US$18 500 (£11 120) in women.

Five general comments are in order here. The first is that costs of this magnitude are within the range usually considered to be acceptable in health economics. They only apply to patients with CHD, however, because these patients are at high risk of death or non-fatal coronary events including requirements for surgery or angioplasty. Costs per year of life saved by treatment with statins, or any lipid-lowering drug, will be much higher if the risk of events including deaths is lower, as in primary prevention.

The second concerns the selective nature of enquiry in clinical science. Costs per year of life saved are incalculable (incalculably higher), if reduction of mortality has not been demonstrated in a randomized clinical trial. In such areas of medicine, diabetology for example, calculations of this kind are, perhaps for that reason, not done.

The third has to do with the delimitation of assumptions on which calculations of cost-effectiveness are based. The health economic studies of the 4S data are, like almost all other studies of this kind, strictly limited to a small number of possible social contexts. Any more comprehensive set of assumptions implies a rapid multiplication of complexities that would make analysis difficult. It is possible to generalize and show, however, that eradication of fatal diseases such as CHD and cancer would increase the total costs of healthcare as more people would survive to develop non-fatal but costly diseases, especially mental and musculoskeletal diseases, before a later death from whatever cause.[13]

The fourth is that a common reaction of health authorities to the results of the statin trials has been alarm that public expenditure on these drugs cannot be controlled.[14] Moreover, many health authorities are sceptical of health economic analyses of the sort referred to above because, in the real world outside the randomized clinical trial, there will rarely be any cost savings. The reason is that such savings require, for example, laying off surgeons and nurses and closing hospital wards. For many reasons, therefore, the advent of the statin drugs have increased health expenses.

The fifth is that these expenses can now be sharply reduced, because patents have already expired for lovastatin and simvastatin, and the patent will soon expire for pravastatin. Not only will prices drop; promotional activity will also decrease. Important as health economics may be, physicians should insist on the legitimacy of the costliness of healthcare. We must prevent disease and care for the sick not because these endeavours are cost-effective but because they are part of a humanitarian culture. And if we think that health economic analyses are important, especially in their more limited applications, then we should be willing to apply those analyses to all areas of medicine, including the well-established ones.

SUBGROUP ANALYSES AND VALIDITY OF TRIAL RESULTS

As in most other trials, the 4S protocol listed criteria for exclusion of patients from participation. The reasons for exclusion criteria differed. It was considered unethical, for example, to include patients with familial hypercholesterolaemia (FH), and tendon xanthomata therefore comprised an exclusion criterion. So did a history of abuse of drugs or alcohol, because participants as well as investigators must be minimally disciplined if the trial is to proceed as planned. Congestive heart failure or other serious disease identified patients unlikely to survive for the duration of the trial for reasons irrelevant to the study, and they were therefore also excluded. There were other reasons for other exclusion criteria but it should be obvious that exclusion criteria are necessary. The problem is that they reduce the external validity of the results of any trial by limiting the extent to which they can be applied to other kinds of patients. Moreover, exclusion criteria are sometimes based on poor thinking. I shall illustrate this point later.

Subgroup analyses can be important in this context. If results are the same across several subgroups of patients, it is more likely that they pertain to a broad range of patients. Subgroup analyses are especially valuable if they have been specified in the protocol. The 4S protocol specified subgroup analysis of results in women (19% of patients) and patients over 60 years at entry (51% of patients) but several analyses of data from subgroups identified after the trial (*post hoc*) have also been performed.

Women

Of the 4444 participants, 827 were women.[15] They were on average 2.3 years older than the men, and more women than men were entered into the trial with angina pectoris as the criterion of CHD (37% vs 17%). Fewer women than men had undergone revascularization procedures but more of them had a history of hypertension. Only 3.7% of simvastatin-treated women and 3.8% of placebo-treated women were treated with oestrogens.

Only 6.0% of placebo-treated women died during the trial (53 deaths), compared with 12.8% of placebo-treated men, and there was no significant difference in rates of either total or coronary death between women in the simvastatin and placebo groups. A much larger proportion of women sustained major coronary events and tertiary end-points (any CHD-related event, any atherosclerosis-related event, and bypass surgery or PTCA), and a significant reduction in relative risk of such an event as a consequence of treatment was virtually identical to that in men (major coronary events in women vs men: 0.66 vs 0.66; any CHD-related event: 0.72 vs 0.69; any atherosclerosis-related event: 0.71 vs 0.74; bypass or PTCA: 0.51 vs 0.64).

Older patients

At entry into the 4S, 1021 patients were between 65 and 70 years of age.[15] They were therefore between 70 and 75 years if they survived to the end of the study. More patients in this group were women (24%) than in the group less than 65 years old at entry (17%), more were qualified for entry because of a MI (67% vs 61%) and more were non-smokers (33% vs 23%). Event rates were, of course, much higher in the older group of patients but the reduction in relative risk of sustaining an event was virtually the same in those older and younger than 65 (deaths: 0.66 vs 0.72; major coronary events: 0.66 vs 0.66; any CHD-related event: 0.66 vs 0.75; any atherosclerosis-related event: 0.67 vs 0.76; bypass surgery or PTCA: 0.59 vs 0.65). The absolute reduction in risk of an event was therefore uniformly greater in the oldest group.

These two pre-specified subgroup analyses therefore showed that cholesterol reduction with a statin drug produced statistically significant risk reductions in women, men and patients older and younger than 65 years for major coronary events and all tertiary end-points that were positive for the whole 4S cohort. Moreover, the magnitudes of the observed relative risk reductions in these subgroups were remarkably similar to those of the whole cohort.

Several analyses of subgroups not specified in the protocol have also been performed. The results of such *post hoc* analyses must be interpreted with care, because chance will produce spurious results if enough analyses are performed. Obvious analyses to do were in patients at particularly high risk and in patients taking other cardiovascular drugs.

Diabetes

One of the most obvious subgroups to study is patients with diabetes. Only 202 of the 4444 participants (4.5%) were diabetic as ascertained from patient records before the baseline examination. Twelve per cent were treated with insulin, 39% with oral hypoglycaemic drugs and 50% with diet only. Since this was not a pre-defined subgroup, the diabetic state had not been characterized in detail but most of these patients had type 2 diabetes.

In one study of unselected patients with CHD, 18% were diabetic.[16] More diabetic patients would have been included in the 4S, had it not been for a decision to exclude patients with triglycerides over 2.5 mmol/1 (221 mg/dl). This decision by the steering committee was an unfortunate one, for which I was largely responsible. Since statins are better at lowering LDL than triglycerides, we reasoned that inclusion of many hypertriglyceridaemic patients would decrease the likelihood of adequately testing our hypothesis. As will be seen from the analysis of diabetic data (and of the lipid results described below) we were probably wrong. I suppose this is as good an example as any of an exclusion criterion unnecessarily limiting the conclusions that can be drawn from a randomized clinical trial.

Despite the triglyceride exclusion criterion, plasma lipids in these patients reflected those characteristic of type 2 diabetes. Triglycerides were significantly higher than in the non-diabetic patients: 1.73 mmol/1 (153 mg/dl) versus 1.49 mmol/1 (132 mg/dl); and HDL cholesterol was significantly lower: 1.13 mmol/1 (44 mg/dl) versus 1.19 mmol/1 (46 mg/dl). Mortality in the diabetic patients was very high: 24 of the 97 diabetic patients in the placebo group died during the study (24.7%). In the simvastatin group, 15 of 105 died (14.7%). The numbers were small, however, and the reduction in deaths was not statistically significant ($p = 0.087$). There were more secondary and tertiary end-points, and treatment significantly reduced the relative risk of a major coronary event to 45%, of any CHD event to 45%, of any atherosclerosis-related event to 63% and of bypass grafting or coronary angioplasty to 68% of that in the control group.[17] These results were, of course, closely consistent with those obtained in the main study cohort. If anything, they suggest that diabetic patients with CHD are particularly likely to benefit from treatment with a statin drug.

Interaction with effects of other cardiovascular drugs

Many, if not most, patients with CHD are receiving some kind of drug treatment. An obvious problem, rarely addressed, is whether treatments known to relieve symptoms or prevent recurrence of disease when given as monotherapy somehow interfere with each other when given in a kind of polypharmaceutical package. Some of the data concerning this problem have been published.[18–19] They showed that the effect of simvastatin on major coronary effects was unaffected by concomitant treatment with aspirin, beta-blockers and calcium channel blockers.

Results of the diabetes and the concomitant treatment subgroup analyses therefore also support the external validity of the main results of the 4S trial.

Non-coronary atherosclerotic events and heart failure

The coronary arteries are not the only arteries susceptible to atherosclerosis, and reduction of plasma concentrations of LDL cholesterol would be expected to alleviate signs and symptoms due to atherosclerosis in non-coronary as well as coronary arteries. The assessment of such symptoms is therefore another way to approach the general problem of external validity of the main trial results.[20]

Clinical examinations at baseline, and annually thereafter, included auscultation of the carotid and femoral arteries. Patients were asked about symptoms of intermittent claudication, details of which could also be extracted from adverse event report forms filed six weeks, 12 weeks and six months after initiation of therapy as well as semi-annually thereafter. Cerebrovascular events were a tertiary end-point.

Treatment reduced the risk of new or worsening claudication by 28%, but an 11% reduction in the development of femoral bruits was not significant. Carotid bruits were reduced significantly by 48%, and fatal plus non-fatal cerebrovascular events (stroke and transient ischaemic attacks) were reduced significantly by 28% (3.4% vs 4.6%).

Yet another way in which to examine the validity of results is to look at cardiac consequences of coronary atherosclerosis. Heart failure was an exclusion criterion in the 4S trial but during the course of the study, heart failure was diagnosed in 10.3% of placebo patients compared with 8.3% of simvastatin patients ($p < 0.015$).[21]

Relationship of changes in plasma lipoproteins to clinical events

In this analysis of the 4S database,[22] we emphasized that the analytic techniques employed were not pre-defined. Rather, they were selected from a large number of exploratory analyses to identify those that were simple, conservative and least likely to be confounded. Ultimately, however, the selection was a matter of judgement.

Major coronary events were preferred to total mortality data for this analysis because major coronary events are not diluted by non-coronary events and because more than 1000 patients had one or more such events, providing greater statistical power. Events were related to concentrations in plasma of various lipoprotein components at baseline and after one year of treatment.

In the placebo group, major coronary events during the trial were associated with higher concentrations of total cholesterol, LDL cholesterol, apolipoprotein B and triglycerides, and lower concentrations of HDL cholesterol, measured at baseline. This was as expected. In the simvastatin group, it was the one-year concentrations, not the baseline concentrations, of total cholesterol, LDL cholesterol and apolipoprotein B that predicted major coronary events. Measurements of HDL cholesterol at baseline and marginally at one year also predicted events but triglyceride concentrations did not.

These findings are compatible with the concept that the effect of simvastatin was determined mainly by the magnitude of change in LDL, measured as cholesterol, but also as reflected in measurements of total cholesterol and apolipoprotein B. The predictive power of baseline triglyceride measurements in the placebo group but not the simvastatin group is compatible with the concept that triglycerides are carried in non-atherogenic as well as atherogenic lipoproteins, and it is only changes in the latter that affect major coronary events.

The relationship of major coronary events with percentage decrease of lipoprotein components (increase for HDL cholesterol) from baseline to one year in the simvastatin group was analysed according to a Cox proportional hazards regression model. Again, the relationship with reductions in total cholesterol, LDL cholesterol and apolipoprotein B was strong but there was no relationship with triglyceride reductions.

For each additional percentage point reduction in total cholesterol, the risk of a major coronary event was reduced by 1.9% ($p = 0.00005$). The data did not allow us to say whether percentage reduction of LDL cholesterol or LDL cholesterol concentration achieved was more important. There was also no indication of a percentage reduction or on-treatment threshold below which further lipid reduction would be futile.

The results of this analysis were therefore consistent with the concept that reduction of LDL, and closely related classes of lipoproteins also known to be affected by simvastatin,[23] could account for the effects on clinical events. They are also consistent with a meta-analysis of trials of statins and other lipid-lowering drugs indicating that the effect of statins on CHD and deaths can be explained by and is directly proportional to the degree of lipid reduction.[24] In contrast, the results of the 4S analysis were at variance with analogous analyses of pravastatin trials, and this difference was discussed in a commentary by Grundy.[25]

SAFETY AND TOLERABILITY

In-trial safety and tolerability analysis

Meta-analyses of trials of older forms of lipid-lowering treatment that produced mean 10% reductions of cholesterol had raised concerns that treatment increased the risk of cancer deaths and traumatic deaths, including suicides and violence.[26,27] In the 4S trial, in which the mean reduction of serum cholesterol was 25%, not only were deaths due to cancer and trauma (including suicides) similar in the two treatment groups; there was also no suggestion of an increase in cancer (fatal plus non-fatal) overall or at any particular site. The only significant difference in the occurrence of serious adverse events was an increase in trauma (9 vs 22) and arthritis (0 vs 6) in the placebo group, almost certainly due to chance. Despite these results, there continues to be concern about violence and low cholesterol.[28,29]

There was one case of myopathy clearly related to use of simvastatin, and simvastatin produced small but consistent mean increases in concentrations of creatine kinase. There was one case of non-viral hepatitis in the simvastatin group and two in the placebo group, but simvastatin produced small but significant increases in alanine aminotransferase and aspartate aminotransferase. There were also small but significant differences between the treatment groups for mean total bilirubin (6% higher in the simvastatin group) and alkaline phosphatase (4% lower in the simvastatin group).[30]

Follow-up study

Safety and tolerability were therefore very good, but five years is a limited period of observation for a treatment that patients may take for several decades. At present, we have had the opportunity to perform a two-year follow-up study demonstrating that treatment with simvastatin continues to be safe and yield survival benefit.[31] The double-blind study had, as mentioned earlier, been stopped on 1 August 1994. The vital status of all patients exactly two years later was ascertained from government records, and the use of cholesterol-lowering drugs and latest cholesterol concentrations were ascertained with a questionnaire sent to 3731 patients reported to be alive in the autumn of 1997. The response rate was 89%. Cholesterol-lowering drugs were used by 80.5% of the original placebo group and by 85.1% of the original simvastatin group. By 1 August 1996, death had claimed 15.9% of the original placebo group and 11.5% of the original simvastatin group, so that the absolute percentage difference in death rates had increased from 3.3% in 1994 to 4.4% in 1996. The difference was due to a lower rate,

not only of coronary deaths (10.8 vs 6.9%) but also of deaths due to cancer (3.1% in the original placebo group vs 2.3% in the original simvastatin group, $p = 0.087$). The latter finding, although not statistically significant ($p = 0.087$), is important because it lessens or dispels concern that lowering cholesterol causes cancer. If anything, it supports an emerging concept of using cholesterol reduction with statins to inhibit cancer growth.[32]

FURTHER STUDIES

Intuition tells us that treatment to prevent disease is most likely to be effective when it is delivered to those at highest risk of getting the disease and, conversely, that modest if any benefit attends treatment of patients who are at low risk. Indeed, this is one of the important concepts underlying guidelines for assessment of risk and prevention of coronary artery disease.[33,34] Yet this idea has been subjected to repeated experimentation, perhaps because, on closer examination, it is not necessarily correct. Therapy could be ineffective if it works by one mechanism, and high risk is mediated by another mechanism. On the other hand, if drug treatment actually does work well in a particular group of high-risk patients, but the disease mechanism increasing risk is apparently unrelated to how the drug is thought to work, then it might reasonably be conjectured that the drug has additional mechanisms of action.

Here, I shall attempt to describe how more recent *post-hoc* analyses of the 4S database illuminate this general problem. The studies concern patients with diabetes or the metabolic syndrome, patients with apolipoprotein E4, and patients with high plasma concentrations of C-reactive protein.

Diabetes and the metabolic syndrome

Ballantyne et al. identified two small subgroups of 4S patients by baseline triglycerides and HDL cholesterol.[35] One group with the 'lipid triad' (high triglycerides; low HDL cholesterol; high LDL cholesterol) was composed of patients who were in the highest quartile of triglycerides as well as in the lowest quartile of HDL cholesterol (n = 458). The other group had 'isolated high LDL cholesterol'. It was composed of patients who simultaneously were in the lowest quartile of triglyceride and in the highest quartile of HDL cholesterol (n = 545). Both groups fulfilled, of course, the general 4S criterion that they must have high LDL. Placebo patients with the 'lipid triad' did much worse than placebo patients with 'isolated high LDL cholesterol', but treatment with simvastatin virtually eliminated the increased risk. Thus, the 5.4-year risk of major coronary events was lowered from 35.9% to 19.0% in the lipid triad group but only from 20.8% to 18.0% in the group with isolated high LDL cholesterol. The lipid triad group tended to have other characteristics of the metabolic syndrome (diabetes; higher body mass index; history of hypertension) but exclusion of the diabetic patients did not affect results or conclusions. Thus, presence of the lipid triad identified patients who were at highest risk of major coronary events and, at the same time, the most likely to benefit from therapy with a statin.

Analogously, the earlier *post-hoc* analysis of the 4S data showed not only that patients with diabetes were at particularly high risk, but also that they were particularly likely to benefit from therapy.[17] Thus, and as already noted, the 5.4-year risk of death was lowered by 3% (from 10.9% to 7.9%) in non-diabetic patients but it was lowered by 10.4% (from 24.7% to 14.3%) in diabetic patients. Similarly, risk of a major coronary event was lowered by 32% in non-diabetic patients and by 55% in the diabetic patients. As ascertained from patient records before the baseline examination, only 202 of the 4444 participants in the 4S were diabetic. Haffner et al. therefore carried out an analysis of a larger segment of the 4S database.[36]

They took their point of departure in the 1997 American Diabetes Association redefinitions of diabetes. The ADA redefined diabetes as fasting plasma glucose ≥7 mmol/l. Patients with fasting glucose levels 6.0–6.9 mmol/l were defined as having 'impaired fasting glucose', a category which, in broad terms, replaced the earlier category of impaired glucose tolerance. Strictly speaking, the name of the new category is nonsense (you can impair a process such as tolerance but you cannot impair a particular molecule like glucose) but Haffner et al. identified 678 patients as having 'impaired fasting glucose', and they identified 483 patients with diabetes. The diabetic group included a group of 281 patients with concentrations of plasma glucose ≥7 mmol/l in the fasting state (the new ADA definition of diabetes) as well as the original 202 patients with a history of diabetes.

Compared with patients with normal fasting glucose, patients were at somewhat higher risk of a major coronary event if they had impaired fasting glucose (relative risk 1.15) or glucose ≥7 mmol/l (relative risk 1.19) but the increase in risk was not statistically significant, as it was in the 202 patients with a history of frank diabetes (relative risk 1.83). Treatment reduced risk of a major coronary event by 32% in patients with normal fasting glucose, by 38% in patients with impaired fasting glucose and by 42% in the 483 patients with diabetes. Thus, once again, there was a trend towards increasing benefit of statin therapy with increasing baseline risk as a function of increasing plasma concentrations of glucose.

There was no great overlap between the 4S subgroups studied by Ballantyne et al. and those studied by Haffner et al., suggesting that different elements of the metabolic syndrome, the lipid triad as well as hyperglycaemia, can be used to identify coronary artery disease patients who are in particular need of treatment of dyslipidaemia. That general impression is consistent with a much larger body of literature based on the other large statin trials and trials of treatment with fibrates.

Apolipoprotein E and Lp(a)

Blood samples were available for genetic studies from most of the Danish and Finnish 4S patients. That enabled Gerdes et al. to study how a polymorphism in the gene for apolipoprotein E (apoE) affected risk of death in patients in the 4S trial.[37] ApoE is a small protein with multiple functions, not only in the metabolism of plasma lipoproteins but also in lipid transport in the brain.[38] A common polymorphism in the gene for apoE determines whether it codes for apoE3, the most common isoform of apoE, or for apoE4, a slightly less common isoform. The two isoforms differ from each other by only one amino acid. Presence of one ε4 allele (coding for apoE4) increases risk of Alzheimer's disease as well as of coronary artery disease in most but not all populations.[39] If both apoE gene alleles are ε4, the risk of getting either disease is even higher. The ε4 allele is probably the ancestral form of the gene, and it is carried by about 15 to 20% of people in most populations.

Lp(a) is an LDL to which is attached an extra protein called apo(a), the gene for which is probably an imperfect duplication of the gene for plasminogen.[40] The gene and its protein come in many sizes. When apo(a) is small, concentrations of Lp(a) in blood are high, and vice versa. High concentrations of Lp(a) in plasma promote arterial deposition of Lp(a)[41] and risk of atherosclerotic disease.[42]

Lp(a) concentrations were measured, and the apoE genotype or protein phenotype were determined, in Danish and Finnish male patients of the 4S trial. In placebo patients, low Lp(a) and absence of apoE4 were associated with a within-trial mortality risk of 6.5%. Risk was approximately doubled to 12.5% if the patient had either apoE4 or high Lp(a), and it was almost quadrupled to 21.3% if the patient had both apoE4 and high Lp(a). Thus, genetically determined variations in these two proteins identified patients with coronary heart disease who were at low, medium and very high risk of dying within the next 5.4 years. Treatment with simvastatin reduced the risk of dying to the same low level (5–7%) in all four groups. LDL cholesterol was lowered similarly in the various groups, and there was therefore no apparent relationship between the degree of benefit and the degree of lowering of LDL. Nevertheless, once again, those at highest risk also had the greatest benefit from treatment.

C-reactive protein

Elevated serum concentrations of C-reactive protein (CRP) are part of the acute-phase reaction to a variety of diseases. The name derives from the ability of CRP to agglutinate pneumococcal C polysaccharide, and CRP belongs to one of several large families of carbohydrate-binding proteins (lectins).[43] It is composed of five identical polypeptide units that have combined to form a doughnut-like structure. The gene for CRP has been stably conserved throughout vertebrate evolution, and the protein appears to have important physiological functions, the most important of which are probably to scavenge cell debris and combat inflammation.

Ridker et al. have used pravastatin, and also lovastatin and cerivastatin, to study the relationships between CRP concentrations, statin therapy and risk. They have shown that elevated CRP identifies patients who simultaneously are at elevated risk of cardiovascular disease and particularly likely to benefit from therapy with statins. They have argued, moreover, that statins lower CRP in a manner that is independent of LDL cholesterol lowering.[43–46] This concept is now so fashionable that some authors incorporate it into the conclusions of their studies, even if they have found that the association between reductions of CRP and LDL is statistically significant.[47] Indeed, the idea has emerged that CRP is 'a mediator as well as a marker of atherothrombotic disease', and a large-scale statin prevention trial, targeting patients with low LDL and high CRP, is about to be launched, perhaps to test this idea.[48]

A 4S sub-study of CRP[49] was not mentioned in a recent review of the literature about CRP and cardiovascular disease prevention and detection.[48] The results of the 4S sub-study led Crea et al. to a conclusion that differed from the pattern we have seen, not only in the 4S sub-studies of the metabolic syndrome and apoE/Lp(a) but also in the studies of CRP performed by Ridker et al. Baseline serum samples were no longer available from all of the 438 patients who died during the 4S, but Crea et al. measured CRP in the 129 available samples and compared these measurements with those in 129 sex-, age- and treatment-matched survivors. Average CRP concentrations were higher in those who later died (2.5 mg/l) than in those who survived the trial period (1.9 mg/l) but the increased risk of death was confined to patients who were in the highest quartile of CRP levels (≥4.1 mg/l). Treatment with simvastatin lowered LDL cholesterol by 39% and CRP by 21%, and Crea et al. did not address whether the latter depended on the former. There was no significant difference between the two treatment groups in the odds ratios for death associated with the top quartile of CRP serum concentrations. Thus, very high concentrations of CRP were associated with increased risk of death, and treatment with simvastatin was associated with a lowering of CRP. Nevertheless, simvastatin did not reduce the enhanced risk associated with high CRP concentrations, and baseline concentrations of CRP therefore did not allow the authors to identify the patients who were particularly likely to benefit from therapy.

Crea et al. also studied whether concentrations of antibody against oxidized LDL and seropositivity for *Chlamydia pneumoniae* or *Helicobacter pylori* at baseline could differentiate between patients destined or not destined to die within the trial period. They could not. Thus, whereas an unequivocal marker of inflammation, elevated CRP, identified patients at increased short-term risk of death, evidence of exposure to possible agents of inflammation (oxidized LDL or two micro-organisms) did not.

The concept that statins lower CRP by a mechanism unrelated to lowering of LDL is only one of many elements of a debate concerning the pleiotropic effects of these drugs. Statins were initially developed to lower LDL cholesterol by the inhibition of the synthesis of cholesterol (see Chapter 3), but they affect a large number of biochemical variables apart from plasma lipoproteins.[50] These other effects are called pleiotropic to indicate that they differ from the effect originally thought to be the primary effect of the drugs. Similarly, triglyceride lowering can be considered a pleiotropic effect of niacin because the ability to prevent pellagra has been considered the primary effect of niacin.

There are at least two levels on which to consider the pleiotropic effects of statins. Myocardial perfusion can, for example, be improved by lowering plasma LDL cholesterol, not only by statin therapy but also by LDL apheresis. Thus, improvement of myocardial perfusion by statin therapy can be considered a pleiotropic effect of the drug in the sense that the effect on perfusion is different from, albeit a consequence of, LDL lowering. In contrast, statins increase the synthesis of nitric oxide in a manner that is clearly not a consequence of LDL-lowering, although it is in fact due to the inhibition of HMG-CoA reductase. Thus it is a pleiotropic effect if the primary effect of statins is considered to be LDL lowering but it is not if the primary effect of statins is considered to be inhibition of HMG-CoA reductase.

At this point it is not known whether reduction of CRP by statins is secondary to LDL lowering, whether it is due to another effect of inhibition of HMG-CoA reductase or whether it is due to an unknown effect of statins on biochemical processes that are unrelated to HMG-CoA reductase. The latter possibility is inherently unlikely because CRP is reduced by most statins, which, by definition, have the inhibition of HMG-CoA reductase as their shared property.

It is certainly possible that statins lower CRP by mechanisms that are not related to the lowering of LDL. It is also possible that the reduction of CRP in itself really does lower risk of cardiovascular disease because CRP could have an atherogenic role as an activator of complement or monocytes. It is not a straightforward hypothesis, however, and the probable functions of CRP (scavenging of cell debris and anti-inflammation) are more consistent with the concept that CRP is an unspecific marker of tissue damage due to cancer, surgery, infection, ischaemia and some autoimmune diseases. Why elevated CRP should be an agent of only one of these diseases, atherothrombotic disease, but a marker of them all, is not obvious. It is also not immediately obvious that it is a good idea to lower CRP by mechanisms independent of, for example, the lowering of LDL. Something is probably burning if fire-engines are racing along the street but taking the fire-engines off the street might not be the best way to fight the fire.

A more parsimonious hypothesis is that statins lower risk of cardiovascular disease by lowering LDL, which is already known to be atherogenic, and that the resulting cooling of the artery lowers CRP. This hypothesis is consistent with the biology of CRP and the results of the 4S sub-study of CRP.

EXTRAPOLATION AND IMPLEMENTATION OF RESULTS

The randomized clinical trial ensures a high degree of validity of results but, as mentioned earlier, it also limits the extent to which results can be applied to patients who would not have met criteria for inclusion in the trial. Analysis of sub-groups, however – pre-specified as well as non-pre-specified – indicated a high degree of consistency with the main results of the 4S trial. The main trial results were also consistent with the hypothesis underlying all the statin trials, namely that the reduction of serum cholesterol prevents atherosclerotic disease.

It is hardly these main points that now attract so much attention at meetings and in the scientific and commercial literature. The issues attracting most attention are not only, or perhaps no longer, fundamentally scientific ones. They are instead the practical issues of implementation, government policy and commerce.

The task that should absorb the physician is the intelligent extrapolation of results of trials to clinical practice. Physicians must, in broad terms, know about results of clinical science. They should know of good evidence, as in the case of the treatment of hypercholesterolaemia with statins, and they should, in spite of medical orthodoxy, know where evidence is poor or absent. But the decision to start or withhold treatment, especially with drugs given for a long time to prevent disease that may not occur anyway, must ultimately depend on judgement.

In randomized clinical trials, aspirin, beta-blockers, warfarin and angiotensin-converting enzyme (ACE) inhibitors reduce rates of deaths and major córonary events after MI. In contrast, calcium antagonists have in general not been shown to reduce events. The 4S database provided insights into how differently results of such trials are exploited in clinical practice in the five participating countries.[19] The use of aspirin increased in all countries during the study, as evidence of its beneficial effects became more generally known, but Norwegian patients continued to be given less aspirin than, in particular, Danish patients. In contrast, the use of beta-blockers, calcium channel blockers, long-acting nitrates and thiazides was stable throughout the study. The use of beta-blockers in Danish patients was in almost all cases less than half that in the other countries. The use of calcium channel blockers in Finnish and Icelandic patients was in most cases more than twice as common as in Norwegian patients.

The percentage of current smokers was high, especially in Norway and Denmark, and it remained high throughout the study, especially in Norway and Denmark. Conversely, the frequency of ex-smokers at the end of the trial was 36% in Denmark, 44% in Finland, 64% in Iceland, 54% in Norway and 56% in Sweden.

There were substantial differences in 4S placebo group rates of mortality, coronary deaths and major coronary events between the five countries. Mortality rates were particularly high in Denmark. It was not possible to ascribe differences in 4S placebo group rates of deaths, coronary deaths and major coronary events between countries to any particular difference in concomitant therapy. The data show, however, that such differences in clinical outcome occur in a setting of very uneven exploitation of the potential for improving survival of patients with ischaemic heart disease.

CONCLUSIONS

In 1994, the 4S trial demonstrated to physicians the potential of statin therapy to lower plasma concentrations of LDL cholesterol, prevent atherosclerotic disease and postpone death. Confirmed externally by a remarkable series of studies with other statins, this result was also internally consistent as tested in a series of sub-group and *post-hoc* analyses of the 4S database. Most importantly, though, it was consistent with the lipid theory of atherogenesis and the corollary proposition that coronary atherosclerotic disease can be effectively and safely prevented by lowering plasma cholesterol. The 4S sub-studies suggest that different elements of the metabolic syndrome, dyslipidaemia and hyperglycaemia each identify patients with coronary artery disease who not only are at significantly increased risk of new major coronary events but who also stand to benefit particularly well from treatment with a statin drug. Similarly, a 4S sub-study of the common apoE polymorphism and Lp(a) showed that the presence of apoE4 and high concentrations of Lp(a) identify patients with coronary artery disease who are at greatly increased risk of an early death. They also identified the patients who benefited most from therapy. In contrast, high concentrations of CRP identified patients at increased risk of death but they did not identify patients who were particularly likely to benefit from therapy. Results of the 4S CRP sub-study are at variance with fashionable ideas about the role of CRP in atherothrombotic disease.

REFERENCES

1. Report of the Committee of Principal Investigators. WHO cooperative trial on primary prevention of ischaemic heart disease with clofinbrate to lower serum cholesterol: final mortality follow-up. *Lancet* 1984; **2**: 600–4.
2. Oliver MF. Reducing cholesterol does not reduce mortality. *J Am Coll Cardiol* 1988; **12**: 814–17.
3. Carlson LA, Danielson M, Ekberg I et al. Reduction of myocardial reinfarction by the combined treatment with clofibrate and nicotinic acid. *Atherosclerosis* 1977; **28**: 81–6.
4. Dählof B, Lindholm LG, Hansson L et al. Morbidity and mortality in the Swedish Trial in Old Patients with Hypertension (STOP-Hypertension). *Lancet* 1991; **338**: 1281–5.
5. Rose G, Hamilton PJS, Colwell L, Shipley MJ. A randomised controlled trial of anti-smoking advice: 10-year results. *J Epidemiol Community Health* 1982; **36**: 102–8.
6. UK Prospective Diabetes Study (UKDPS) Group. Intensive blood-glucose control with sulphonylureas or insulin compared with conventional treatment and risk of complications in patients with type 2 diabetes. *Lancet* 1998; **352**: 837–53.
7. Pedersen TR. The Norwegian multicenter study of timolol after myocardial infarction. *Circulation* 1983; **67**: 149–53.
8. The Scandinavian Simvastatin Survival Study Group. Design and baseline results of the Scandinavian Simvastatin Survival Study (4S) of patients with stable angina pectoris and/or previous myocardial infarction. *Am J Cardiol* 1993; **71**: 393–400.
9. The Scandinavian Simvastatin Survival Study Group. Randomised trial of cholesterol lowering in 4444 patients with coronary heart disease: the Scandinavian Simvastatin Survival Study (4S). *Lancet* 1994; **344**: 1383–9.
10. Jönsson B, Johannesson M, Kjekshus J et al. Cost-effectiveness of cholesterol lowering, *Eur Heart J* 1996; **17**: 1001–7.
11. Pedersen TR, Kjekshus J, Berg K et al. Cholesterol lowering and the use of healthcare resources. *Circulation* 1996; **93**: 1796–802.
12. Johannesson M, Jönsson B, Kjekshus J et al. Cost effectiveness of simvastatin treatment to lower cholesterol levels in patients with coronary heart disease. *N Engl J Med* 1997; **336**: 332–6.
13. Bonneaux L, Barendregt JJ, Nusselder WJ, van der Maas PJ. Preventing fatal diseases increases healthcare costs: cause elimination life table approach. *BMJ* 1998; **316**: 26–9.
14. Haq IU, Ramsay LE, Pickin DM et al. Lipid-lowering for prevention of coronary heart disease: what policy now? *Clin Sci* 1996; **91**: 399–413.
15. Miettinen TA, Pyörälä K, Olsson AG et al. Cholesterol-lowering therapy in women and elderly patients with myocardial infarction or angina pectoris. *Circulation* 1997; **96**: 4211–18.
16. Euroaspire Study Group. Euroaspire. A European Society of Cardiology survey of secondary prevention of coronary heart disease: principal results. *Eur Heart J* 1997; **18**: 1569–82.
17. Pyörälä K, Pedersen TR, Kjekshus J et al. Cholesterol lowering with simvastatin improves prognosis of diabetic patients with coronary heart disease. *Diabetes Care* 1997; **20**: 614–20.
18. Kjekshus I, Pedersen TR. Reducing the risk of coronary events: evidence from the Scandinavian Simvastatin Survival Study (4S). *Am J Cardiol* 1995; **76**: 64C–68C.
19. Faergeman O, Kjekshus J, Cook T et al. Differences in the treatment of coronary heart disease between countries as revealed in the Scandinavian Simvastatin Survival Study (4S). *Eur Heart J* 1998; **19**: 1531–7.

20. Pedersen TR, Kjekshus J, Pyörälä K et al. Effect of simvastatin on ischemic signs and symptoms in the Scandinavian Simvastatin Survival Study (4S). *Am J Cardiol* 1998; **81**: 333–35.

21. Kjekshus J, Pedersen TR, Olsson AG et al. The effects of simvastatin on the incidence of heart failure in patients with coronary heart disease. *J Card Fail* 1997; **3**: 249–54.

22. Pedersen TR, Olsson AG, Faergeman O et al. Lipoprotein changes and reduction in the incidence of major coronary heart disease events in the Scandinavian Simvastatin Survival Study (4S). *Circulation* 1998; **97**: 1453–60.

23. Gaw A, Packard CJ, Murray ET et al. Effects of simvastatin on apoB metabolism and LDL subfraction distribution. *Arterioscler Thromb* 1993; **13**: 170–89.

24. Gould AL, Rossouw IE, Santanello NC et al. Cholesterol reduction yields clinical benefit: impact of statin trials. *Circulation* 1998; **97**: 946–52.

25. Grundy S. Statin trials and goals of cholesterol-lowering therapy. *Circulation* 1998; **97**: 1436–9.

26. Muldoon MF, Manuck SB, Matthews KA. Lowering cholesterol concentrations and mortality: a quantitative review of primary prevention trials. *BMJ* 1990; **301**: 309–14.

27. Smith GD, Pekkanen J. Should there be a moratorium on the use of cholesterol-lowering drugs? *BMJ* 1992; **304**: 431–4.

28. Kaplan JR, Muldoon MF, Manuck SB, Mann JJ. Assessing the observed relationship between low cholesterol and violence-related mortality: implications for suicide risk. *Ann NY Acad Sci* 1997; **836**: 57–80.

29. Golomb BA. Cholesterol and violence: is there a connection? *Ann Intern Med* 1998; **128**: 478–87.

30. Pedersen TR, Berg K, Cook TJ et al. Safety and tolerability of cholesterol lowering with simvastatin during 5 years in the Scandinavian Simvastatin Survival Study. *Arch Intern Med* 1996; **156**: 2085–92.

31. Pedersen TR, Wilhelmsen L, Faergeman O et al. Follow-up study of patients randomized in the Scandinavian Simvastatin Survival Study (4S) of cholesterol lowering. *Am J Cardiol* 2000; **86**: 257–62.

32. Buchwald H. Cholesterol inhibition, cancer and chemotherapy. *Lancet* 1992; **339**: 1154–6.

33. Wood D, de Backer G, Faergeman O et al. Prevention of coronary heart disease in clinical practice. Recommendations of the Second Joint Task Force of European and Other Societies on Coronary Prevention. *Eur Heart J* 1998; **19**: 1453–503.

34. National Cholesterol Education Program Expert Panel. *Third Report of the Expert Panel on Detection, Evaluation, and Treatment of High Blood Cholesterol in Adults (Adult Treatment Panel III) Full Report.* World Wide Web 2001 (17.5.2002).

35. Ballantyne CM, Olsson AG, Cook TJ et al. Influence of low high-density lipoprotein cholesterol and elevated triglyceride on coronary heart disease events and response to simvastatin therapy in 4S. *Circulation* 2001; **104**: 3046–51.

36. Haffner SM, Alexander CM, Cook TJ et al. Reduced coronary events in simvastatin-treated patients with coronary heart disease and diabetes or impaired fasting glucose levels: subgroup analyses in the Scandinavian Simvastatin Survival Study. *Arch Intern Med* 1999; **159**: 2661–7.

37. Gerdes LU, Gerdes C, Kervinen K et al. The apolipoprotein ε4 allele determines prognosis and the effect on prognosis of simvastatin in survivors of myocardial infarction. A substudy of the Scandinavian Simvastatin Survival Study. *Circulation* 2000; **101**: 1366–71.

38. Mahley RW, Rall SC Jr. Apolipoprotein E: far more than a lipid transport protein. *Ann Rev Genom Human Gen* 2000; **1**: 507–37.

39. Liu S, Ma J, Ridker PM et al. A prospective study of the association between APOE genotype and the risk of myocardial infarction among apparently healthy men. *Atherosclerosis* 2003; **166**: 323–9.

40. Hobbs HH, White AL. Lipoprotein(a): intrigues and insights. *Curr Opin Lipidol* 1999; **10**: 225–36.

41. Reblin T, Meyer N, Labeur C et al. Extraction of lipoprotein(a), apo B, and apo E from fresh human arterial wall and atherosclerotic plaques. *Atherosclerosis* 1995; **113**: 179–88.

42. Danesh J, Collins R, Peto R. Lipoprotein(a) and coronary heart disease. Meta-analysis of prospective studies. *Circulation* 2000; **102**: 1082–5.

43. Kilpatrick DC. Animal lectins: a historical introduction and overview. *Biochim Biophys Acta* 2002; **1572**: 187–97.

44. Ridker PM, Rifai N, Pfeffer MA et al. Inflammation, pravastatin, and the risk of coronary events after myocardial infarction in patients with average cholesterol levels. Cholesterol and Recurrent Events (CARE) Investigators. *Circulation* 1998; **98**: 839–44.

45. Ridker PM, Rifai N, Clearfield M et al. Measurement of C-reactive protein for the targeting of statin therapy in the primary prevention of acute coronary events. *N Engl J Med* 2001; **344**: 1959–65.

46. Albert MA, Danielson E, Rifai N, Ridker PM. Effect of statin therapy on C-reactive protein levels: the pravastatin inflammation/CRP evaluation (PRINCE): a randomized trial and cohort study. *JAMA* 2001; **286**: 64–70.

47. Van de Ree MA, Huisman MV, Princen HM et al. Strong decrease of high-sensitivity C-reactive protein with high-dose atorvastatin in patients with type 2 diabetes mellitus. *Atherosclerosis* 2003; **166**: 129–35.

48. Ridker PM. Clinical application of C-reactive protein for cardiovascular disease detection and prevention. *Circulation* 2003; **107**: 363–9.

49. Crea F, Monaco C, Lanza GA et al. Inflammatory predictors of mortality in the Scandinavian Simvastatin Survival Study. *Clin Cardiol* 2002; **25**: 461–6.

50. Davignon J, Laaksonen R. Low-density lipoprotein-independent effects of statins. *Curr Opin Lipidol* 1999; **10**: 543–59.

8

Primary prevention of coronary heart disease with statins

James Shepherd

INTRODUCTION

Among all of the risk factors which have been linked to coronary artery disease (CAD), hypercholesterolaemia appears to be pre-eminent. Populations whose plasma cholesterol levels are inherently low can withstand exposure to high levels of tobacco consumption and arterial hypertension without developing significant coronary disease. Conversely, in Western industrialized countries, where hypercholesterolaemia is endemic, coincidence of the other two risk factors is linked to more extensive aortic atherosclerosis[1,2] and to a multiplicative increase in coronary morbidity and mortality. The lipid hypothesis, formulated more than 20 years ago, proposed that the reduction of plasma – or more specifically low-density lipoprotein (LDL) – cholesterol would lead to a fall in coronary disease. This chapter assesses the current status of that hypothesis in the light of recent clinical trial evidence derived from the use of statins in clinical practice.

Prior to the introduction of the 3-hydroxy-3-methylglutaryl coenzyme A (HMG-CoA) reductase inhibitors (statins), three major primary prevention trials had already reported on attempts to prevent coronary heart disease by lowering blood cholesterol levels. The first, the World Health Organization (WHO) clofibrate trial,[3,4] demonstrated a reduction in the rate of non-fatal myocardial infarction (MI) in the drug-treated group but also suggested that clofibrate therapy was associated with a rise in total mortality. This finding raised doubts over the benefits of widespread use of lipid-lowering agents. The publication of the Lipid Research Clinic's Coronary Primary Prevention Trial (LRC-CPPT) in 1984[5–7] and the Helsinki Heart Study (HHS) in 1987[8,9] reversed this attitude to some extent but many still remained skeptical because of the inability of all three trials to show a significant benefit with regard to coronary or total mortality. In the LRC-CPPT, an 11% decrease in the level of LDL cholesterol was associated with a significant reduction (of 19%) in cardiac events (fatal plus non-fatal MI). The performance of this study was less than predicted due to compliance problems. In the HHS, gemfibrozil was less potent but was palatable, and compliance among subjects at trial visits was high. The drug lowered LDL cholesterol and triglyceride levels by 8% and 35%, respectively, and increased levels of high-density lipoprotein (HDL) cholesterol by about 10%. These lipid changes were associated with a significant reduction (34%) in the incidence of CAD as measured by the combined fatal plus non-fatal MI end-point.

Neither the LRC-CPPT nor the HHS had the statistical power to address the question of the benefits of lipid-lowering agents in preventing coronary death. To do this, it is necessary to:

- study a population with higher event rates
- increase the sample size and
- use a more effective lipid-lowering agent.

The West of Scotland Coronary Prevention Study (WOSCOPS), using pravastatin, set out in 1988 to address each of these issues. Pravastatin, one of the newly developed HMG-CoA reductase inhibitors, is a powerful cholesterol-reducing agent that is easily tolerated and uniformly effective.[10–16] The increase in sample size and the recruitment of older men in a high-risk area (Scotland had, at the time, the world's highest incidence of CAD mortality) with associated higher event rates increased the power of the study to assess the impact of an improved lipid profile on CAD. The project reported in 1995.[17,18] Following hard on the heels of this development, Downs et al. established a second primary prevention trial, differing in design from WOSCOPS[19] and based in San Antonio, Texas. Their project, the Air Force or Texas Coronary Atherosclerosis Prevention Study (AFCAPS/TexCAPS) employed lovastatin[20–24] as the cholesterol-lowering agent, and was conducted between 1991 and 1997. Its preliminary findings were first presented at the American Heart Association meeting in November 1997 and appeared in print in 1998.[25] WOSCOPS and AFCAPS together sweep away resistance to and concerns over the value of cholesterol lowering in the prevention of the first MI and help refocus the debate on the issue of which subjects to treat in order to gain optimal benefit from the intervention strategy. The merits of the two studies are highlighted below.

WOSCOPS: PRIMARY PREVENTION OF CORONARY HEART DISEASE IN MIDDLE-AGED, HYPERCHOLESTEROLAEMIC MEN

WOSCOPS recruited 6595 men aged 45–64 who had never had a MI but were at risk because their average total cholesterol was 7.0 mmol/l (270 mg/dl) and their LDL cholesterol 4–6 mmol/l (155–232 mg/dl). Five percent of the participants had evidence of angina as determined by a positive Rose questionnaire but none had been hospitalized for investigation of this problem within the previous 12 months, nor did they demonstrate any major ECG abnormalities such as the presence of Q waves, significant ST-T wave changes or left bundle branch block. The participants were randomized to receive pravastatin 40 mg at

night or placebo and followed up in the community at three-monthly intervals for an average of 4.9 years. Smoking and dietary advice were provided throughout the study. The primary end-point in the trial was combined definite non-fatal MI and coronary heart disease (CHD) death. Other (secondary) endpoints included definite non-fatal MI, CHD death, all cardiovascular deaths, the need for revascularization procedures, death from noncardiovascular causes and all-cause mortality.

AFCAPS/TexCAPS: PRIMARY PREVENTION OF CORONARY HEART DISEASE IN MEN AND WOMEN WITH 'AVERAGE' PLASMA CHOLESTEROL LEVELS

Like WOSCOPS, AFCAPS was a randomized, double-blind, placebo-controlled trial designed to test the benefit of cholesterol reduction in the primary prevention of CHD. There were, however, minor but important design differences between the two trials. For example, men and women were admitted to AFCAPS, the latter accounting for 15% of the total recruits. The age range of the subjects also differed. Men aged 45–73 years and post-menopausal 55- to 73-year-old women were eligible for participation so long as they met the lipid entry criteria and had no history or clinical evidence of MI, angina, claudication, cerebrovascular accident or TIA. Also, it was necessary that their total cholesterol lay between 4.65 and 6.83 mmol/l (180–264 mg/dl), LDL cholesterol between 3.36 and 4.91 mmol/l (130–190 mg/dl), HDL cholesterol ≤1.16 mmol/l (45 mg/dl) in men or ≤1.22 mmol/l (47 mg/dl) in women and triglyceride was below 4.52 mmol/l (400 mg/dl), as measured on two occasions no more than one month prior to randomization. Higher risk individuals with uncontrolled hypertension, obesity (defined as more than 50% above the desirable limit for height according to the Metropolitan Life Insurance tables) or diabetics receiving insulin therapy or with glycated haemoglobin values greater than 50% above the upper normal limit were specifically excluded. The cholesterol-lowering treatment strategy was also different inasmuch as dietary advice was

Table 8.1 Design features of WOSCOPS and AFCAPS		
	WOSCOPS	AFCAPS/TexCAPS
Study design	**Double-blind, placebo-controlled**	
Drug (dose, mg/day)	Pravastatin (40 mg at night)	Lovastatin (20–40 mg, depending on response)
Subjects	6595, (100% male)	6605 (85% male)
Age	45–64 years	males 45–73 years; females 55–73 years
Target lipid reduction	None	LDL cholesterol ≤2.84 mmol/l (110 mg/dl)
Subject years of follow-up	32 216	32 300

continued with lovastatin (20 mg/day), whose dose was doubled if LDL cholesterol did not reach a target value of 2.84 mmol/l (110 mg/dl) within three months of initiating therapy. The average baseline total, LDL and HDL cholesterol values were 5.71 ± 0.54 mmol/l (211 ± 21 mg/dl), 3.88 ± 0.44 mmol/l (150 ± 17 mg/dl) and 0.96 ± 0.16 mmol/l (37 ± 6 mg/dl) – all lower than in the WOSCOPS cohort. This, in conjunction with the lower level of other coronary risk factors, reduced the expectation of events in the AFCAPS participants and led the trialists to expand their primary end-point from the narrower constraints of the WOSCOPS definition to include, in addition, the development of unstable angina pectoris and sudden cardiac death.

Secondary end-points focused on cardiovascular episodes, and incorporated fatal or non-fatal MI, fatal or non-fatal coronary events, fatal or non-fatal cardiovascular events, cardiovascular mortality, CHD mortality, fatal or non-fatal coronary revascularization procedures and unstable angina pectoris.

Finally, safety issues were dealt with in the tertiary end-points of incident and fatal cancers, non-cardiovascular death and death from any cause.

THE COMPLEMENTARITY OF AFCAPS AND WOSCOPS

There are remarkable similarities and interesting points of difference between WOSCOPS and AFCAPS. Table 8.1 encapsulates the design features of both studies. WOSCOPS, which pio-

neered primary CHD prevention with statins, specifically targeted high-risk males from a population in which CHD was prevalent and resistance to cholesterol lowering among clinicians was the norm. Conversely, AFCAPS focused on lower-risk Air Force men and women (15% of the total cohort) or civilians from the vicinity without clinical evidence of atherosclerotic disease and with substantially lower baseline lipid levels, simply because there is a much greater enthusiasm among American physicians for intervention against hypercholesterolaemia, even in individuals who are otherwise healthy. This arrangement presumably was responsible for the decision to admit older participants (up to 75 years) into the AFCAPS trial with a view to increasing the number of end-points expected throughout its course. Both studies recruited virtually identical numbers of subjects and followed them for an average of 4.9 years, the decision being taken to terminate AFCAPS prematurely for reasons based on issues other than safety. One unique feature of AFCAPS was the decision to aim for an on-treatment plasma LDL cholesterol value of ≤2.84 mmol/l (110 mg/dl). This necessitated upward titration of the dose of administered lovastatin form 20 mg to 40 mg/day in those individuals who failed to achieve the desired LDL cholesterol at the basal drug dose. Approximately 50% of the actively treated participants were prescribed the higher dosage, so that on average the mean prescribed lovastatin dose was 30 mg/day.

Partly for the reasons noted above, the baseline lipid profile of the AFCAPS cohort was

Table 8.2 Baseline and on-treatment lipids of the WOSCOPS and AFCAPS/TexCAPS actively treated cohorts

Variable (mmol/l)	WOSCOPS lipids (± 1 SD)		AFCAPS/TexCAPS lipids (± 1 SD)	
	Baseline	Mean % change	Baseline	Year 1 % change
Total cholesterol*	7.03 ± 0.59	20↓	5.71 ± 0.54	18↓
Total triglyceride**	1.83 ± 0.79	12↓	1.84 ± 0.76	15↓
LDL cholesterol	4.96 ± 0.44	26↓	3.88 ± 0.44	25↓
HDL cholesterol	1.14 ± 0.23	5↑	0.96 ± 0.16	6↑

* To convert to mg/dl, multiply by 38.7.
** To convert to mg/dl, multiply by 88.5.

Table 8.3 Baseline non-lipid coronary risk factors in WOSCOPS and AFCAPS/TexCAPS

Risk factor	Percent cohort affected at baseline	
	WOSCOPS	AFCAPS/TexCAPS
Diagnosed hypertension	16	22
Diabetes mellitus	1	2
Family history of premature CHD	6	16
Smokers	44	12

significantly lower than in WOSCOPS (Table 8.2). Starting values for total, LDL and HDL cholesterol values in AFCAPS were 19%, 22% and 16% lower than in the pravastatin cohort of the West of Scotland Study at baseline. Moreover, only 12% of the Texas recruits smoked, versus 44% in WOSCOPS (Table 8.3). Conversely, in AFCAPS there were twice as many diabetics, 37% more diagnosed hypertensives and almost three times as many recruits with a family history of premature ischaemic heart disease. Despite these increases in non-lipid risk factors the absolute risk of the typical AFCAPS recruit is significantly less than in WOSCOPS, as reflected in the recorded event rates in the placebo-treated cohorts in each study. In WOSCOPS, the absolute risk of CHD death or non-fatal MI recorded at five years in the placebo group was 7.9% whereas in AFCAPS less than 5% of the control cohort had experienced CHD death, non-fatal MI or

had developed unstable angina. Consequently, AFCAPS incorporated a broader aggregate primary end-point (Table 8.4) in its design as a means of increasing the number of end-points recorded over the five years of the project and strengthening the power calculations within the study.

The main findings of WOSCOPS and AFCAPS are remarkably concordant (Fig. 8.1). Intention-to-treat analysis shows (see Table 8.2) that both drugs produced virtually identical percentage reductions in total and LDL cholesterol. This corresponds to an average 1.41 and 1.03 mmol/l absolute reduction in total cholesterol and a 1.29 and 0.97 mmol/l fall in LDL on pravastatin and lovastatin, respectively. As a consequence (see Fig. 8.1), the incidence of combined CHD death and non-fatal MI fell by 31% ($p < 0.001$) or 74 events in WOSCOPS while the aggregate of unstable angina/CHD

Table 8.4	Comparative end-points in WOSCOPS and AFCAPS/TexCAPS	
End-point	*WOSCOPS*	*AFCAPS/TexCAPS*
Primary	• Definite CHD death or non-fatal MI	• Unstable angina pectoris or CHD death or non-fatal MI or sudden cardiac death

Others	• Definite non-fatal MI
	• Definite and suspect CHD death and/or non-fatal MI
	• Strokes (fatal or non-fatal)
	• Coronary angiography
	• PTCA or CABG
	• Death from:
	  CHD
	  cardiovascular causes
	  non-cardiovascular causes
	  all causes
	• Cancer (incident and fatal)
		• CHD death or non-fatal MI
		• Unstable angina
		• Coronary events
		• Cardiovascular events
		• Death from:
		  CHD
		  cardiovascular causes
		  non-cardiovascular causes
		  All causes
		• Cancer (incident and fatal)

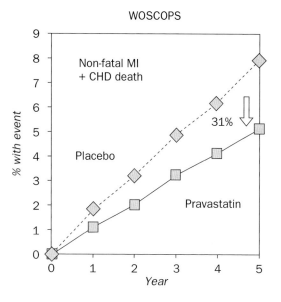
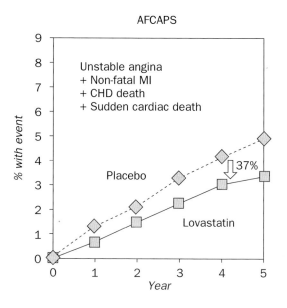

Fig. 8.1 Primary end-points in WOSCOPS and AFCAPS.

death/non-fatal MI/sudden cardiac death was reduced by 37% (57 events; $p < 0.001$) in AFCAPS. These benefits from statin administration in both studies began to appear within about six months of initiation of therapy and continued as long as treatment was maintained.

LESSONS FROM AFCAPS AND WOSCOPS

While it is clear that both lovastatin and pravastatin help reduce the risk of a first MI without producing significant side-effects or increasing the risk of morbidity or mortality from other causes, it is inappropriate to conclude that all individuals who meet the entry criteria for WOSCOPS and AFCAPS should automatically be offered lipid-lowering drug therapy. Implementation of such a liberal strategy is clearly economically impractical in most cost-challenged health services. Instead, it is more rational to identify and intervene only in those individuals whose risk of an event exceeds an accepted specified value. In 1998, the Joint Task Force of the European Atherosclerosis Society, the European Society of Cardiology and the European Society for Hypertension ruled[26] that a 20% risk of a vascular event over the next ten years (or, broadly, a 2% risk per annum) warranted consideration for intervention, fully aware that such an arbitrary decision required enough flexibility in its interpretation to meet the circumstances of populations with differing financial and healthcare constraints. With that caveat in mind, how can one target patients for treatment on the basis of their prospective risk of an event? Consideration of the frequency and distribution of cardiovascular events in the placebo groups of WOSCOPS and AFCAPS permit such a selection to be made. Individuals with a 10% risk of an ischaemic event over the five years of the trial warrant active intervention. In WOSCOPS only one quarter of the placebo group had a risk of definite CHD death or non-fatal MI which exceeded this 10% treatment threshold, and undoubtedly the percentage of the AFCAPS population who would be targeted would be even less. Detailed examination of the top-risk quartile in WOSCOPS showed that it encapsulated 45% of the coronary events in the study. In other words, application of the European Joint Guidelines to WOSCOPS or AFCAPS will successfully identify 45% (or fewer) of the incipient infarcts in this mild-to-moderate risk group and disregard the majority of all first MI victims. The simplest way to locate the highest-risk patients is on the basis of their non-lipid risk factor profiles, which is a cogent argument that cholesterol screening of asymptomatic individuals should be limited to middle-aged or older individuals at high short-term risk of a coronary event, with treatment restricted to this group and to those who present with atherosclerotic disease.

Compared with a strategy of untargeted screening and treatment, this approach would ensure the maximum absolute benefit and cost-effectiveness of therapy. However, adoption of this strategy would result in the majority of events being missed, even though it is clear that the two statins induced the same relative reduction in coronary risk across the entire spectrum of the WOSCOPS and AFCAPS cohorts. So, the number of people needed to be treated to prevent one major coronary event (Fig. 8.2 and Table 8.5) is considerable in the low-risk WOSCOPS subjects and even greater in AFCAPS. Treatment targeted to higher-risk individuals in WOSCOPS improves this situation (see Table 8.5) and makes more economic sense. Table 8.6 underscores the differences in absolute risk which pertained in the WOSCOPS and AFCAPS cohorts. In order to avoid one primary end-point (non-fatal MI plus CHD death) in WOSCOPS, 42 individuals required pravastatin therapy over the study duration. In AFCAPS, the number needed to treat with lovastatin to avoid one was 47, but to strengthen the power of the study the end-point had been expanded to include, *inter alia*, unstable angina. A truer picture is obtained of the absolute vascular risk of the two cohorts when comparison is made of the same end-point. The AFCAPS trialists, for example, needed to treat two to three times as many individuals to avoid a combination of non-fatal MI plus CHD or a fatal cardiovascular event (Table 8.6). It is curious but interesting to note that 125 individuals required treatment over the five-year WOSCOPS duration to avoid one revascularization procedure versus 63 individuals in AFCAPS. These unexpected figures reflect the differences in cardiological practice between Scotland and the USA and highlight the more aggressive approach to interventional cardiology in Texas.

The need for discrimination in using statins for the primary prevention of CHD makes a strong case for the kind of aggressive lifestyle intervention proposed by the Task Force of the European Societies of Cardiology, Atherosclerosis and Hypertension[26] and the National Cholesterol Education Program Adult Treatment Panel[27]

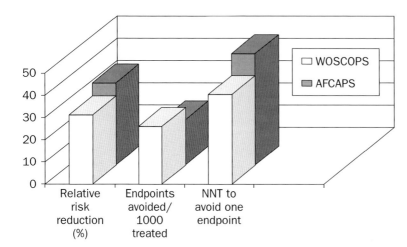

Fig. 8.2 Primary end-point comparisons in WOSCOPS and AFCAPS. The primary end-point in WOSCOPS (non-fatal MI plus CHD death) was expanded in AFCAPS in order to increase the number of primary events recorded.

Table 8.5 Numbers of subjects needing treatment to avoid one primary end-point event

Trial	Total cohort	High-risk subjects (>10% risk over 5 yrs)
WOSCOPS	40	20
AFCAPS	56	Not available

before any consideration is given to drug therapy. The relative merits of targeted versus generalized approaches to cholesterol screening and treatment are the subject of current debate[28,29] which hopefully will lead to enlight-ened guidance for the average clinician. Both WOSCOPS and AFCAPS were initiated prior to publication of the NCEP[27] or original joint European Task Force[30] guidelines. According to the latter, as noted above, only one quarter of the WOSCOPS participants had a high enough absolute risk at baseline to warrant statin intervention but, reflecting the more liberal approach to therapy in the USA, three-quarters of the group (Table 8.7) lay within the NCEP drug treatment watershed. Inevitably, economic constraints will continue to wield an ever-growing influence on clinical decision making, but for these 25% high-risk individuals in Europe and 77% in the USA, pravastatin therapy can be recommended on the firm evidence base of WOSCOPS as a safe and effective means of

Table 8.6 Numbers of subjects needing treatment to avoid vascular events in AFCAPS and WOSCOPS*

	WOSCOPS			AFCAPS		
	Placebo rate (%)	Statin rate (%)	NNT	Placebo rate (%)	Statin rate (%)	NNT
Primary end-point	7.9	5.5	42	5.7	3.5	47
Non-fatal MI/CHD death	7.9	5.5	42	2.9	1.7	83
Fatal cardiovascular event	2.3	1.6	143	0.8	0.5	333
Revascularization	2.5	1.7	125	4.8	3.2	63

* Over study duration.

Table 8.7 Correspondence of the WOSCOPS population with NCEP guidelines

Clinical category	Baseline LDL (mg/dl)	Number (%)
No CHD		
<2 risk factors	≥190	1249 (18.9)
	<190	1545 (23.4)
≥2 risk factors	≥160	3187 (48.3)
	<160	0
Clinical CHD	≥130	614 (9.3)
	<130	0
Total		**6595 (100)**

annum, would have saved more than half of the avoidable events by only treating one-third of the cohort. So, it is efficient in clinical terms to set levels of intervention at a value which makes economic sense to society as a whole. Primary prevention of CHD with statins is cost-effective. Treatment can be monitored to meet the expectations of society while at the same time maximizing economic efficiency. A detailed risk–benefit analysis of the AFCAPS patients, currently underway, will allow clinicians to judge how best to target lovastatin therapy at lower-risk subjects in order to help avoid a first MI.

SHOULD WE TREAT TO TARGET LIPID LEVELS?

There is heated ongoing debate over the value of aggressive total and LDL cholesterol reduction in the prevention of CHD.[32] The protagonists assert that increasing benefit will accrue from greater lipid lowering, implying that there is a linear association between plasma cholesterol values and coronary risk. However, the Multiple Risk Factor Intervention Trial,[33] the largest observational study of its kind, and other similar large-scale prospective projects make it clear that populations experience a curvilinear rise in coronary events with increasing plasma cholesterol. By inference, then, cholesterol-lowering strategies would most effectively reduce events in individuals with more severe hypercholesterolaemia and would become attenuated in their capacity to do so as individual plasma cholesterol values fell. In other words, a patient will receive greater absolute cardioprotection from the first, say, 25% cholesterol reduction than from efforts to lower cholesterol by 25%

reducing the risk of major coronary events, if lifestyle intervention fails to achieve the expected benefits. It is instructive to review the relative merits of applying the various treatment guideline recommendations to vascular disease prevention in, for example, the WOSCOPS cohort. Over the 4.9 years of the study, 460 cardiovascular events of all types were recorded in the 3293 placebo-treated subjects. Pravastatin therapy achieved a relative risk reduction of 22% when applied to the totality of these events, thereby avoiding 101 of the 460 events (Table 8.8). Application of the NCEP guidelines would have limited treatment to 81% of the placebo cohort and avoided 92% of the possible number of events prevented. Application of the European guidelines triggering action at a 2% per annum risk would have treated two-thirds of the placebo group with the avoidance of 83% of the events, while the even more conservative Sheffield risk tables,[31] based on a 3% risk per

Table 8.8 Guideline selection influences efficiency of therapy

Guidelines	Subjects (%)	Events avoided
WOSCOPS selection criteria	3293 (100)	101
NCEP (LDL cholesterol <160 mg/dl + 2 risk factors)	2669 (81)	92
European (2% risk p.a.)	2187 (66)	83
Sheffield (3% risk p.a.)	1135 (34)	55

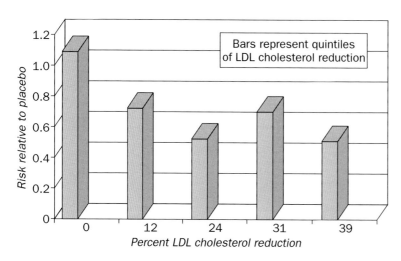

Fig. 8.3 LDL cholesterol reduction and event reduction in WOSCOPS. Pravastatin-treated individuals in WOSCOPS were grouped into quintiles of increasing on-treatment LDL cholesterol reduction. Individuals whose LDL did not fall in the trial (compliance was a likely cause) saw no benefit. Maximal benefit in terms of cardiovascular disease reduction was achieved when LDL cholesterol was reduced by 25%. Individuals who recorded a 40% fall in LDL cholesterol saw no additional benefit.

more. Comparison of AFCAPS with WOSCOPS exemplifies this point. Both studies produced approximately a one-third relative reduction in risk of a cardiovascular event, but this benefit translated into an avoidance of 74 fatal and non-fatal MIs in WOSCOPS versus 57 avoided aggregate cases of unstable angina, fatal and non-fatal infarcts and sudden cardiac deaths in AFCAPS, despite the more aggressive drive to achieve a lower target on-treatment LDL cholesterol value. Of course, the average absolute risk of an event in AFCAPS was about 30% lower than in WOSCOPS and so the absolute gain from intervention was, not unexpectedly, less.

This principle of diminishing returns was tested in the WOSCOPS population using the following approach.[34] First, the percentage reduction of LDL cholesterol from baseline was calculated for each individual in the pravastatin-treated group. To provide the most accurate measure of plasma lipid concentration during follow-up, on-treatment lipid values were calculated as the mean of all lipid measurements made after randomization until the patient had an event or reached the end of the study. If a lipid value was missing at a visit but study medication had been issued at the previous visit (three months earlier), the most recent measurement that had been preceded by a medication issue was carried forward. If before the visit no such on-treatment measurement existed then the baseline value was imputed. Baseline value was also imputed if no medication had been

issued at the previous visit and the present lipid level was missing. Not unexpectedly, the response of the pravastatin-treated individuals varied substantially. Some experienced virtually no change in their plasma LDL cholesterol while in others it fell by 50% or more. The cohort was therefore divided into quintiles of achieved LDL reduction and the diminution in risk of a coronary event calculated for each quintile. The men in quintile 1, who showed no LDL cholesterol fall, experienced the same rate of coronary events as the placebo-treated WOSCOPS cohort. Quintiles 2 to 5, which had mean percentage LDL reductions of 12%, 24%, 31% and 39%, exhibited 28%, 47%, 31% and 43% fewer coronary events, respectively (Fig. 8.3). In other words, an LDL reduction of 25% in WOSCOPS (as seen in quintile 3) yielded as much benefit as was seen in quintile 5, where the achieved LDL cholesterol was almost 40% lower than the baseline value.

A second analysis compared the event rates of subjects in the placebo group and in the pravastatin-treated group who had the same LDL cholesterol for the duration of the study. The majority of individuals on placebo had LDL cholesterol levels of about 4.4 mmol/l (170 mg/dl) and the majority of individuals on pravastatin had values below 3.0 mmol (50 mg/dl) but there existed an overlap where the two groups were similar. The 446 individuals on the placebo group with an average LDL cholesterol of 4.2 mmol/l (162 mg/dl)

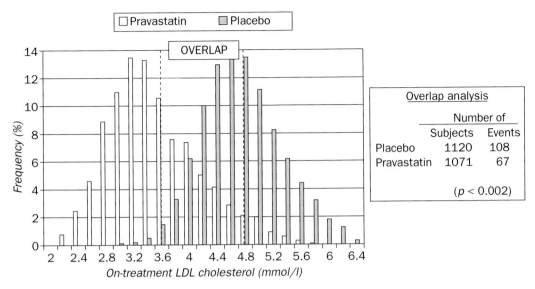

Fig. 8.4 WOSCOPS overlap analysis. Approximately 1100 individuals in each arm of the WOSCOPS trial maintained the same LDL cholesterol over the duration of the study. Those receiving pravastatin suffered significantly fewer (38%) events, suggesting that the benefits of statin therapy may extend beyond their cholesterol-lowering capability.

had a risk of a coronary event over the duration of the study of 5.6%. The 466 pravastatin users, with a similar LDL cholesterol of 4.1 mmol (159 mg/dl), had a significantly lower risk of 3.88%. In other words, receiving pravastatin resulted in 32% less risk of a coronary event than receiving placebo, despite the subjects having the same LDL level. Selection of a broader overlap group (Fig. 8.4) produced the same result, reinforcing the more precise findings of the narrow overlap analysis. What factors can account for this benefit? Statins may confer value beyond LDL cholesterol reduction such as, for example, reducing blood viscosity, stabilizing plaques, suppressing inflammatory responses, decreasing the probability for lipoprotein oxidation, and so on (see Chapter 5). *Post-hoc* analyses of this kind are, of course, fraught with difficulties and must be viewed with caution, but these trends in the WOSCOPS data were consistent with the general outcome of the trial and with the early benefit seen in response to treatment. It will be instructive to determine whether a similar analysis of AFCAPS reveals the same benefit.

THE PROSPECTIVE STUDY OF PRAVASTATIN IN THE ELDERLY AT RISK (PROSPER)

In November 2002 *The Lancet* carried the primary results of a new trial of the benefits of pravastatin in an elderly cohort of subjects at high risk of cardiovascular disease.[35] In distinction to the WOSCOPS/AFCAPS comparison outlined above, the uniqueness of the PROSPER study design (see Chapter 12) allows for a direct within-trial assessment of individual responsiveness to statin therapy (in this case pravastatin) used in primary and secondary prevention mode.

PROSPER differed from all of the other statin end-point trials by recruiting individuals (44% of the total) who had either had a vascular event in the past (MI; stroke; peripheral vascular disease) or who were at high risk of developing one (56% of the total) because they were diabetic, hypertensive or smokers.

Senior citizens represent the most rapidly growing segment of society. They expect, after years of contributing to the economy, to carry on receiving continuing benefit in terms of health, honour and dignity. This is only possible if policy-makers and the healthcare industry

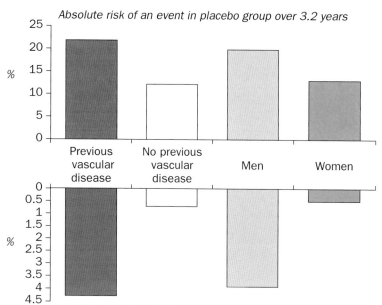

Absolute risk of an event in placebo group over 3.2 years

Absolute benefit from pravastatin over 3.2 years

Fig. 8.5 Primary versus secondary vascular disease prevention: an analysis from PROSPER. Although men and those with existing vascular disease were at greatest risk of a vascular event in PROSPER and gained most from pravastatin treatment, tests for interaction revealed no significant differences between these subgroups.

recognize their impending problems and make provision for the inevitable explosive expansion, which will occur in coronary, peripheral and cerebrovascular disease. PROSPER aimed to identify effective treatment strategies for these problems.

The 5804 patients who participated in PROSPER contained proportionately more women than any other statin-based trial, and this, combined with the breadth of acceptability of risk factors at baseline, ensured that the risk of vascular events in this cohort was wide-ranging (Fig. 8.5). As might be expected, women with no previous history of overt vascular disease had the lowest risk while risk was significantly higher in men harbouring existing disease. Unsurprisingly again, those at the highest level of risk experienced the greatest absolute benefit from statin intervention (see Fig. 8.5). Note, however, that this does not imply differences in responsiveness to treatment on the basis of absolute risk or gender since statistical testing for intervention revealed no significant differences between these sub-groups. The take-home message, therefore, is that neither gender nor degree of risk should be a barrier to the use of statin therapy in vascular disease prevention; and, as indicated in Chapter 12, elderly individu-

als, who clearly are at the greatest risk of an event, deserve as much consideration as the middle-aged when it comes to the design of national prevention strategies.

REFERENCES

1. McGill HC, McMahan CA, Malcolm GT et al. Effects of serum lipoproteins and smoking on atherosclerosis in young men and women. *Arterioscler Thromb Vasc Biol* 1997; **17**: 95–106.
2. McGill HC, Strong JP, Tracy RE et al. Relation of a post mortem renal index of hypertension to atherosclerosis in youth. *Arterioscler Thromb Vasc Biol* 1995; **15**: 2222–8.
3. Committee of Principal Investigators. WHO Clofibrate Trial. A co-operative trial in the primary prevention of ischaemic heart disease using clofibrate: report from the Committee of Principal Investigators. *Br Heart J* 1978; **40**: 1069–118.
4. Committee of Principal Investigators. WHO Clofibrate Trial. Co-operative Trial on primary prevention of ischaemic heart disease using clofibrate to lower serum cholesterol: mortality follow-up report. *Lancet* 1980; **ii**: 379–85.
5. The Lipid Research Clinics Program. The Coronary Primary Prevention Trial: design and implementation. *Chron Dis* 1979; **32**: 609–31.

6. The Lipid Research Clinics Coronary Primary Prevention Trial Results. I. Reduction in incidence of coronary heart disease. *JAMA* 1984; **251**: 351–64.

7. The Lipid Research Clinics Coronary Primary Prevention Trial Results. II. The relationship of reduction in incidence of coronary heart disease to cholesterol lowering. *JAMA* 1984; **251**: 365–74.

8. Mantarri O, Elo O, Frick, MH et al. The Helsinki Heart Study: basic design and randomisation procedure. *Eur Heart J* 1987; **9** (Suppl 1): 1–29.

9. Frick MH, Elo O, Haapa K et al. Helsinki Heart Study: primary prevention trial with gemfibrozil in middle-aged men with dyslipidemia: safety of treatment, changes in risk factors, and incidence of coronary heart disease. *N Engl J Med* 1987; **317**: 1237–245.

10. Pan HY. HMG-CoA reductase inhibitors: clinical pharmacology. In: Gotto AM Jr, Mancini M, Richter WO, Schwandt P, eds. *Treatment of Severe Hypercholesterolemia in the Prevention of Coronary Heart Disease. Proceedings of the 2nd International Symposium, Munich 1989.* Basel: Karger, 1990: 66–70.

11. Tsujita Y, Juroda M, Shimada Y et al. CS–514, a competitive inhibitor of 3-hydroxy-3-methylglutaryl coenzyme A reductase: tissue-selective inhibition of sterol synthesis and hypolipidemic effect on various animal species. *Biochim Biophys Acta* 1986; **877**: 50–60.

12. Tsujita Y, Watanabe Y. Pravastatin sodium: novel cholesterol-lowering agent that inhibits HMG-CoA reductase. *Cardiovasc Drug Rev* 1989; **7**: 110–26.

13. Reihner E, Rudling M, Stahlberg D et al. Influence of pravastatin, a specific inhibitor of HMG-CoA reductase on hepatic metabolism of cholesterol. *N Engl J Med* 1990; **3223**: 224–8.

14. Singhvi SM, Pan HY, Morrison RA, Willard DA. Disposition of pravastatin sodium, a tissue-selective HMG-CoA reductase inhibitor, in healthy subjects. *Br J Clin Pharmacol* 1990; **29**: 239–42.

15. Vega GL, Krauss RM, Grundy SM. Pravastatin therapy in primary moderate hypercholesterolaemia: changes in metabolism of apolipoprotein B-containing lipoproteins. *J Intern Med* 1990; **227**: 81–94.

16. Mosley ST, Kalinowski SS, Shafer BL, Tanaka RD. Tissue-selective acute effects of inhibitors of 3-hydroxy-3-methylglutaryl coenzyme A reductase on cholesterol biosynthesis in the lens. *J Lipid Res* 1989; **30**: 1411–20.

17. The West of Scotland Coronary Prevention Study Group. A coronary primary prevention study of Scottish men aged 45–74 years: trial design. *J Clin Epidemiol* 1992; **45**: 849–60.

18. Shepherd J, Cobbe SM, Ford I et al. Prevention of coronary heart disease with pravastatin in men with hypercholesterolemia. *N Engl J Med* 1995; **333**: 1301–7.

19. Downs JR, Beere PA, Whitney E et al. Design and rationale of the Air Force/Texas Coronary Atherosclerosis Prevention Study (AFCAPS/TexCAPS). *Am J Cardiol* 1997; **80**: 287–93.

20. Alberts AW. Discovery, biochemistry and biology of lovastatin. *Am J Cardiol* 1988; **62**: 10J–15J.

21. Alberts AW, Chen J, Juron G et al. Mevinolin: a highly potent competitive inhibitor of hydroxymethylglutaryl-coenzyme A reductase and a cholesterol-lowering agent. *Proc Natl Acad Sci USA* 1980; **77**: 3957–61.

22. Albers-Schonberg G, Joshua H, Lopez MB et al. Dihydromevinolin, a potent hypocholesterolemic metabolite produced by *Aspergillus terreus. J Antibiotics* 1981; **34**: 507–12.

23. MacDonald JS, Gerson RJ, Kornburst DJ et al. Preclinical evaluation of lovastatin. *Am J Cardiol* 1988; **62**: 16J–27J.

24. Henwood JM, Heel RC. Lovastatin, a preliminary review of its pharmacodynamic properties and therapeutic use in hyperlipidaemia. *Drugs* 1988; **36**: 429–54.

25. Downs JR, Clearfield M, Weis S et al. Primary prevention of acute coronary events with lovastatin in men and women with average cholesterol levels. *JAMA* 1998; **279**: 1615–22.

26. Wood D, DeBacker G, Faergeman O et al., on behalf of the Task Force. Prevention of coronary heart disease in clinical practice. Recommendations of the Second Task Force of European and Other Societies on Coronary Prevention. *Atherosclerosis* 1998; **140**: 199–270.

27. National Cholesterol Education Program. Adult Treatment Panel II. Second report of the expert panel on detection, evaluation and treatment of high blood cholesterol in adults. *Circulation* 1994; **89**: 1329–445.

28. Garber AM, Browner WS, Hulley SB. Cholesterol screening in asymptomatic adults, revisited. *Ann Intern Med* 1996; **124**: 518–31.

29. LaRosa JC. Cholesterol agnostics. *Ann Intern Med* 1996; **124**: 505–8.

30. Pyörälä K, DeBacker G, Poole-Wilson P, Wood D, on behalf of the Task Force. Prevention of

coronary heart disease in clinical practice. Recommendations of the Task Force of the European Society of Cardiology, European Atherosclerosis Society and European Society of Hypertension. *Atherosclerosis* 1994; **110**: 121–61.

31. Haq IV, Jackson PR, Yeo WW, Ramsay LE. Sheffield risk treatment table for cholesterol lowering for primary prevention of coronary heart disease. *Lancet* 1995; **346**: 1467–71.

32. Shepherd J. Resource management in prevention of coronary heart disease: optimising prescription of lipid-lowering drugs. *Lancet* 2002; **359**: 2271–3.

33. Martin MJ, Hulley SB, Browner WS et al. Serum cholesterol blood pressure and mortality: implications from a cohort of 361,662 men. *Lancet* 1986; **ii**: 933–6.

34. West of Scotland Coronary Prevention Study Group. Influence of pravastatin and plasma lipids on clinical events in the West of Scotland Coronary Prevention Study (WOSCOPS). *Circulation* 1998; **97**: 1440–5.

35. Shepherd J, Blauw GJ, Murphy MB et al. Pravastatin in elderly individuals at risk of vascular disease (PROSPER): a randomised controlled trial. *Lancet* 2002; **360**: 1623–30.

9

The CARE trial: the effect of pravastatin on coronary events after myocardial infarction in patients with average cholesterol levels

J Wayne Warnica

INTRODUCTION

The Cholesterol and Recurrent Events (CARE) trial was a secondary prevention trial designed to test the effects of lowering cholesterol levels in patients with a history of myocardial infarction (MI) and average initial cholesterol levels.[1] The direct association between serum cholesterol levels and coronary disease risk is well established. As serum cholesterol levels rise within a population, so too does the coronary disease risk. The highest risk is borne by those individuals with the highest cholesterol levels.[2–5]

The relationship between cholesterol levels and risk appears to be attenuated at lower levels of total cholesterol, such that the line describing this relationship is curvilinear rather that straight (Fig. 9.1).[2–6]

The landmark studies described in the preceding chapters have proven conclusively that lowering both serum total cholesterol and low-density lipoprotein (LDL) cholesterol with HMG-CoA reductase inhibitors in patients with hypercholesterolaemia reduces the rate of ischaemic cardiac events and reduces cardiac mortality.[7,8] This is true whether cholesterol levels are reduced as a primary or as a secondary intervention strategy.[7,8] It is important to remember, however, that an earlier meta-analysis by Holme[9] found that the initial serum cholesterol level is an important determinant of the effects of cholesterol reduction. Higher cholesterol levels, particularly those greater than 7.1 mmol/l (275 mg/dl), predicted the patients who would benefit most from cholesterol lowering. The fact remains that the majority of patients with coronary heart disease (CHD), including those who have suffered an acute MI, do not have elevated levels of total or LDL cholesterol when compared with the general population.[10,11] It was therefore not clear whether plasma cholesterol reduction would be of clinical benefit in patients with established CHD who have cholesterol levels of less than 6.2 mmol/l (240 mg/dl) and who have experienced less reduction in recurrent events than did sub-groups with elevated cholesterol levels (6.4–7.9 mmol/l; 247–305 mg/dl) in earlier trials.[12–15]

In most earlier clinical trials, both elderly patients and female patients were either excluded or relatively under-represented.[16] From these trials it was not possible to draw conclusions about the effectiveness of cholesterol lowering in reducing the cardiovascular risk in either group, and particularly so for the majority of patients who have average cholesterol levels.

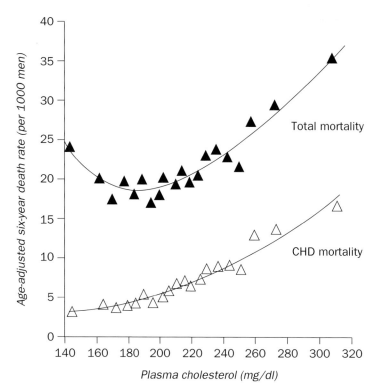

Fig. 9.1 Age-adjusted six-year coronary heart disease (CHD) and total mortality per 1000 men screened for MRFIT in relation to plasma cholesterol level at baseline examination. (Adapted with permission from ref. 3.)

The CARE trial was designed to answer the question of the effectiveness of cholesterol lowering in the largest population of patients with coronary artery disease, namely those with average cholesterol levels, and to assess the effectiveness of such therapy in the elderly and in females.[1] The hypothesis on which this randomized, double-blind, placebo-controlled trial was based was that cholesterol reduction with pravastatin would reduce subsequent coronary events in survivors of a MI with total cholesterol levels less than 6.2 mmol/l (240 mg/dl). This is a descriptor that applies to approximately 75% of the North American population who suffer from coronary disease.[11,17]

The rationale and design of the CARE trial has been described in detail by Sacks et al.[18] The trial, with a planned median follow-up period of five years, comprised men and woman from 80 centres: 13 in Canada and 67 in the USA (approximately one-third of the total trial population were from Canada). Eligible patients were between 21 and 75 years of age, and had suffered an acute MI between three and 20 months before randomization. Total cholesterol levels less than 6.2 mmol/l (240 mg/dl) and LDL levels between 3.0 and 4.5 mmol/l (116–174 mg/dl) were required. The requirements for triglyceride levels were fairly liberal: (triglyceride levels less than 4.05 mmol/l (359 mg/dl). Exclusion criteria included the use of lipid-lowering drugs, clinical congestive heart failure or a left ventricular ejection fraction less than 25% despite therapy, the presence of renal, hepatic or immune disorders, treatment-requiring malignancy, and the use of other investigative drugs. Following study entry, patients were randomized to receive either pravastatin 40 mg/day or placebo.

MAJOR END-POINTS

The major outcome variable was a composite (end-point) of fatal CHD or confirmed non-fatal recurrent MI. Other major parameters for analysis included fatal CHD and non-fatal recurrent MI (components of the primary end-

Table 9.1 Baseline characteristics of CARE participants

Characteristic	Placebo (n = 2078)	Pravastatin (n = 2081)
Age (years)	59 ± 9	59 ± 9
Women/men	14/86	14/86
Non-white/white	8/92	7/93
History of hypertension (%)	43	42
History of diabetes (%)	15	14
Current cigarette smoker (%)	21	21
Blood pressure (mmHg)		
systolic	129 ± 18	129 ± 18
diastolic	79 ± 10	79 ± 10
Months since index MI (range)	10 (3–20)	10 (3–20)
First MI (%)	83	84
Coronary procedures (%)		
angiography	78	78
angioplasty	32	34
CABG	28	26
Angioplasty or CABG	54	54
Angina pectoris (%)	20	21
Left ventricular ejection fraction (%)	53 ± 12	53 ± 12

MI, myocardial infarction; CABG, coronary artery bypass graft.
Adapted with permission from ref. 1.

point), cause-specific mortality, total MI (fatal + non-fatal), coronary artery revascularization by surgery and/or angioplasty, stroke, and an expanded end-point: a composite of fatal CHD, non-fatal MI or coronary revascularization.

CARE PATIENTS AT BASELINE

Randomization began on 18 November 1989 and was concluded on 31 December 1991. During this two-year period, 4159 patients were enrolled, with 2078 being placed in the placebo group and 2081 in the pravastatin treatment group. The characteristics of the two groups at randomization were virtually identical (Table 9.1). The patients' mean age was 59 years, and they were an average of 10 months post-MI at the time of randomization. The majority of MIs were first infarctions but a significant proportion of patients (16%) had suffered a previous event. Only 14% in both groups were female, less than would have been

expected from the population in most coronary care units, but presumably reflecting the age ceiling of 75 years for the trial, and the presence of other illness as exclusion criteria.

Current cigarette smoking, at 21%, was lower than that seen in any other trial to that date. The rate of post-MI investigation/revascularization procedures (percutaneous transluminal coronary angioplasty, PTCA, 33%; coronary artery bypass grafting, CABG, 27%), with 54% having either PTCA or CABG, was somewhat higher than in other trials. Approximately 25% of the patients were still suffering from angina. The average ejection fraction was 53%, most likely related to the *a priori* exclusion of patients with low ejection fractions. Eighty-three percent of both groups were taking aspirin, 40% were on beta-blocker therapy and 40% were receiving calcium channel blocker therapy. Plasma lipid levels were identical in both groups. The levels of total cholesterol (5.4 mmol/l; 209 mg/dl), LDL (3.6 mmol/l; 139 mg/dl) and

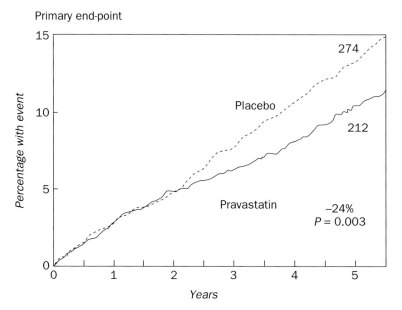

Primary end-point

Fig. 9.2 Incidence of fatal coronary heart disease or non-fatal MI in pravastatin-treated versus placebo-treated CARE participants. (Adapted with permission from ref. 1.)

triglycerides (1.8 mmol/l; 159 mg/dl) were remarkably consistent with the average seen in the adult North American population.[10] The initial preserved left ventricular function, the high rate of aspirin use, as well as average lipid levels, describes a population at much lower expected risk of recurrent ischaemic events than that described in earlier similar clinical trials.

RESULTS

The mean initial LDL cholesterol level of 3.6 mmol/l (139 mg/dl) was lowered by 32% by pravastatin therapy. Levels were maintained at a mean of 2.5 mmol/l (97 mg/dl) during the five-year follow-up of the trial. During follow-up, the LDL cholesterol level was 28% lower in the pravastatin group than in the placebo group, the mean total cholesterol level was 20% lower, the high-density lipoprotein (HDL) cholesterol level was 5% higher and the triglyceride level was 14% lower ($p < 0.001$ for all comparisons). For the primary end-point, fatal CHD or non-fatal recurrent MI, 274 patients (13.2%) in the placebo group experienced an event during the trial, compared with 212 (10.2%) of the pravastatin-treated group. This is a 24% lower incidence of fatal CHD or non-fatal MI ($p = 0.003$) (Fig. 9.2) in patients treated with pravastatin. Similarly, a reduction in

the risk of total MI (non-fatal and fatal) was noted, with 207 placebo-treated patients (10%) experiencing such an event, compared with only 157 pravastatin-treated patients (7.5%, risk reduction 15%, $p = 0.007$). The rate of MI was 37% lower in the pravastatin group (38 or 1.8% in the placebo group vs 24 or 1.2% in the pravastatin group; $p = 0.007$). A surprisingly low number of fatal myocardial reinfarctions may explain the lack of statistical significance of these differences.

As previously noted, 54% of the patients in the CARE trial had undergone a revascularization procedure between the index MI and randomization. During follow-up of five years, 391 placebo-treated patients (18.8%) required a first or repeat revascularization procedure (either angioplasty or coronary bypass surgery) compared with only 294 pravastatin-treated patients (14.4%). Cholesterol lowering in these patients with average cholesterol levels at baseline reduced the need for revascularization procedures by 27% ($p < 0.007$) (Fig. 9.3).

Over five years of therapy, pravastatin reduced the risk of every event examined, including CHD death/non-fatal MI (24% decrease), CHD death (20% decrease), fatal MI (37% decrease), non-fatal MI (23% decrease), CABG (26% decrease), PTCA (23% decrease), unstable angina (13% decrease) and stroke (31% decrease).

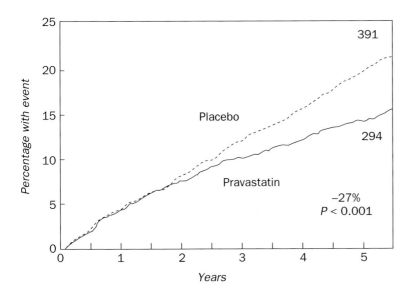

Fig. 9.3 Rate of first or repeat revascularization procedures (coronary bypass surgery or angioplasty) in pravastatin-treated versus placebo-treated CARE participants. (Adapted with permission from ref. 1.)

All reductions were statistically significant except for those of CHD death, unstable angina and fatal MI. These fall short of significance at least in part because of the relatively small number of events that occurred in the trial. This relatively low event rate is illustrated by comparing the combined end-point rate of 13% in the placebo group in the CARE trial with the 28% event rate in the placebo group in the 4S trial.[7]

RISK REDUCTION IN PATIENT SUBGROUPS

A number of sub-groups were pre-specified in the trial design, including women and men, age less than or greater than 60 years, ejection fraction less than or greater than 40%, smoking, hypertension, diabetes and prior revascularization. No one sub-group failed to benefit from treatment with pravastatin. Both men and women treated with pravastatin had significantly lower rates of major coronary events, with women benefiting even more than men (46% risk reduction for women vs 20% for men, $p < 0.001$ for both reductions; $p = 0.05$ for the interaction between patients' gender and treatment group). This is illustrated in Fig. 9.4, where the benefit of cholesterol lowering is evident earlier in the female patients and becomes more dramatic with time.

Notably, patients with ejection fractions of 25–40% benefited as much as did patients with ejection fractions >40%, suggesting that even for patients who suffer substantial loss of left ventricular function post infarction, cholesterol-lowering therapy can still significantly reduce event risks. In addition, pravastatin yielded risk reductions in hypertensive patients, diabetic patients and patients who had undergone revascularization procedures that were equivalent to reductions achieved in the non-smoking, normotensive, non-diabetic and procedure-naïve counterparts. Age did not alter the pravastatin effect on the rate of major coronary events: patients between the ages of 60 and 75 years benefited as much as, or more than, patients who were younger than 60 years of age at randomization. A more detailed analysis of the effects of pravastatin in patients >65 years of age in the CARE trial has since been published.[19] This age-grouping better encompasses the 'elderly' as defined in North America and in other clinical studies. In this subset analysis of CARE, the effects of pravastatin compared with placebo were studied in 1283 patients aged 65–75 years. These results are shown in Table 9.2.

The number of patients over 65 years of age who needed to be treated with pravastatin for five years to prevent a major coronary event was 11, and the equivalent number to prevent a coronary death was 22. For every 1000 older patients treated, 225 cardiovascular hospital-

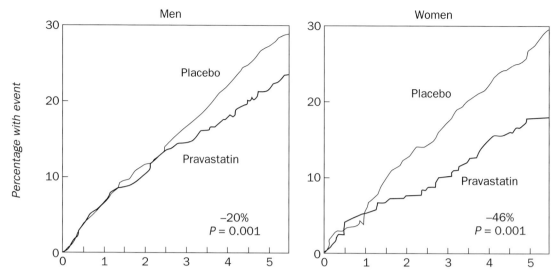

Fig. 9.4 Major coronary events in male and female CARE participants. (Adapted with permission from ref. 20.)

Table 9.2	The effects of pravastatin on clinical events in patients 65–75 years of age				
Cardiovascular events in patients 65–75 years of age	Placebo group	Pravastatin group	Relative risk reduction	Absolute risk reduction	p-value
Major coronary events	181 (28.1%)	126 (19.7%)	32 (15–46)	9.0 (4.2–12.9)	0.001
CAD death or non-fatal MI	111 (17.3%)	69 (10.8%)	39 (18–55)	6.7 (3.1–9.5)	0.001
CAD death	66 (10.3%)	37 (5.8%)	45 (18–63)	4.6 (1.9–6.5)	0.004
Non-fatal MI	57 (8.9%)	41 (6.4%)	30 (–5–53)	2.7 (–0.4–4.7)	0.09
Fatal or non-fatal MI	73 (11.4%)	50 (7.8%)	33 (4–53)	3.8 (0.5–6.0)	0.03
Stroke	47 (7.3%)	29 (4.5%)	40 (4–62)	2.9 (0.3–4.5)	0.03

izations would be prevented compared with 121 hospitalizations similarly prevented in 1000 younger patients. Pravastatin was thus associated with a clinically important reduction in risk for major coronary events and stroke. Given the higher cardiovascular event rate in older patients, the potential for absolute benefit in this age group is substantial.

WOMEN IN CARE

The effects of pravastatin on cardiovascular events in women after MI have been examined

as an important pre-specified sub-group of the CARE study.[20] In the CARE trial, 576 post-menopausal women were randomized to receive pravastatin 40 mg/day or matching placebo. As group, the women enrolled were somewhat different from the men in the CARE trial at entry. Women were older than the men in the study (61 vs 58 years). Several major risk factors were also more prevalent in women than in men. These include hypertension (54% versus 41%), diabetes (20% versus 13%), current smoking (30% versus 20%) and a family history of coronary disease (45% versus 40%). Women

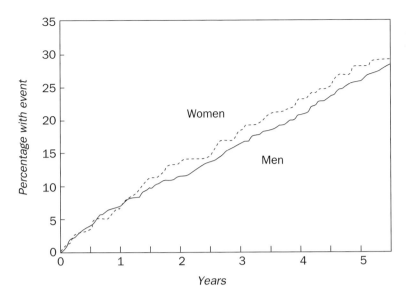

Fig. 9.5 Combined coronary events in women and men treated with placebo. (Adapted with permission from ref. 20.)

Table 9.3   The effects of pravastatin on clinical events in women CARE participants

Cardiovascular events in women	Placebo group	Pravastatin group	Relative risk reduction	Absolute risk reduction	p-value
Major coronary events	181 (28.1%)	126 (19.7%)	32 (15–46)	9.0 (4.2–12.9)	0.001
CAD death or non-fatal MI	111 (17.3%)	69 (10.8%)	39 (18–55)	6.7 (3.1–9.5)	0.001
CAD death	66 (10.3%)	37 (5.8%)	45 (18–63)	4.6 (1.9–6.5)	0.004
Non-fatal MI	57 (8.9%)	41 (6.4%)	30 (–5–53)	2.7 (–0.4–4.7)	0.09
Fatal or non-fatal MI	73 (11.4%)	50 (7.8%)	33 (4–53)	3.8 (0.5–6.0)	0.03
Stroke	47 (7.3%)	29 (4.5%)	40 (4–62)	2.9 (0.3–4.5)	0.03

were more likely than men to have multiple risk factors for coronary disease. Women had a slightly higher mean total cholesterol concentration than men, primarily resulting from a higher HDL cholesterol concentration. Pravastatin had an almost identical effect on plasma lipids in women compared with men and with the total trial population as described earlier. During the trial, there were no differences in the risk of coronary events occurring in the placebo group between men and women (Fig. 9.5). There were, however, significant differences apparent between the women and the men in CARE and on pravastatin.

Details of the effects of pravastatin on recurrent clinical events in women CARE participants are shown in Table 9.3.

The CARE trial has demonstrated that women with an MI show an early reduction in recurrent coronary events during therapy with pravastatin, with the benefits becoming apparent by the first year of treatment. For the risk reductions shown, it may be anticipated that for every 1000 women fulfilling CARE trial entry criteria, and treated for five years, 228 cardiovascular events would be prevented.[1] Lipid-lowering therapy in the majority of women with CHD who have average levels of total and LDL cholesterol is clearly effective in reducing risk.

DIABETES

Although diabetes is a major risk factor for CHD, little information has been available on

Non-diabetic by history

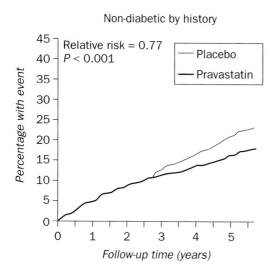

Diabetic by history

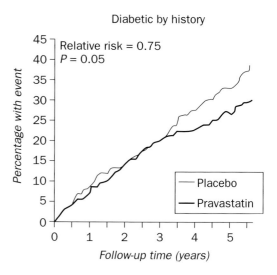

Fig. 9.6 Kaplan–Meier plots for expanded coronary end-point in placebo- and pravastatin-treated patients in diabetes and non-diabetes groups (n = 586 and 3573, respectively). Expanded end-point was CHD death, non-fatal MI, CABG or PTCA. (Adapted with permission from ref. 21.)

the effects of lipid lowering in diabetic patients with proven disease. The effects of lipid-lowering treatment with pravastatin on preventing recurrent cardiovascular events in diabetic patients with an MI and average cholesterol levels has been examined in a sub-study analysis of the CARE trial;[21] 586 patients (14.1% of the total) had a clinical diagnosis of diabetes mellitus. The participants with diabetes were older, more obese and more hypertensive than the non-diabetic participants in the study. Mean baseline lipid concentrations in the group with diabetes, and the responses to therapy with pravastatin, were similar in the diabetic and non-diabetic groups. Not surprisingly, in the placebo-treated group, the diabetics suffered more recurrent coronary events (CHD death, non-fatal MI, CABG and PTCA) than did the non-diabetic patients (37% vs 25%). Pravastatin treatment over five years reduced the absolute risk of coronary events for the diabetics by 8.1%, compared with 5.2% in the non-diabetics, with relative risk reductions of 25% ($p < 0.001$) and 23% ($p = 0.05$), respectively (Fig. 9.6). Pravastatin reduced the relative risk for revascularization procedures by 32% ($p = 0.004$) in diabetic patients. Importantly, in the 3553 patients who were not diagnosed as diabetic,

342 had impaired fasting glucose at entry as defined by the American Diabetes Association. These 'non-diabetic patients' with impaired fasting glucose had a higher rate of recurrent coronary events than did those with a normal fasting glucose (e.g. 13% vs 10% non-fatal MI, respectively). The recurrent event rates tended to be lower in the pravastatin group compared with the placebo group; for example, for the primary end-point the relative risk was 0.77, for non-fatal MI it was 0.50 and for revascularization procedures it was 0.71.

It is apparent that diabetic and non-diabetic patients with impaired fasting glucose who have suffered an MI are at high risk of recurrent coronary events. This risk of recurrent coronary events can be substantially reduced by pravastatin treatment, even in the very large group of patients with MIs and cholesterol levels in the average range as illustrated in the CARE trial.

STROKE

The relationship between serum cholesterol and stroke has not been well established. At very low levels of serum cholesterol, there appears to be a slight increase in the risk for haemor-

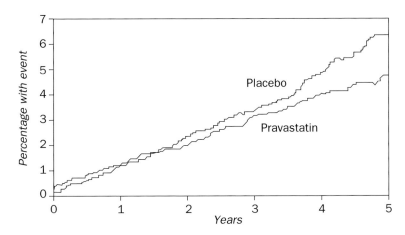

Fig. 9.7 Kaplan–Meier estimates of all-cause stroke or TIA incidence. (Adapted with permission from ref. 23.)

rhagic stroke, particularly among the elderly.[22] CARE was the first large-scale secondary prevention trial of cholesterol reduction with an HMG-CoA reductase inhibitor following MI in which stroke was a pre-specified end-point. Stroke and transient ischaemic attack (TIA) incidence were evaluated over the median five-year follow-up period by the CARE end-points committee using prospectively defined criteria in a review of all reported cerebrovascular events.[23]

Patients on placebo and pravastatin were well matched for stroke risk factors, and 85% of subjects in each group were taking concurrent anti-aspirin therapy. In addition, 82% in each group were on anti-hypertensive medication (ACE inhibitors, beta-blockers and/or calcium antagonists). One hundred and twenty-eight strokes (72 on placebo and 52 on pravastatin) and 216 TIAs (124 on placebo and 92 on pravastatin) were confirmed by committee adjudication. This represented an overall 32% reduction ($p = 0.03$) in all-cause stroke, and a 27% reduction in stroke or TIA ($p = 0.02$) (Fig. 9.7). Stroke was reduced in all categories, and treatment effect was similar when adjusted for age, sex, history of hypertension, cigarette smoking, diabetes, left ventricular ejection fraction and baseline total, HDL and LDL cholesterol, and triglyceride levels. A trend towards an increase in treatment effect was observed in patients with baseline LDL cholesterol >3.9 mmol/l (151 mg/dl). Importantly, there was no increase in haemorrhagic stroke in patients on pravastatin compared with placebo (two vs six,

respectively). The investigators concluded that pravastatin significantly reduced stroke or TIA incidence following MI in patients with serum cholesterol levels in the average range for the North American adult population. This was despite the concurrent use of antiplatelet and/or anti-hypertensive therapy in a high proportion of these patients in the CARE study. Patients with LDL cholesterol exceeding 3.9 mmol/l (151 mg/dl) may receive increased therapeutic benefit from this therapy.

REVASCULARIZATION

A high proportion of the patients in the CARE study underwent coronary angiography (79%), and 54% of these patients had received either CABG or PTCA prior to randomization. These patients were evaluated to determine whether revascularized patients derived benefit from the HMG-CoA reductase inhibitor pravastatin.[24] Of the 2245 patients in the CARE study who underwent revascularization before randomization, 1154 had PTCA, 876 had CABG and 215 patients had both PTCA and CABG. Clinical events in these revascularized patients were compared between patients on placebo and patients on pravastatin. In the 2245 patients with pre-study revascularization, the primary end-point of CHD or non-fatal MI was reduced by 4.1% with pravastatin (relative risk reduction 36%, 95% confidence interval (CI) 17–51, $p = 0.001$). Fatal or non-fatal MI was reduced by 3.3% (relative risk reduction 39%, 95% CI 16–55, $p = 0.002$), post-randomization repeat revascularization was reduced by 2.6% (relative risk reduction 18%, 95% CI 1–33, $p = 0.068$) and stroke was reduced by 1.5% (relative risk reduction 39%, 95% CI 3–62, $p = 0.037$) with pravastatin. PTCA patients in the pravastatin group had significantly fewer MIs, less repeat revascularization and fewer strokes. Of the 1914 patients in CARE who had not undergone pre-randomization revascularization, those assigned to pravastatin had significantly fewer revascularization procedures, but did not have significantly fewer primary end-points or fewer MIs or strokes. It is interesting to compare the results for the revascularization subset of patients with the results of the Post Coronary Artery Bypass Trial (PostCABG).[25] Patients in the PostCABG trial with elevated LDL cholesterol values (mean 4.0 mmol/l; 155 mg/dl) were randomized to one of two groups: a moderately aggressively treated group, designed to reduce LDL to 3.36–3.62 mmol/l and an aggressively treated group with an LDL target of 1.55–2.20 mmol/l.

Patients in the moderately aggressive arm were treated with lovastatin and achieved LDL cholesterol values of 3.4–3.5 mmol/l (133–135 mg/dl), very similar to the baseline LDL cholesterol value of 3.6 mmol/l in the CARE study. Patients in the aggressive arm received more intensive therapy with lovastatin and cholestyramine, achieving LDL cholesterol values of 2.4–2.5 mmol/l (93–94 mg/dl). The aggressively treated patients were found to have reduced graft atherosclerosis compared with the patients who were treated in the moderately aggressive therapy arm. In the CARE revascularization sub-study, pravastatin patients achieved an on-treatment LDL cholesterol level of 2.53 mmol/l (98 mg/dl), very similar to the aggressively treated arm in the PostCABG trial. In contrast to the PostCABG results, CARE demonstrated a reduction in 'hard' coronary end-points, including CHD death and total mortality in CABG-treated patients with monotherapy using the usual doses of pravastatin (40 mg/day).

The favourable effects of pravastatin therapy in patients who had undergone coronary revascularization became obvious over an extended period of time. Based on these data, it appears that HMG-CoA reductase inhibitors should be considered in most patients who have undergone coronary revascularization.

As was discussed earlier, the relationship between cholesterol, particularly LDL cholesterol, and the risk of ischaemic coronary events is non-linear, with both the absolute and relative increases in risk being greater at the higher end of the cholesterol distribution.[1–5] Randomized, controlled clinical trials with HMG-CoA reductase inhibitors in hypercholesterolaemic patients with and without overt coronary disease have proven definitively that these agents reduce CHD events (deaths, MIs and the need for revascularization procedures) without an off-setting increase in non-cardiovascular events. An analysis of the Scandinavian Simvastatin Survival Study (4S) demonstrated that for hypercholesterolaemic patients (total cholesterol 5.5–8.0 mmol/l; 213–309 mg/dl), the relative risk reduction for major coronary events attributed to simvastatin was not influenced by the baseline cholesterol value.[26] The CARE study extended the benefits of cholesterol-lowering therapy to a broader range of patients with average cholesterol, a range that includes the great majority of patients with CHD. An analysis of the CARE data has been conducted to determine the effect of baseline lipid values on the coronary event rates of the groups assigned to placebo and to pravastatin, with particular emphasis on the patients with lower total and LDL cholesterol values.[27] This cohort has been under-represented in previous trials. To evaluate the possible influence of baseline lipid values on the coronary event rates, quartile ranges were constructed based on the distribution of pre-randomization values for total cholesterol, LDL cholesterol, HDL cholesterol and triglyceride levels. Within the cholesterol range of the CARE patients – total cholesterol <6.2 mmol/l (240 mg/dl) and LDL between 3.0 and 4.5 mmol/l (116–174 mg/dl) – the baseline value for total cholesterol did not significantly influence the risk of experiencing a coronary event subsequent to randomization. This was true even in the placebo-assigned patients, where a significant relationship between base-

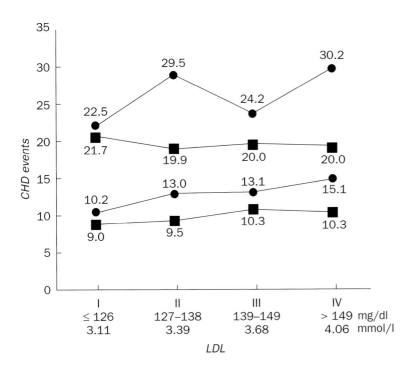

Fig. 9.8 Relationship between quartiles of LDL cholesterol and subsequent coronary events for placebo (●——●) and pravastatin (■——■) groups. The upper two lines are the cumulative event rates for the secondary end-point of fatal CHD, non-fatal MI, coronary artery bypass graft surgery or angioplasty. The lower two lines are the primary cumulative event rates for either CHD or non-fatal MI. (Adapted with permission from ref. 27.)

line cholesterol and the primary study end-point (CHD, death or non-fatal MI) or an expanded coronary end-point which includes revascularization procedures was not detected. On the other hand, there was a significant relationship between baseline LDL cholesterol levels and the risk of experiencing a coronary event. In the placebo group, a 0.6 mmol/l (23 mg/dl) increment in baseline LDL cholesterol was associated with a 28% increase in risk of coronary death or MI (p = 0.0015, 95% CI 5–56). For the expanded end-point, there was a significant influence of baseline LDL cholesterol on coronary events only in the placebo group, with every 0.6 mmol/l (23 mg/dl) increment in LDL cholesterol being associated with an 18% increase in risk (95% CI 3–36, p = 0.021) (Fig. 9.8) For pravastatin-assigned patients, a 0.6 mmol/l (23 mg/dl) increase in baseline LDL cholesterol was not associated with a significant increase in risk of either coronary death or non-fatal MI, or the expanded end-point. This differential influence of baseline LDL cholesterol between the placebo and pravastatin groups on coronary event rates resulted in a convergence of event rates between the placebo and pravastatin

groups in the lower LDL cholesterol levels. This is consistent with the results reported in the original CARE publication, which demonstrated no reduction in risk with pravastatin therapy in those with baseline LDL below 3.2 mmol/l (124 mg/dl).[1]

HDL cholesterol levels did not vary across LDL cholesterol quartiles, and the fasting triglyceride levels decreased with increasing LDL cholesterol quartiles. In the combined treatment arms, there was an important inverse relationship between the baseline HDL values for each LDL cholesterol level and coronary event rates. For example, for each 0.25 mmol/l (10 mg/dl) decrement in baseline HDL cholesterol values, there was an 11% greater likelihood of experiencing a coronary death or non-fatal MI (p = 0.049, 95% CI 0–23). The influence of baseline HDL cholesterol and coronary events was similar in the placebo and pravastatin groups, with no trend for an interaction. In each quartile of HDL cholesterol, the benefits of pravastatin were comparable.

Within the range of fasting triglyceride levels at baseline (1–4.05 mmol/l; 89–359 mg/dl), no significant linear relationship between baseline

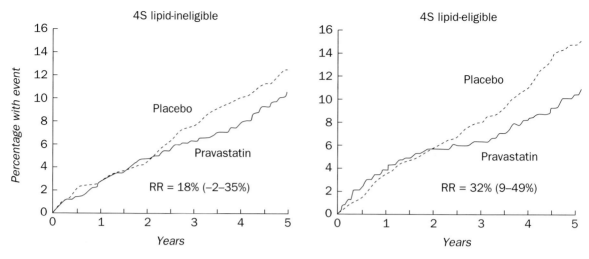

Fig. 9.9 Kaplan–Meier estimates of the incidence of coronary heart disease death or non-fatal MI in subgroups of CARE patients, constructed by baseline lipids for eligibility in 4S. RR, relative risk reduction. (Adapted with permission from ref. 27.)

levels and the primary or expanded end-points was observed in the overall cohort, or within the treatment groups. Although the risk reduction for coronary events was not significantly altered by baseline triglycerides, the lowest quartiles demonstrated the greatest risk reduction with pravastatin.

A *post-hoc* analysis was also conducted utilizing the lipid-eligibility criteria in the 4S study to designate the CARE patients as either '4S lipid-eligible' or '4S-ineligible'.[28] Utilizing 4S lipid criteria, 34% of the CARE population (*n* = 1409) could have been considered as eligible for the 4S trial. In the placebo group, the selection of 4S lipid criteria resulted in a greater likelihood of experiencing coronary death or non-fatal MI. In the CARE patients, the risk reduction for coronary deaths and MI with pravastatin therapy tended to be of a greater magnitude in the 4S lipid-eligible patients (risk reduction 32%) than in 4S lipid-ineligible patients (risk reduction 18%) (Fig. 9.9). A smaller group (*n* = 574) of the CARE cohort fulfilled 4S lipid criteria and other inclusion criteria (age <70 years, no MI in the past six months, no past cerebrovascular event or current anti-arrhythmic therapy); a striking 48% risk reduction was observed for coronary death or MI compared with a 20% risk reduction

observed in the remaining 3555 non-4S-eligible CARE patients.

These data are hypothesis-generating and not definitive. They suggest that further lowering of LDL cholesterol in the group with low LDL cholesterol and coronary artery disease may not have a major clinical impact. The additive and interactive nature of atherosclerotic risk factors complicated the use of arbitrary threshold values for the initiation of therapy. In patients with clinically apparent coronary artery disease, the greater likelihood of a recurrent cardiovascular event justifies an intensive individual approach to their risk factor management. 'Although the CARE study demonstrates that therapy would be anticipated to reduce clinical events in a broad group of patients with coronary artery disease who receive modern management, this study also indicates that the cohort with atherosclerosis and low LDL cholesterol levels appear to benefit less with this form of therapy and thus constitutes an important focus for new investigative efforts.'[27]

After considering the effects of baseline lipid levels on risk, which may suggest a threshold for the initiation of therapy, other important questions remain. While clearly there is value in lowering cholesterol, how much cholesterol lowering is enough? Is it the absolute reduction in LDL level that is important, or is it the percentage reduction in LDL? Does greater reduction in cholesterol yield greater benefit? A meta-analysis of trials in hypercholesterolaemic patients has suggested that the reduction in cardiovascular events and in total mortality is directly proportional to the mean percentage reduction of elevated plasma cholesterol concentrations.[9] The studies evaluated in this analysis had predominantly high pre-treatment LDL concentrations, and mean LDL cholesterol concentrations on treatment which were also relatively high, corresponding to the average pre-treatment range for the average North American and European populations with CHD. No direct information is available on the relationship between the LDL level, treatment and coronary events with LDL concentrations <3.2 mmol/l (124 mg/dl). The CARE trial provided the opportunity to study the effect of lowering LDL to levels not previously achieved in large-scale clinical trials in coronary events. The pretreatment LDL concentrations of 3.0–4.5 mmol/l (116–174 mg/dl), which encompassed approximately the 20th to 80th percentile of the North American population with CHD, and the average reduction of LDL of 32% in the on-treatment group, produced LDL concentrations during the trial ranging from 1.8 to 3.6 mmol/l (70–139 mg/dl). The relationship between plasma LDL concentrations during treatment with pravastatin and recurrent coronary events in the CARE trial has recently been published.[29] In this study, to explore the possibility of non-linearity of the relationship between lipid concentrations and coronary event rates, the lipid concentrations were divided into deciles. As previously described, in the total cohort, the average LDL concentrations during treatment correlated significantly with the risk of a primary or expanded coronary end-point. The relationship between the follow-up average concentration and coronary events in the total cohort was determined to be non-linear by the use of time-dependent decile analysis. As illustrated in Fig. 9.10, the relative risk for both the primary end-point and the expanded end-point declined progressively from the 10th decile (median LDL 4.2 mmol/l;

162 mg/dl) to the 6th decile (median LDL 3.12 mmol/l; 121 mg/dl), and thereafter there was no further reduction. A sequence of Cox proportional hazards models was evaluated for the total cohort. When the maximum likelihood criterion was used, the best model had a cut-point of 3.2 mmol/l (124 mg/dl). The relative risk of a primary end-point for patients who had follow-up LDL >3.2 mmol/l (124 mg/dl) (mean 3.8 mmol/l; 147 mg/dl), whether in the pravastatin or placebo group, was 43% greater than for those with follow-up LDLs <3.2 mmol/l (124 mg/dl) ($p < 0.01$). The average decrease in LDL concentration that resulted in the median LDL concentration during follow-up of 3.2 mmol/l (124 mg/dl) was 0.65 mmol/l (25 mg/dl) or 17% of the pre-treatment concentration. Lower LDL concentrations that were produced by larger decreases in LDL by up to 1.37 mmol/l (53 mg/dl), or by 53% from baseline, were not associated with reductions in coronary event rates below that associated with an LDL concentration of 3.2 mmol/l (124 mg/dl). Whereas pravastatin also has beneficial effects on plasma HDL levels, the HDL level during follow-up was not significantly associated with the coronary event rate after adjustment for baseline non-lipid risk factors. In contrast, the triglyceride level during follow-up was a significant predictor of coronary events, although less strongly so than LDL levels. From the CARE trial, then, the non-linear relationship that was found between LDL during treatment and coronary events with a cut-point of 3.2 mmol/l (124 mg/dl) is consistent with the previously reported finding that a baseline LDL of >3.2 mmol/l (124 mg/dl) identified the portion of the population in which we could expect a reduction in coronary events with treatment. The authors went on to conclude that the CARE trial established that the majority of patients with CHD, namely those with average cholesterol concentrations, should receive lipid-lowering treatment to reduce the risk of recurrent ischaemic events. This analysis suggests that the effect of pravastatin in lowering LDL cholesterol to <3.2 mmol/l (124 mg/dl) was responsible for most of the reduction of coronary events. Since

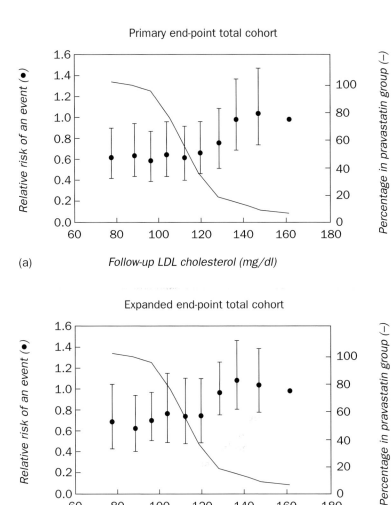

(a)

(b)

Fig. 9.10 LDL cholesterol concentrations during follow-up and coronary events. Placebo and pravastatin groups combined (n = 4159 patients). (a) Primary end-point: coronary death or non-fatal MI (n = 486 patients with end-point, 55 in the 10th decile). (b) Expanded end-point: coronary death, non-fatal MI, CABG or PTCA (n = 979 patients with end-point, 111 in 10th decile). Relative risk determined by Cox proportional hazards analysis with time-dependent covariates (see text). Data points show relative risks with 95% CIs or coronary events for deciles of follow-up LDL concentration. Percentages of patients in each decile of LDL concentration who are in the pravastatin group are indicated by the solid line, corresponding to the right vertical axis. (Adapted with permission from ref. 28.)

it is unlikely that coronary risk will change abruptly at any specific cut-point, the LDL concentration of 3.2 mmol/l (124 mg/dl) must represent an approximate rather than an exact boundary for clinical effectiveness. These clinical findings suggest that a range of optimal LDL concentrations during lipid therapy of 2.6–3.2 mmol/l (101–124 mg/dl) is reasonable. This would be consistent with the results of a recent meta-analysis that used the overall results of published lipid trials.[30]

What is the magnitude of clinical benefit that can be expected from the results of the CARE trial? If 1000 unselected MI survivors with total cholesterol levels <6.2 mmol/l (240 mg/dl)

were treated with pravastatin for five years, we calculated that 150 cardiovascular events could be prevented and 51 patients could be spared from having at least one such event. This projected benefit would be even greater in older patients and in women.

ADVERSE EVENTS

In the CARE trial, there were no significant differences in adverse events in the pravastatin-treated patients compared with the placebo-treated patients. In fact, adverse events were more commonly reported in the placebo group. Seventy-four patients in the placebo group

(3.6%) discontinued the study medication because of an adverse event, compared with 45 (2.2%) in the pravastatin group ($p = 0.007$). In particular, there were no significant differences in aminotransferase elevations, creatine kinase elevations, or myositis. Rhabdomyolysis did not occur in either group.

The possibility of an effect of lipid-lowering therapy on cancer risk was also examined. There were no significant differences in the cancer incidences between the two groups, except in the rate of breast cancer. More patients on pravastatin than on placebo developed breast cancer ($p = 0.002$).[1] In the placebo group, given current rates of breast cancer in the general population for women of similar age and race, we would have expected five cases to have occurred. To evaluate this potential concern, the treatment of 1508 women in the LIPID trial with pravastatin was evaluated and combined with the CARE experience. The totality of the evidence suggests that the findings of the CARE trial were an anomaly. There was no overall increased risk of breast cancer with the combined groups.

Since the publication of the CARE results, several more detailed evaluations of the wealth of data accrued from this large clinical study have added to our understanding of the role of pravastatin in secondary prophylaxis after an acute coronary event. These have included mechanistic studies for the laboratory, and more clinical assessments such as cost and effectiveness. A cost-effectiveness analysis of pravastatin therapy for patients in the CARE study (in the USA) has been published.[31] This was based upon actual clinical events, costs (in US$), and health-related quality-of-life data available from the CARE study. Pravastatin therapy increased quality-adjusted life expectancy at an incremental cost of US$16 000–32 000 per quality-adjusted life-year (QALY) gained. For patients >60 years, the cost-effectiveness ratio was more favourable (US$9100–12 000). More favourable cost-effectiveness ratios were also noted with increasing baseline LDL levels (US$16 000–18 000 per QALY when pre-study LDL levels were 3.2–3.9 mmol/l (125–150 mg/dl), and US$7900–20 000 per QALY when LDL levels

were greater than 3.8 mmol/l (>150 mg/dl)). The cost-effectiveness of pravastatin in survivors of MI with average cholesterol levels thus compares favourably with other common interventions such as haemodialysis.

The majority of subsequent studies utilizing the CARE data may be characterized as either mechanistic or risk assessment.

Mechanistic studies

The role of inflammation in the precipitation of cardiac ischaemic events is a topic of considerable current interest. This interest was further stimulated by several recent publications utilizing custody data from the CARE population. In the first, a nested case-control design was used to compare C-reactive protein (CRP) and serum amyloid A (SAA) levels in pre-randomization blood samples from 391 CARE participants who subsequently developed either a recurrent non-fatal infarction or fatal MI and from an equal number of age- and sex-matched participants who remained free of these events during follow-up.[32] Overall, levels of both CRP and SAA were higher in those with a subsequent recurrent cardiac ischaemic event (for CRP, $p = 0.05$; for SAA, $p = 0.006$). For this group with pre-randomization CRP levels in the highest quintile, the relative risk of developing disease was 77% (RR = 1.77, $p = 0.02$) (Fig. 9.11). Similar relative risk was noted for the highest quintile of pre-randomization SAA levels (RR = 1.74, $p = 0.02$). To investigate a potential inter-relationship between inflammation and pravastatin, the 708 study patients with concomitant CRP and SAA levels were divided into four groups on the basis of the presence or absence of high levels of both markers, and on randomization to pravastatin or placebo. The study group at highest risk was that with high levels of both CRP and SAA assigned to placebo (RR = 2.81, $p = 0.007$). The risk estimate was greater than the product of individual risk associated with inflammation, or the placebo assignment alone (Fig. 9.12). In stratified analysis, there is an association between inflammation and risk among those assigned to placebo (RR = 2.11, $p = 0.048$) but this is attenuated and non-

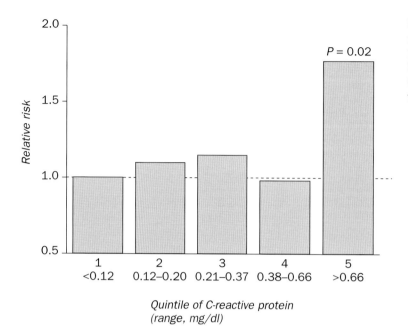

Fig. 9.11 Relative risks of recurrent coronary events among post-MI patients according to baseline plasma concentration of CRP. (Adapted with permission from ref. 31.)

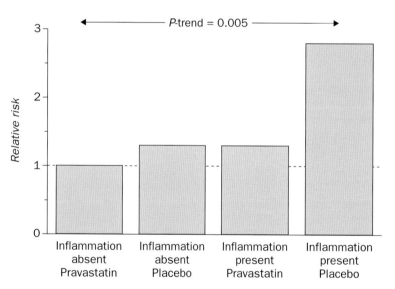

Fig. 9.12 Relative risks of recurrent coronary events among post-MI patients according to presence (both CRP and SAA levels 90th percentile) or absence (both CRP and SAA levels <90th percentile) of evidence of inflammation and by randomized pravastatin assignment. (Adapted with permission from ref. 31.)

significant among those assigned to pravastatin (RR = 1.29, p = 0.5). Evidence of inflammation after MI is thus associated with increased risk of recurrent coronary ischaemic events. These data suggest that markers of inflammation may provide a mechanism to stratify post-MI patients into relatively high-risk and low-risk groups. They also suggest that the effect of inflammation on coronary risk may be attenuated with pravastatin therapy. The possibility of an anti-

inflammatory effect of pravastatin as well as a lipid-lowering effect is also suggested.

A follow-up report by the same authors reported on the long-term effects of pravastatin on CRP. CRP levels were measured at baseline and at five years in 472 randomly selected CARE participants who remained free of recurrent cardiac ischaemic events during follow-up. Overall, CRP levels at baseline and at five years were highly correlated (r = 0.60, p = 0.001).

Among those assigned to placebo, CRP levels tended to increase over time. By contrast, median CRP levels and the mean change in CRP decreased over time among those allocated to pravastatin. These effects persisted in analysis stratified by age, body mass index, smoking status, blood pressure and baseline lipid levels. There appeared to be no obvious relationship between the magnitude of change in CRP and the magnitude of change in lipids in both the pravastatin and placebo groups. The general stability of CRP over long follow-up periods supports the use of this inflammatory marker as a novel means for cardiac risk detection. Long-term HMG-CoA reductase therapy with pravastatin appears to result in significantly reduced levels of CRP, suggesting that CRP may be a modifiable marker of risk. The efficacy of pravastatin in reducing recurrent events is greater among those with elevated levels of CRP, an effect independent of baseline lipid levels, similar to the pravastatin-induced changes in CRP, which also did not correlate with changes in LDL cholesterol. These data have provided additional insights into the role of inflammation in atherogenesis, and the potential mechanisms by which the HMG-CoA reductase therapy may reduce the risk of recurrent ischaemic events.

Another apparent marked of inflammation is tumour necrosis factor-α (TNF-α), a multifunctional circulating cytokine derived from endothelial and smooth muscle cells, and from macrophages associated with coronary atheroma. TNF-α levels are markedly elevated in advanced heart failure[33] and are upgraded in myocardium in response to transient ischaemia or reperfusion.[34,35] To investigate whether potential elevations of TNF-α levels measured several months after an MI are associated with increased risk of recurrent coronary events, TNF-α levels obtained in participants in the CARE trial were compared in patients who subsequently suffered a cardiovascular death or non-fatal MI with an equal number of age- and sex-matched participants who did not suffer such an event during follow-up.[36] All TNF-α levels were drawn an average of 8.9 months after the index MI, and the 272 CARE partici-

pants who subsequently developed either non-fatal MI or cardiovascular death (cases) were compared with an equal number of those without such events (controls) during the five-year follow-up. TNF-α levels were higher overall in cases than in controls (2.84 vs 2.57 pg/ml, $p = 0.02$). The excess risk was predominantly among those with the highest TNF-α levels (>4.17 pg/ml, the 95th percentile of the control distribution), who had an approximate three-fold increase in risk (RR = 2.7, 95% CI 1.4–5.2, $p = 0.004$) (Fig. 9.13). These risk estimates were independent of other risk factors, including CRP and SAA, and were similar in sub-group analysis limited to cardiovascular death (RR = 2.1) or to recurrent non-fatal MI (RR = 3.2). From these observations, it is possible to conclude that persistently elevated TNF-α concentrations among post-MI patients identify a group at increased risk for recurrent coronary events. These data also support the hypothesis that persistent inflammatory instability is present among stable patients at increased risk.

Risk assessment

A further analysis of the lipid data obtained from the CARE participants has explored the major components of plasma triglycerides as potential risk factors for recurrent coronary events.[37] The VLDL group, the major carriers of plasma triglycerides, vary in triglyceride and cholesterol content, apolipoprotein apoC and apoE, and in their metabolism. ApoCIII and apoE are the major determinants of VLDL metabolism in plasma. In animal studies, the former accelerates and the latter protects against atheroma. The apolipoprotein component of lipoprotein may be more closely linked to CHD than conventional lipoprotein measurements of content and density. Participants in the CARE trial had average LDL levels at baseline. Baseline concentrations of VLDL-apoB (the VLDL particle concentration), VLDL lipids, and apoCIII and apoE in VLDL + LDL and in HDL were compared in patients (those who subsequently suffered a recurrent non-fatal MI, or death (cases = 418)) with those who did not have a cardiovascular event (control = 370) in

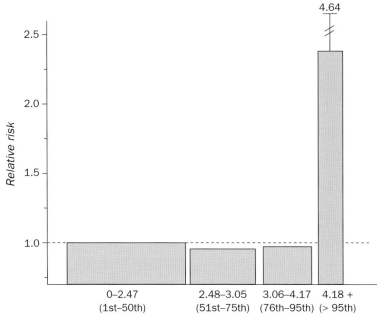

Fig. 9.13 Relative risk of death and recurrent non-fatal MI among participants in the CARE trial according to baseline levels of TNF-α. Data are analyzed in four groups, with the referent group being those with levels of TNF-α less than or equal to the 50th percentile of the control distribution. (Adapted with permission from ref. 32.)

five years' follow-up. The significant independent predictors were VLDL-apoB (RR = 3.2 for highest to lowest quintiles, p = 0.04), apoCIII in VLDL and LDL (RR = 2.3, p = 0.04) and apoE in HDL (RR = 1.8, p = 0.02). Plasma triglycerides, a univariate predictor of coronary events (RR = 1.6, p = 0.03), were no longer related to such events when apoCIII in VLDL + LDL was included in the model, whereas apoCIII remained significant. Adjustment for LDL and HDL cholesterol did not affect these results. In summary, VLDL-apoB concentration, the apoCIII concentration in VLDL + LDL, and apoE in HDL are all independent predictors of recurrent coronary events, and explain the weaker relationship of plasma triglycerides and recurrent events. These results are consistent with the known metabolic properties of VLDL particles which link them to atherosclerosis, and with the newly recognized properties of apoE, suggesting that plasma triglyceride levels are an imperfect marker for these specific lipoprotein measurements in VLDL + LDL.

The next logical step using the CARE data was to evaluate the effects of pravastatin on VLDL-

apoB and apo CIII.[38] At baseline, 788 participants had measurements of apolipoprotein and VLDL. Of these, 100 who were randomized to pravastatin and 100 to placebo were chosen at random to have the same measurements one year after treatment to evaluate the potential effects of pravastatin. At baseline, the concentrations of lipid risk factors were similar between the two groups, and to the entire trial population. Pravastatin had a significantly greater effect in lowering apoCIII in VLDL and LDL, and VLDL-apoB in patients whose triglycerides were elevated above the median at baseline (1.7 mmol/l). Pravastatin compared with placebo lowered plasma VLDL-apo B by 27% (p < 0.001) and apoCIII VLDL/LDL by 19% (p < 0.001). For those patients with initially elevated plasma triglycerides above the median (mean 2.2 mmol/l) versus those below the median (mean 1.2 mmol/l), pravastatin lowered VLDL-apoB by 35% versus –13%, and apo-CIII in VLDL and LDL by 34% versus 2%. Pravastatin lowered plasma triglycerides by 24% in those with baseline triglycerides above the median compared with only 3% in those with initial triglycerides below the median. This substantial reduction in

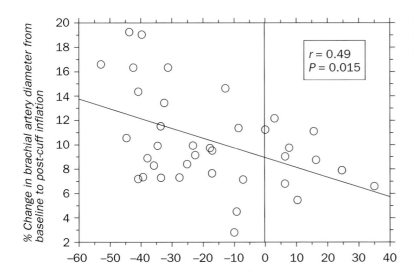

Fig. 9.14 Relation between LDL-C change and endothelium-dependent vasodilation (both sub-groups combined, $n = 36$). (Adapted with permission from ref. 39.)

apolipoprotein risk factors related to hyper-triglyceridaemia may be an important mechanism for reducing coronary events.

Lipoprotein particle size has also been considered important when considering progression of coronary artery disease, with small dense LDL of particular concern. A prospective nested case-control study in the CARE trial examined the potential role of LDL particle size on risk for current ischaemic events.[39] Interestingly, large LDL size was shown to be an independent predictor of coronary events in this population but this adverse effect was not present among patients who were treated with pravastatin. It appears then that identifying patients at risk on the basis of LDL particle size may not be useful clinically. Effective treatment of elevated LDL cholesterol also effectively treats risk associated with large LDL.

Finally, several studies have discussed the relationship of lipid levels to vascular reactivity and to recurrent cardiac ischaemic events. In a sub-group of participants in the CARE trial, the impact of lipid-lowering therapy on vascular reactivity was evaluated to determine if an effect on endothelial function is a viable mechanism for the observed reduction in clinical events.[40] Patients were randomized to either placebo or pravastatin 40 mg/day, and fol-

lowed for over five years. In the final six months of the trial, vascular reactivity was assessed using ultrasound brachial artery diameters in response to ischaemia and to nitroglycerine. There was significantly greater endothelium-dependent vasodilatation in the pravastatin group compared with the placebo group (13% vs 8%, $p = 0.0002$), with no difference observed between the two groups in their response to nitroglycerine. The magnitude of the endothelium-dependent vasoreactivity correlated significantly with the percent change in LDL cholesterol from baseline to final visit ($r = 0.49$, $p = 0.015$) (Fig. 9.14).

CONCLUSION

The CARE study has made an important contribution to our management of the majority of patients in North America who have survived a MI. Most patients have cholesterol levels which do not differ from those of the average adult population, yet treatment with pravastatin is effective in reducing rates of recurrent ischaemic events. It is especially important in sub-groups such as diabetics, women, the elderly and those who have been revascularized. The CARE study also raises important questions with regard to the degree of cholesterol lowering necessary to produce the treatment effect. Subsequent analysis of the data from the CARE trial and its pre-specified substudies have contributed in an important way to our knowledge of the mechanisms of atherosclerotic coronary artery disease and to potential novel methods of risk assessment and treatment modalities. The role of inflammatory markers in disease progression and risk prediction may become the most important legacies of the CARE trial.

REFERENCES

1. Sacks F, Pfeffer MA, Moye LA et al. The effects of pravastatin on coronary events after myocardial infarction in patients with average cholesterol levels. *N Engl J Med* 1996; **335**: 1001–9.
2. Rose G, Hamilton PJ, Keen H et al. Myocardial ischaemic risk factors and death from coronary heart disease. *Lancet* 1977; **1**: 105–9.
3. Martin MJ, Hully SB, Brownes WS et al. Serum cholesterol, blood pressure, and morbidity: implication from a cohort of 361,667 men. *Lancet* 1986; **ii**: 933–6.
4. Pekkanen J, Linn S. Heiss G et al. Ten-year mortality from cardiovascular disease in relation to cholesterol levels among men with and without pre-existing cardiovascular disease. *N Engl J Med* 1990; **322**: 1700–7.
5. Kannel WB. Range of serum cholesterol values in the population developing coronary heart disease. *Am J Cardiol* 1995; **76**: 69C–77C.
6. Stamler J, Wentworth D, Neaton JD. Is the relationship between serum cholesterol and risk of premature death from coronary heart disease continuous and graded? Findings in 356,272 primary screenees of the Multiple Risk Factor Intervention Trial (MRFIT). *JAMA* 1986; **256**: 2823–8.
7. Scandinavian Simvastatin Survival Study Group. Randomized trial of cholesterol lowering in 4444 patients with coronary heart disease: the Scandinavian Simvastatin Survival Study (4S). *Lancet* 1994; **344**: 1383–9.
8. Shepherd J, Cobbe SM, Ford I et al. Prevention of coronary heart disease with pravastatin in men with hypercholesterolemia. *N Eng J Med* 1995; **333**: 1301–7.
9. Holme I. An analysis of randomized trial evaluating the effect of cholesterol reduction on total mortality and coronary heart disease incidence. *Circulation* 1990; **82**: 1916–24.
10. Johnson CL, Rifkind BM, Sempos CT et al. Declining serum total cholesterol levels among US adults. The National Health and Nutrition Examination Surveys. *JAMA* 1993; **269**: 3002–8.
11. Rubins HB, Robins SJ, Collins D et al. Distribution of lipids in 8500 men with coronary artery disease. *Am J Cardiol* 1995; **75**: 1196–201.
12. Dayton S, Pearce ML, Hashimoto S et al. A controlled clinical trial of a diet high in unsaturated fat in preventing complications of atherosclerosis. *Circulation* 1969; **39, 40** (Suppl II): II-1–II-63.
13. Research Committee of the Scottish Society of Physicians. Ischaemic heart disease: a secondary prevention trial using clofibrate. *BMJ* 1971; **iv**: 775–84.
14. Canner PL, Berge KG, Wenger NK et al. Fifteen-year mortality in Coronary Drug Project patients: long-term benefit with niacin. *J Am Coll Cardiol* 1986; **8**: 1224–5.
15. Report of the Committee of Principal Investigators. WHO Cooperative Trial on primary prevention of ischaemic heart disease using clofibrate to lower serum cholesterol: mortality follow-up. *Lancet* 1980; **ii**: 379–85.
16. Gurwitz JH, Col NF, Avorn J. The exclusion of the elderly and women from clinical trials in acute myocardial infarction. *JAMA* 1992; **268**: 1417–22.
17. Genest J Jr, McNamara JR, Ordovas JM et al. Lipoprotein cholesterol, apolipoprotein A-I and B and lipoprotein (a) abnormalities in men with premature coronary heart disease. *J Am Coll Cardiol* 1992; **19**: 792–802.
18. Sacks FM, Pfeffer MA, Moye L et al. Rationale and design of a secondary prevention trial of lowering normal plasma cholesterol levels after acute myocardial infarction: the Cholesterol and Recurrent Events trial (CARE). *Am J Cardiol* 1991; **68**: 1436–46.
19. Lewis SJ, Moye LA, Sacks FM et al. Effect of pravastatin on cardiovascular events in older patients with myocardial infarction and cholesterol levels in the average range. Results of the Cholesterol and Recurrent Events (CARE) trial. *Ann Intern Med* 1998; **129**: 681–9.
20. Lewis SJ, Sacks FM, Mitchell JS et al. Effects of pravastatin on cardiovascular events in women after myocardial infarction: the Cholesterol and Recurrent Events (CARE) trial. *J Am Coll Cardiol* 1998; **32**: 140–6.
21. Goldberg RB, Melliers MJ, Sacks FM et al. Cardiovascular events and their reduction with pravastatin in diabetic and glucose-intolerant

myocardial infarction survivors with average cholesterol levels. Subgroup analysis in the Cholesterol and Recurrent Events (CARE) trial. *Circulation* 1998; **98**: 2513–19.

22. Law MR, Thompson SA, Waid NJ. Assessing possible hazards of reducing serum cholesterol. *BMJ* 1994; **308**: 373–9.

23. Plehn JF, Doris BR, Sacks FM et al. Reduction of stroke incidence after myocardial infarction with pravastatin. *Circulation* 1999; **99**: 216–23.

24. Flaker GC, Warnica JW, Sacks FM et al. Pravastatin prevents clinical events in revascularized patients with average cholesterol concentration. *J Am Coll Cardiol* 1999; **34**: 106–12.

25. The Post Coronary Artery Bypass Trial Investigation. The effect of aggressive lowering of low-density lipoprotein cholesterol levels and low-dose anticoagulation on obstructive change in saphenous vein coronary-artery bypass grafts. *N Engl J Med* 1997; **336**: 153–62.

26. Pederson T, Kjekshus J, Berg K et al. Baseline serum cholesterol and treatment effect in the Scandinavian Simvastatin Survival Study (4S). *Lancet* 1995; **345**: 1274–5.

27. Pfeffer MA, Sacks FM, Moye LA et al. Influence of baseline lipids and effectiveness of pravastatin in the CARE trial. *J Am Coll Cardiol* 1999; **33**: 125–36.

28. Sacks FM, Moye LA, Davis BR et al. Relationship between plasma LDL concentrations during treatment with pravastatin and recurrent coronary events with cholesterol and recurrent events trial. *Circulation* 1998; **97**: 1446–52.

29. Fager G, Wiklund O. Cholesterol reduction and clinical benefit: are there limits to our expectation? *Arterioscler Thromb Vasc Biol* 1997; **17**: 3527–33.

30. Tsevat J, Kuntz KM, Orav EJ et al. Cost-effectiveness of pravastatin therapy for survivors of myocardial infarction with average cholesterol levels. *Am Heart J* 2001; **141**: 727–34.

31. Ridker PM, Rifai N, Pfeffer MA et al. for the Cholesterol and Recurrent Events (CARE) Investigators. Inflammation, pravastatin, and the risk of coronary events after myocardial infarction in patients with average cholesterol levels. *Circulation* 1998; **98**: 839–44.

32. Ridker PM, Rifai N, Pfeffer MA et al. for the Cholesterol and Recurrent Events (CARE) Investigators. Long-term effects of pravastatin on plasma concentration of C-reactive protein. *Circulation* 1999; **100**: 230–5.

33. Levine B, Kalman J, Mayer L et al. Elevated circulating levels of tumor necrosis factor in severe chronic heart failure. *N Engl J Med* 1990; **323**: 236–41.

34. Vaddi K, Nicolini FA, Mehta P, Mehta JL. Increased secretion of tumour necrosis factor-alpha and interferon-gamma by mononuclear leukocytes in patients with ischemic heart disease: relevance in superoxide anion generation. *Circulation* 1994; **90**: 694–9.

35. Kulkeilka GL, Smith CW, Maning AM et al. Induction of interleukin synthesis in the myocardium. *Circulation* 1995; **92**: 1866–75.

36. Ridker PM, Rifai N, Pfeffer MA et al., for the Cholesterol and Recurrent Events (CARE) Investigators. Evaluation of tumour necrosis factor-α and increased risk of recurrent coronary events after myocardial infarction. *Circulation* 2000; **101**: 2149–53.

37. Sacks FM, Alaupovic P, Moye LA et al. VLDL, apolipoproteins B, CIII, and E, and risk of recurrent coronary events in the Cholesterol and Recurrent Events (CARE) trial. *Circulation* 2000; **102**: 1886–92.

38. Sacks FM, Alaupovic P, Moye LA. Effect of pravastatin on apolipoproteins B and C-III in very low-density lipoproteins and low-density lipoproteins. *Am J Cardiol* 2002; **90**: 165–7.

39. Campos H, Moye LA, Glasser SP et al. Low-density lipoprotein size, pravastatin treatment, and coronary events. *JAMA* 2001; **286**: 1468–74.

40. Cohen JD, Drury JH, Ostdiek J et al. Benefits of lipid lowering on vascular reactivity in patients with coronary artery disease and average cholesterol levels: a mechanism for reducing clinical events? *Am Heart J* 2000; **139**: 734–8.

10

The LIPID study: results and implications for clinical practice

Andrew M Tonkin, on behalf of the LIPID Study Group

INTRODUCTION

Manifestations of atherosclerosis are already the leading cause of death in most developed countries.[1] Furthermore, it is predicted that ischaemic heart disease will rapidly impose the major global public health burden[2] because of its epidemicity in developing countries related to epidemiological transitions associated with urbanization and globalization.[3]

Among other risk factors, compelling epidemiological data has related cholesterol levels to the risk of coronary heart disease (CHD).[4] However, until the last decade, although there was evidence for a decrease in CHD mortality and CHD events,[5,6] there was no evidence that cholesterol-lowering therapy prolonged survival and indeed these were concerns about the safety of such treatment.[6] This was partly because older trials had tested interventions which only lowered cholesterol by an average of about 10%[7] and typically in cohorts which often had a relatively low risk of future events. Accordingly, until recent years, the use of lipid-modifying therapy was controversial.

However, the robustness of the clinical trial data that now exist to support the use of lipid-modifying therapy is comparable to that of any other cardiovascular drug group. The Long-term Intervention with Pravastatin in Ischaemic Disease (LIPID) study[8] was one of the large-scale trials of the 3-hydroxy-3-methylglutaryl coenzyme A (HMG-CoA) reductase inhibitors which has provided such data.

THE LIPID STUDY

Study design

The LIPID study was a randomized placebo-controlled trial. The design and management have been described in detail.[9,10] A total of 9014 patients (7498 men and 1516 women) aged 31–75 years were recruited in 87 centres, 67 in Australia and 20 in New Zealand, between June 1990 and December 1992.

All patients had had an acute myocardial infarction (MI) or a hospital discharge diagnosis of unstable angina pectoris 3–36 months before randomization.

Patients had a plasma total cholesterol level of 4.0–7.0 mmol/l (155–271 mg/dl) and fasting triglycerides <5.0 mmol/l (445 mg/dl) after an eight-week single-blind placebo run-in phase during which they received standard dietary advice, particularly to limit saturated fat intake, according to the guidelines of the National Heart Foundation of Australia. Major exclusion criteria included a significant medical or surgical event within three months before study entry, significant cardiac failure, renal or hepatic disease, and current use of any cholesterol-lowering agents.

After stratification according to the qualifying diagnosis and clinical centre, participants were randomly assigned to receive 40 mg of pravastatin or matching placebo once daily. Both groups continued to receive dietary advice. Their usual care continued with their own doctors, including commencement of

Table 10.1   Baseline characteristics of patients randomly assigned to receive pravastatin or placebo in the LIPID trial

Characteristic	Pravastatin group (%) n = 4052	Placebo group (%) n = 4512
Age (years)		
median	62	62
>65	39	39
Sex, female	17	17
Qualifying event		
myocardial infarction	64	64
unstable angina	36	36
Medication		
aspirin	83	82
beta-blocker	46	48
nitrate	35	36
Median lipid levels (mmol/l (mg/dl))		
total cholesterol	5.6 (218)	5.6 (218)
LDL cholesterol	3.9 (150)	3.9 (150)
HDL cholesterol	0.9 (36)	0.9 (36)
triglycerides	1.6 (142)	1.6 (138)

other cholesterol-lowering therapy if considered appropriate. This allowed for the uptake into clinical practice of results from other statin trials and removed ethical concerns following the publication of results of these trials, which were actually disseminated to patients, their treating doctors and to ethics committees.[10]

The primary end-point of the study was CHD mortality. Secondary outcomes included all-cause mortality, cardiovascular mortality, death from CHD or non-fatal MI (the end-point used for pre-specified sub-group analysis), MI, stroke, non-haemorrhagic stroke, coronary revascularization, number of days of hospitalization, lipid changes and the relation of changes in these to cardiovascular outcomes. All end-points were pre-specified. All deaths, MI and strokes were assessed by outcomes assessment committees, blinded to the treatment allocations. All patients gave written informed consent and the trial was approved by the ethics committee for each participating centre.

Results and principal outcomes

Final patient visits took place between June and September 1997, when the mean duration of follow-up was 6.1 years. This followed notification from the independent Data and Safety Monitoring Committee that the pre-specified boundary rule for stopping, a difference of three standard deviations in total mortality between the two groups, had been exceeded. At the end of follow-up, 19% of patients assigned to pravastatin had stopped this and 24% of those assigned to placebo had begun open-label therapy with a cholesterol-lowering drug.

Full results have been published.[8] The pravastatin- and placebo-assigned patient groups were very well matched in terms of baseline characteristics. Median age was 62 years but 39% of the cohort were older than 65 years; 83% were male, 82% were taking aspirin, 47% were taking beta-blockers, 36% were receiving chronic nitrate therapy, and 41% had had prior revascularization – either coronary artery bypass grafting, coronary angioplasty or both (Table 10.1).

Averaging the changes in lipid fractions over five years, treatment with pravastatin resulted in a decrease in plasma total cholesterol of 1.0 mmol/l (39 mg/dl) from the median baseline of 5.6 mmol/l (218 mg/dl) (an 18% reduction when compared with placebo); a decrease in low-density lipoprotein (LDL) cholesterol of 25% from 3.9 mmol/l (150 mg/dl); a decrease in triglycerides of 11% from 1.6 mmol/l (142 mg/dl); and an increase in high-density lipoprotein (HDL) cholesterol of 5% from 0.9 mmol/l (36 mg/dl) ($p < 0.001$ for all comparisons).

Over the period of follow-up of 6.1 years, there was a highly significant difference in the rate of death from CHD (the primary study endpoint) from 8.3% in the placebo group to 6.4% in the pravastatin group ($p = 0.0004$). Overall mortality was significantly lower in the pravastatin group (11.0%) than in the placebo group (14.1%, $p = 0.00002$). Rates of all pre-specified cardiovascular events were also significantly lower in the pravastatin treatment group.

There were fewer deaths from cancer in those assigned to pravastatin (128) than in those assigned placebo (141) ($p = $ not significant), and fewer deaths from trauma and suicide in the pravastatin-treated group, although numbers were small (6 and 11, respectively).

Treatment with pravastatin was very safe. A total of 403 newly diagnosed cancers occurred in 379 patients assigned to receive pravastatin, compared with 417 cancers in 399 patients assigned to placebo ($p = 0.43$). Organ-specific analysis of cancers, including breast cancer (ten invasive cancers in the placebo group and nine invasive cancers and one carcinoma *in situ* in the pravastatin group) showed no significant differences. There were no differences in other serious adverse events. Eight compared with ten patients assigned pravastatin and placebo, respectively, developed myopathy. Also, there was no significant difference in major liver enzyme abnormalities nor in other laboratory results, particularly in creatine kinase levels. A total of 2.1% of the pravastatin group and 1.9% of the placebo group had an elevation in serum alanine and aspartate aminotransferase levels greater than three times upper limit of normal ($p = 0.41$).

Further follow-up of the LIPID cohort

After early closure of the placebo-controlled trial, all patients still alive were offered open-label 40 mg pravastatin, whether or not they had originally been assigned blinded pravastatin or placebo at randomization in 1990–92. The only exceptions were those patients who had contraindications such as previous discontinuation because of an adverse effect.

A total of 7680 patients (6361 men, 1319 women; 97% of those still alive at the randomized trial completion in 1997) consented to two years of further follow-up. In all, 86% and 88% of those randomized initially to receive placebo and pravastatin, respectively, commenced open-label pravastatin during this further period of follow-up.[11]

During this two-year period, the groups initially randomized to pravastatin and placebo had almost identical lipid levels. Despite this, those originally randomized to pravastatin had a lower risk of death from all causes (5.6% vs 6.8%, $p = 0.03$), death from CHD (2.8% vs 3.6%, $p = 0.03$) and CHD death or non-fatal MI (4.5% vs 5.2%, $p = 0.08$) than those originally assigned placebo.[11] These observations were probably most consistent with a delay in onset of treatment effect with pravastatin.

This extended period of follow-up (a total of eight years) thus provided even stronger evidence of benefit of pravastatin therapy than the placebo-controlled trial (six years). Absolute benefits are shown in Table 10.2.

IMPLICATIONS OF THE LIPID STUDY FOR CLINICAL PRACTICE

Generalizability of the benefits

The LIPID study results have major implications for the clinical management of patients who are known to have CHD. The patients enrolled in this study were representative of those currently seen in usual practice. The 'average' cholesterol range at baseline closely reflected levels of typical patients,[12] and benefits of pravastatin were demonstrated on a background of therapy such as aspirin, beta-blockers and myocardial revascularization,

Table 10.2   Absolute benefits of pravastatin

End-point	RCT (6 years)		RCT + OL phase (8 years)	
	Events prevented per 1000	NNT	Events prevented per 1000	NNT
CHD death	19	52	26	39
Death, all causes	30	33	38	26
CHD event	35	28	40	25
Myocardial infarct	28	36	30	33
Stroke	8	127	11	93
Death, MI or stroke	47	21	58	17

RCT, randomized controlled trial; OL, open-label extended follow-up; NNT, number needed to treat; CHD, coronary heart disease; MI, myocardial infarction.

which represent usual practice in the management of CHD patients. The study extended previous benefits shown in other trials to now include reduction in mortality and not only CHD events in those with relatively normal cholesterol levels.

Furthermore, beneficial effects were consistent across all pre-specified sub-groups. The LIPID study was not designed to have adequate power to demonstrate reliably the effects in such sub-groups. However, coronary events (fatal CHD and non-fatal MI), the pre-specified end-point for sub-group analyses, were reduced consistently in all sub-groups pre-defined according to age, sex, qualifying diagnosis, other coronary risk factors and baseline lipid parameters, with no evidence of any statistical heterogeneity in effects according to these sub-groups.[8] Similar relative risk reductions then translate to greater overall benefit in those at highest absolute risk of further events, such as those over 65 years.[13] The higher rate of events with pravastatin in older patients and greater reduction in events in older patients is shown in Fig. 10.1.

Specifically, among patients with cholesterol levels <5.5 mmol/l (<215 mg/dl) there were separately significant beneficial effects of pravastatin that were consistent with the overall result. The benefits seen during extended follow-up strengthened the evidence for benefit in important sub-groups such as women, the elderly and those with low cholesterol levels.

Inclusion of patients with previous unstable angina

LIPID included patients with either previous MI or unstable angina. Similar significant reductions in the risk of CHD events, including MI, unstable angina and myocardial revascularization, and also in mortality were observed in both groups.[14] The inclusion in the LIPID study of patients with unstable angina and delay in randomization of patients until at least three months after their acute coronary syndrome (when the risk of further CHD events approximates that in patients with stable angina)[15] probably allow the results to be extrapolated to all patients who are known to have CHD.

Prevention of stroke in CHD patients

Stroke is the second leading cause of death in the world and the leading cause of long-term disability. Its relationship to cholesterol levels is not straightforward. A meta-analysis has shown no relationship between cholesterol levels and stroke of all types.[16] However, rates of non-haemorrhagic stroke increase with increased plasma cholesterol levels.[17,18] In contrast, rates of haemorrhagic stroke might be increased in those with low cholesterol levels, particularly if they also have hypertension, the major risk factor for this outcome.[17,18] The background use of aspirin by 82% of patients and their average range of

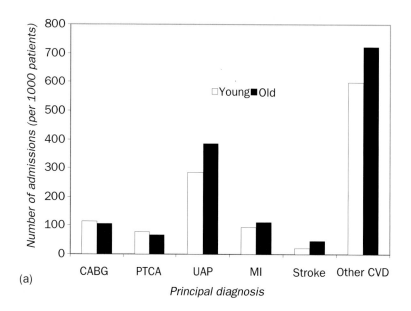

(a)

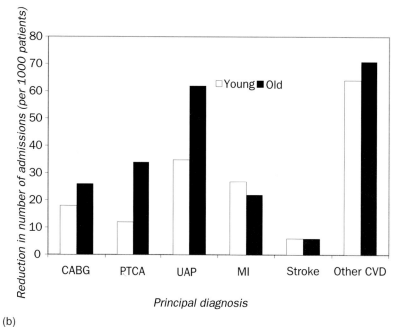

(b)

Fig. 10.1 Cardiovascular admissions in placebo-assigned patients during the placebo-controlled phase of LIPID (a) and reduction in admissions with pravastatin by diagnosis (b), comparing in both panels patients older or younger than 65 years. CABG, coronary artery bypass graft; PTCA, percutaneous transluminal coronary angioplasty; UAP, unstable angina pectoris; MI, myocardial infarction; CVD, cardiovascular disease.

cholesterol levels at baseline made the findings of the LIPID study important.

A total of 419 strokes were verified in the main LIPID study. Total strokes were significantly reduced by 19% by pravastatin (3.7% in the pravastatin group and 4.5% in the placebo group, $p = 0.048$).[19] There was a 23% reduction in non-haemorrhagic stroke (3.4% in

the pravastatin group and 4.4% in the placebo group, $p = 0.022$), which was consistent across the different types of ischaemic stroke. The evidence for benefit was even greater with extended follow-up.[11] Many factors may have contributed to stroke reduction. These include the reduction in cardiac events such as acute MI and consequent left ventricular thrombus formation and cerebral embolism, less heart failure and atrial fibrillation, decreased need for coronary bypass surgery and percutaneous intervention, as well as possibly effects of pravastatin on the cerebral circulation and aortic arch atheroma. In a LIPID sub-study, 522 patients had serial evaluations of carotid thickness.[19] At four years, the mean carotid intimal–medial thickness was significantly less in the pravastatin group than in the placebo group ($p < 0.001$).[20]

Safety

Safety is an important consideration, particularly with the long-term use of medications. Pravastatin was well tolerated with no significant increase in important adverse events during the double-blind randomized trial follow-up of six years. This favourable safety experience was reinforced during the extended follow-up of two further years. Including this additional experience, in all 1035 patients developed new cancers over eight years with no increased risk with pravastatin in either all cancers or any specific cancer type.[9,11] In particular, there was no increase in risk of breast cancer (as observed in the CARE study)[21] nor gastrointestinal malignancy (seen in the PROSPER study).[22] A further sub-study in 1130 patients in the placebo-controlled phase of LIPID showed no adverse effect on psychological well-being.[23] This is important because of previous concerns about a possible increase in violent deaths in those receiving cholesterol-lowering therapy.

Cost-effectiveness

Cardiovascular disease imposes the largest portion of direct health expenditure in many developed countries. Typically, much of this relates to hospitalization and related interventions and a lesser but still significant amount to nursing home care. Because a large proportion of these hospitalizations and costs relate to care of the elderly, in whom the burden of CHD is projected to increase further,[24] cost-effectiveness assessments are important.

During the six years of the LIPID study, pravastatin cost AUS\$ 4913 per patient but reduced total hospitalization costs by AUS\$ 1385 per patient and other long-term medication costs by AUS\$ 360 per patient.[25] The estimated cost per life-year saved was AUS\$ 7695 (and AUS\$ 10 938 with costs and life-years discounted at an annual rate of 5%). This is at least comparable to other accepted therapies in developed countries. Treatment is even more cost-effective when the increased absolute benefit during extended follow-up is considered.

Mechanisms

The extent to which LDL cholesterol should be lowered by treatment had been somewhat controversial. Epidemiological studies have shown a continuous association between cholesterol levels, particularly LDL cholesterol and the risk of subsequent CHD events.[4] However, analyses of some studies, such as the Cholesterol and Recurrent Events (CARE) trial suggested a possible threshold, with little or no treatment effect with LDL cholesterol below 3.2 mmol/l (125 mg/dl).[21]

The LIPID investigators analysed the relationship between baseline and on-study lipid parameters at 12 months and CHD event rates.[26] Baseline lipids in those assigned placebo, including total cholesterol (relative risk 1.24, $p = 0.004$), LDL cholesterol (relative risk 1.28, $p = 0.002$) and HDL cholesterol (relative risk 0.52, $p = 0.004$) were significant predictors of subsequent events, as also were apolipoproteins A and B. The most important lipid parameters at 12 months on treatment in the trial for explaining subsequent reduction CHD events were apolipoprotein B, LDL cholesterol and the combination of total and HDL cholesterol.[26] However there were wide confidence intervals about these estimates.

CONCLUSIONS

The LIPID study provides compelling evidence for the benefits, safety and cost-effectiveness of pravastatin 40 mg daily in secondary prevention in patients with previous acute coronary syndromes. A further LIPID analysis provides a model for quantifying risk in CHD patients.[27] However, overall the study adds to the body of data supporting the need for the more widespread use of HMG-CoA reductase inhibitors in such patients.[28] What were outstanding questions in the minds of some concerning the need for demonstration in placebo-controlled trials of significant reduction in events in sub-groups such as those with low HDL cholesterol levels, women or people with diabetes were answered by the Heart Protection Study, which was reported subsequently.[28]

REFERENCES

1. World Health Organization. *World Health Report 2002. Reducing Risks, Promoting Healthy Life.* Geneva: World Health Organization, 2002.
2. Murray CJL, Lopez AD. *The Global Burden of Disease: A Comprehensive Assessment of Mortality and Disability from Diseases, Injuries and Risk Factors in 1990 and Projected to 2020.* Boston: Harvard School of Public Health, 1996.
3. Yusuf S, Reddy S, Ounpou S, Anand S. Global burden of cardiovascular diseases. Part 1. General considerations, the epidemiologic transition, risk factors and impact of urbanisation. *Circulation* 2001; **104**: 2746–53.
4. Law MR, Wald NJ, Wu T et al. Systematic underestimation of association between serum cholesterol concentration and ischaemic heart disease in observational studies. *BMJ* 1994; **308**: 363–6.
5. Rossouw JE, Lewis B, Rifkind BM. The value of lowering cholesterol after myocardial infarction. *N Engl J Med* 1990; **323**: 1112–19.
6. Muldoon MF, Manuck SB, Mathews KA. Lowering cholesterol concentrations and mortality: a quantitative review of primary prevention trials. *BMJ* 1990; **301**: 309–14.
7. Peto R, Yusuf S, Collins R. Cholesterol-lowering trial results in their epidemiological context. *Circulation* 1985; **72** (Suppl III): 451 (abst).
8. The LIPID Study Group. Prevention of cardiovascular events and death with pravastatin in patients with coronary heart disease and a broad range of initial cholesterol levels. *N Engl J Med* 1998; **339**: 1349–57.
9. The LIPID Study Group. Design features and baseline characteristics of the LIPID (Long-Term Intervention with Pravastatin in Ischaemic Disease) Study: a randomized trial in patients with previous acute myocardial infarction and/or unstable angina pectoris. *Am J Cardiol* 1995; **76**: 474–9.
10. Tonkin AM for the LIPID Study Group. Management of the Long-term Intervention with Pravastatin in Ischaemic Disease (LIPID) study after the Scandinavian Simvastatin Survival Study (4S). *Am J Cardiol* 1995; **76**: 107C–112C.
11. The LIPID Study Group. Long-term effectiveness and safety of pravastatin in 9014 patients with coronary heart disease and average cholesterol levels: the LIPID trial follow-up. *Lancet* 2002; **359**: 1379–87.
12. Kannel WB. Range of serum cholesterol values in the population developing coronary artery disease. *Am J Cardiol* 1995; **76**: 69C–77C.
13. Hunt D, Young P, Simes J et al., for the LIPID investigators. Benefits of pravastatin on cardiovascular events and mortality in older patients with coronary heart disease are equal to or exceed those seen in younger patients: results from the LIPID trial. *Ann Intern Med* 2001; **134**: 931–40.
14. Tonkin AM, Colquhoun D, Emberson J et al., for the LIPID Study Group. Effects of pravastatin in 3260 patients with unstable angina: results from the LIPID study. *Lancet* 2000; **355**: 1871–5.
15. Braunwald E, Mark PB, Jones RH et al. *Unstable Angina: Diagnosis and Management. Clinical Practice Guideline Number 10.* AHCPR Publication 94–0602. Rockville, MD: US Department of Health and Human Services, 1994.
16. Prospective Studies Collaboration Cholesterol. Diastolic blood pressure and stroke: 13,000 strokes in 450,000 people in 45 prospective cohorts. *Lancet* 1995; **346**: 1647–53.
17. Iso SH, Jacobs DR Jr, Wentworth D et al. Serum cholesterol levels and six-year mortality from stroke in 350,977 men screened for the Multiple Risk Factor Interventional Trial. *N Engl J Med* 1989; **320**: 904–10.
18. Eastern Stroke and Coronary Heart Disease Collaborative Research Group. Blood pressure, cholesterol and stroke in eastern Asia. *Lancet* 1998; **352**: 1801–17.
19. White HD, Simes RJ, Anderson NE et al. Pravastatin therapy and the risk of stroke. *N Engl J Med* 2000; **343**: 317–26.
20. MacMahon S, Sharpe N, Gamble G et al. Effects of lowering average or below-average cholesterol levels on the progression of carotid athero-

sclerosis: results of the LIPID Atherosclerosis Substudy. *Circulation* 1998; **97**: 1784–90.

21. Sacks FM, Pfeffer MA, Moye LA et al. The effect of pravastatin on coronary events after myocardial infarction in patients with average cholesterol levels. *N Engl J Med* 1996; **335**: 1001–9.

22. Shepherd J, Blauw GJ, Murphy MB et al. Pravastatin in elderly individuals at risk of vascular disease (PROSPER): a randomised controlled trial. *Lancet* 2002; **360**: 1623–30.

23. Stewart RA, Sharples KJ, North FM et al. for the LIPID Study Investigators. Long-term assessment of psychological well-being in randomised placebo-controlled trial of cholesterol reduction with pravastatin. *Arch Intern Med* 2000; **160**: 3144–52.

24. Kelly DT. Paul Dudley White International Lecture. Our future society. A global challenge. *Circulation* 1997; **95**: 2459–64.

25. Glasziou PP, Eckermann SD, Mulray SE et al. Cholesterol-lowering therapy with pravastatin in patients with average cholesterol levels and established ischaemic heart disease. Is it cost-effective? *Med J Aust* 2002; **177**: 428–34.

26. Simes RJ, Marschner IC, Hunt D et al. Relationship between lipid levels and clinical outcomes in the Long-Term Intervention with Pravastatin in Ischaemic Disease (LIPID) trial: to what extent is the reduction in coronary events with pravastatin explained by on-study lipid levels. *Circulation* 2002; **105**: 1162–9.

27. Marschner IC, Colquhoun D, Simes RJ et al. on behalf of the LIPID Study Investigators. Long-term risk stratification for survivors of acute coronary syndromes. Results from the Long-term Intervention with Pravastatin in Ischaemic Disease (LIPID) Study. *J Am Coll Cardiol* 2001; **38**: 56–63.

28. Euroaspire Study Group. A European Society of Cardiology survey of secondary prevention of coronary heart disease. *Eur Heart J* 1997; **18**: 1569–82.

11

Mega-trials: the Prospective Pravastatin Pooling (PPP) Project and the Heart Protection Study (HPS)

Robert P Byington and Curt D Furberg

HISTORICAL BACKGROUND

By the middle of the 1960s it had been generally accepted that elevated blood cholesterol was a risk factor for experiencing a coronary heart disease (CHD) event, such as acute myocardial infarction (MI). However, whether this association was causal, and therefore whether treatment of hypercholesterolaemia would reduce the risk, had yet to be demonstrated. This crucial question was referred to as the 'lipid hypothesis'.

In a span of 22 years, from 1965 to 1987, a series of large, long-term clinical trials were conducted in high-risk patients to test this hypothesis. Four of the trials are now considered classic and pivotal to our understanding of the relationships among lipids, clinical disease and appropriate treatment. These are the Coronary Drug Project (CDP),[1-3] the WHO Clofibrate trial,[4-6] the Coronary Primary Prevention Trial (CPPT),[7-9] and the Helsinki Heart Study (HHS).[10] The first was a secondary prevention trial in men with electrocardiographic evidence of a prior MI, while the last three were primary prevention trials in hypercholesterolaemic men. The trials all demonstrated that major coronary events could be reduced in high-risk men with modest total cholesterol lowering (about 10%). Taken together, and with the results of about 20 smaller trials, these trials ultimately led to the acceptance of the lipid hypothesis.

However, some of the results of these early trials were disturbing. For example, although the use of clofibrate in the WHO trial was associated with a 20% reduction in major coronary events, there was a 25% increase in all-cause mortality. (Subsequent pooled analyses of other trials demonstrated that this was a function of clofibrate, not 'lipid-lowering', per se.)[11,12] In CDP other lipid-lowering agents (two oestrogen regimens and dextrothyroxine) were also tested but were discontinued early because of adverse events.[13,14] In CPPT, there were almost three times as many accidental and violent deaths in the cholestyramine group compared with placebo (11 vs 4).[8]

In addition, the restrictive eligibility criteria of these early trials (e.g. high-risk men) left many questions unanswered. Could women benefit from lipid lowering? Older individuals? Diabetic patients? Hypertensive patients? Individuals with less than markedly elevated lipids? Also, and as brought to our attention in CDP and the WHO trial, are all lipid-lowering drugs safe?

In the early 1980s, at which point the first generation of lipid trials were beginning to publish results, there was a movement away from the large, long-term 'events' trials, which were very resource- and time-consuming. The notion of studying atherosclerosis itself was explored and thus the second generation of lipid-lowering trials began, which included many angiographic (e.g. CLAS,[15] MARS,[16] CCAIT,[17] PLAC-I,[18] REGRESS[19]) and B-mode ultrasonographic (e.g. ACAPS,[20] PLAC-II,[21] CAIUS[22]) trials. The advantages of these trials were that they could be conducted in a shorter period of time (e.g. two to three years) with a much smaller sample size (e.g. ≤500 participants).

As intriguing as these trials were, and although they very often provided evidence of a slowing down (and sometimes a halting) of atherosclerotic processes, the results they provided were not 'bottom-line'. Although a drug may favourably alter lipid levels and may slow down atherosclerosis, do these (surrogate) effects translate to a reduction in events?

Thus the third generation of lipid-lowering trials, now with event outcomes again, began in the late 1980s. For the most part, these trials were testing the effects of a new class of agents, the HMG-CoA reductase inhibitors (the 'statins'), which had lipid-lowering effects greater than the agents used in the earliest trials: typically 20–40% reductions in low-density lipoprotein cholesterol (LDL-C). (Many of the angiographic and ultrasonographic trials also used statins.) The trials were designed to answer the clinical questions that remained unanswered from the first generation of trials, namely effects of lipid lowering on all-cause mortality, effects in more generalizable sub-groups of patients (including women) and safety.

The major trials of this generation include the Scandinavian Simvastatin Survival Study (4S,[23] begun in 1988), the West of Scotland Coronary Prevention Study (WOSCOPS,[24] begun in 1989), the Cholesterol and Recurrent Events trial (CARE,[25] begun in 1989), the Long-term Intervention with Pravastatin in Ischaemic Disease trial (LIPID,[26] begun in 1990) and the Heart Protection Study (HPS,[27] begun in 1994). WOSCOPS was the only purely primary prevention trial; HPS was both primary and secondary; all others were secondary prevention. The 4S trial was designed to test the effects of 20–40 mg simvastatin on all-cause mortality in 4444 participants followed for 5.4 years. WOSCOPS, CARE and LIPID are described below; all tested the effect of 40 mg pravastatin

on non-fatal and/or fatal CHD. HPS, also described below, was a factorial trial designed to test the independent effects of 40 mg simvastatin and antioxidant vitamin supplementation on all-cause mortality.

A special characteristic of the HPS was that it was designed *a priori* as a mega-trial, randomizing, treating and following 20 536 high-risk individuals, with over 100 000 patient-years of experience. As noted below, the extremely large sample size was selected to address the questions regarding lipid-lowering therapies by assessing the long-term effects of simvastatin on vascular and non-vascular mortality and major morbidity among a wide range of patients.

Although WOSCOPS, CARE and LIPID were not individually mega-trials, during the early phases of these trials the investigators organized themselves as the Prospective Pravastatin Pooling (PPP) Project.[28] This endeavour established *a priori* that upon the completion of the three trials, a pooled mega-trial database of 19 768 participants, also with over 100 000 patient-years of experience, would be created to address questions similar to those posed by HPS.

THE PROSPECTIVE PRAVASTATIN POOLING PROJECT

Background to the project

The Prospective Pravastatin Pooling (PPP) Project was a prospectively defined collaboration of three randomized, placebo-controlled, long-term, large-scale, monotherapy trials of pravastatin. The three constituent trials were WOSCOPS, CARE and LIPID. Although the first generation of trials of cholesterol-lowering therapies (most of which had only modest reductions in lipids) had clearly demonstrated reductions in coronary events in high-risk populations,[1–10] the question of the effects of cholesterol lowering on overall mortality remained unresolved, as did the effects of cholesterol lowering in many population sub-groups (such as older patients, women, diabetics, etc.).[29–31] The introduction of the statins (with their greater reductions in cholesterol) also provided the intriguing possibility of greater reductions in events than observed earlier.

PPP design

PPP was initiated before the completion of any of the three trials.[28] In 1992, the investigators from the three trials met to discuss the advantages of creating a single pooled database of their trials to provide increased power overall and for sub-group analyses. The stated goal for this collaboration was to pool data from three large randomized clinical trials of pravastatin to address questions for which there may be inadequate power from within the individual trials.

The primary objectives of PPP were to determine the effect of pravastatin on all-cause mortality and on cause-specific mortality. The two specific secondary objectives were to determine the effect of pravastatin on total coronary incidence (defined as the first occurrence of non-fatal MI or fatal CHD), both overall and by sub-group, and on total (fatal plus non-fatal) incidence of specific non-coronary events, including cancer, trauma and stroke.

The trials were selected because of their common design features, including drug, dose and duration of treatment or follow-up. Organizationally, the investigators agreed that there should be an independent trialist who would chair the PPP Steering Committee and an independent epidemiologist/trialist responsible for assisting the investigators with the analyses. Neither of these individuals – the authors of this chapter – was associated with any of the three trials.

Collectively, there would be 19 768 randomized patients in the PPP database with a mean of 5.2 years of follow-up, providing over 100 000 patient-years of follow-up. This sample size would also permit analyses of the effects of pravastatin on outcomes with lower event rates, such as stroke. A PPP protocol was assembled, pre-specifying the primary and secondary outcomes of interest and the primary methods of analyses, including the decision that all analyses would be based on the intention-to-treat principle. It was important to the

PPP investigators that each research question be asked a priori, without knowledge of treatment effect by trial. In this manner, the pooled results from PPP would provide much stronger evidence than simply carrying out a retrospective meta-analysis on published results. Also, because the trials may have used slightly different definitions for any particular outcome (e.g. MI), a PPP sub-committee of investigators from all three trials reviewed the definitions and agreed on a common PPP definition. For this reason, some numbers of events in PPP may not match the sum of the events from the three individual trials.

PPP: the trials

Each of the three trials was a randomized, double-masked, placebo-controlled trial of 40 mg/day pravastatin. Two trials were secondary prevention and one was primary prevention. WOSCOPS was the primary prevention trial evaluating the effectiveness of pravastatin in preventing fatal and non-fatal coronary events in 6595 men aged 45–64 years with hyperlipidaemia (specifically, an LDL-C of 155–174 mg/dl, 4.0–4.5 mmol/l) and no history of MI.[24,32] In contrast to the first generation of primary prevention trials that used lipid-lowering agents with only a modest effect on lipids, WOSCOPS was designed to address the lipid hypothesis using the more powerful pravastatin. WOSCOPS participants were followed for a mean of 4.9 years, providing over 32 000 patient-years of experience. In the final WOSCOPS results paper,[24] the investigators reported that pravastatin reduced the incidence of MI and cardiovascular disease (CVD) death in men with moderate hypercholesterolaemia and no history of MI.

CARE, conducted in the USA and Canada, was a secondary prevention trial evaluating the effectiveness of pravastatin in preventing fatal and non-fatal coronary events in 4159 men and women aged 21–75 years with average lipid levels and an MI 3–20 months before randomization.[25,33] In contrast to most of the first generation of lipid-lowering trials, in which patients with hyperlipidaemia were studied, the CARE investigators, acknowledging that most coronary patients had average (not elevated) lipid levels, designed CARE to evaluate the effect of lipid lowering in coronary patients who had average lipid levels. The lipid eligibility criteria for CARE were a total cholesterol less than 240 mg/dl (6.2 mmol/l) and an LDL-C between 115 and 174 mg/dl (3.0–5.5 mmol/l), inclusive. CARE patients were followed for a mean of 5.0 years, providing almost 21 000 patient-years of experience. In the CARE final results paper,[25] the investigators reported that pravastatin reduced the rate of fatal and non-fatal coronary events in coronary patients who had average cholesterol levels.

LIPID, conducted in Australia and New Zealand, was the other secondary prevention trial and the largest of the three pravastatin trials.[26,34] It was designed to examine the effects of lipid lowering on CHD mortality in coronary patients with a broad range of cholesterol values, and, as a secondary outcome, all-cause mortality. It evaluated the effectiveness of pravastatin in 9014 men and women aged 31–75 years with a history of MI or unstable angina and a wider lipid range than CARE – total cholesterol in the range 155–270 mg/dl (4.0–7.0 mmol/l). LIPID patients were followed for a mean of 6.1 years, providing almost 55 000 patient-years of experience. In the LIPID final results paper,[26] the investigators reported that pravastatin reduced CHD and all-cause mortality in coronary patients who had a broad range of cholesterol levels.

PPP: baseline description

Table 11.1 describes the baseline characteristics of the three trials and demonstrates the overall comparability of the pravastatin and placebo groups in the pooled PPP database. LIPID participants made up 45% of the PPP population, WOSCOPS 33% and CARE 21%. The overall mean age was 58 years (with the WOSCOPS participants being four to six years younger on average than the other participants) and 11% of the participants were female (all from CARE and LIPID). As expected from the design features of the trials, the mean LDL-C level in the primary

prevention trial (WOSCOPS) was much greater than in either of the secondary prevention trials, with CARE having the lowest mean. The secondary trials had higher prevalences of clinical disease, including (as expected) MI and angina, but also diabetes, stroke and hypertension.

PPP: adherence to study medications and effect of pravastatin on lipids

The drop-in and drop-out rates were never large among the three PPP trials.[35] For example, 2% of the placebo group participants in CARE + LIPID were on an open-labeled statin at one year post randomization and only 13% were on a statin at five years. (These data were unavailable for WOSCOPS.) Between LIPID and CARE, the rate of beginning active statin therapy among placebo participants (the 'drop-in' rate) was greater in LIPID.

Conversely, an average of 9% of the participants assigned to pravastatin in all three trials were off their masked study medication at one year, and this only rose to 18% at five years post randomization. Most of these drop-outs were clustered in WOSCOPS, the primary prevention trial.

There was more than a moderate effect of pravastatin on lipid levels among the PPP trials over time.[35] Using an intention-to-treat analysis and compared with placebo participants in the overall PPP database, there was a 37.5 mg/dl (0.97 mmol/l) greater mean drop in total cholesterol levels among the pravastatin participants over five years of follow-up. Among these pravastatin participants, there was also a 36.3 mg/dl (0.94 mmol/l) greater decrease in LDL-C, a 1.9 mg/dl (0.05 mmol/l) greater increase in high-density lipoprotein cholesterol (HDL-C), and a 15.9 (0.18 mmol/l) greater decrease in triglycerides. Among the PPP participants who took their assigned medications for five years, the pravastatin participants had (at five years) a 41.4 mg/dl (1.07 mmol/l) greater mean drop in total cholesterol, a 39.8 mg/dl (1.03 mmol/l) greater decrease in LDL-C, a 2.3 mg/dl (0.06 mmol/l) greater increase in HDL-C, and a 17.7 mg/dl (0.20 mmol/L) greater drop in triglycerides.[35]

Table 11.1   Baseline descriptions of PPP trials

| Baseline characteristic | Clinical trial | | | Pool of three trials | |
	WOSCOPS (n = 6595)	CARE (n = 4159)	LIPID (n = 9014)	Pravastatin (n = 9895)	Placebo (n = 9873)
Mean age (years)	54.7	58.6	60.8	58.3	58.4
Female (%)	0.0	13.9	16.8	10.5	10.6
Qualifying event/condition (%)					
myocardial infarction (CARE + LIPID)	–	100.0	63.8	50.1	50.2
unstable angina (LIPID)	–	–	36.2	16.5	16.5
hyperlipidaemia (WOSCOPS)	100.0	–	–	33.4	33.4
Cigarette smoking status (%)					
current	35.2	16.1	9.6	19.4	19.7
former	39.2	61.5	63.7	55.6	54.5
never	25.6	22.4	26.7	25.0	25.9
Mean diastolic BP (mmHg)	83.9	78.6	80.5	81.2	81.3
Mean systolic BP (mmHg)	135.5	128.9	134.1	133.3	133.6
Mean heart rate (beats/min)	72.8	67.2	68.9	69.7	70.0
Mean cholesterol level (mg/dl)	271.8	208.5	218.7	234.3	234.3
(mmol/l)	(7.0)	(5.4)	(5.7)	(6.1)	(6.1)
Mean LDL-C level (mg/dl)	191.9	138.6	150.0	161.4	161.7
(mmol/l)	(5.0)	(3.6)	(3.9)	(4.2)	(4.2)
Mean HDL-C level (mg/dl)					
Men	44.1	37.9	35.9	39.3	39.4
(mmol/l)	(1.1)	(1.0)	0.9	(1.0)	(1.0)
Women	–	44.8	42.5	43.0	43.2
(mmol/l)	–	(1.2)	(1.1)	(1.1)	(1.1)
LDL-C/HDL-C ratio	4.5	3.7	4.3	4.2	4.3
Mean triglyceride level (mg/dl)	163	156	160	161	159
(mmol/l)	(1.8)	(1.8)	(1.8)	(1.8)	(1.8)
Mean body mass index (kg/m^2)	26.0	27.6	26.8	26.7	26.7
History of stroke (%)	1.0	2.9	4.1	2.7	2.9
History of angina (%)	5.1	20.7	99.9	51.7	51.5
History of diabetes (%)	1.2	14.1	8.7	7.3	7.3
On insulin (%)	0.1	4.6	1.2	1.5	1.6
History of hypertension (%)	15.7	42.6	41.7	33.1	33.4
On a medication that reduces BP* (%)	15.8	81.2	75.7	56.7	57.0
On aspirin (%)	2.9	83.6	82.4	56.4	55.9

BP, blood pressure; LDL-C, low-density lipoprotein cholesterol; HDL-C, high-density lipoprotein cholesterol; NA, not available.
* Includes beta-blockers, calcium channel blockers, ACE inhibitors, diuretics.
Adapted with permission from ref. 52.

PPP: effect of pravastatin on mortality

The PPP mortality results are presented in Table 11.2.[35] As expected in these trials of high-risk participants, 65% of all deaths were cardio-vascular. When the three trials are combined and with a mean 5.2 years of follow-up, there were 784 deaths among the 9895 patients randomized to the pravastatin groups (= 152 deaths

Table 11.2   Mortality rates by treatment group in PPP

Cause of death	Pravastatin group (n = 9895)		Placebo group (n = 9873)		Percent reduction in relative risk (95% CI)	p-value
	No. of Deaths	Rate/10 000/yr	No. of Deaths	Rate/10 000/yr		
Fatal CHD	425	82.6	555	108.1	24% (33% to 14%)	<0.001
definite MI	62		124			
possible MI	32		36			
sudden death	253		287			
cardiac failure	45		61			
other CHD	33		47			
Other fatal CVD	68	13.2	81	15.8	17% (40% to − 14%)	0.25
stroke	38		36			
other CVD	30		45			
Total CVD	493	95.8	636	123.9	24% (32% to 14%)	<0.001
Total non-CVD	291	56.6	328	63.9	12% (25% to − 3%)	0.10
cancer	221		235			
trauma/suicide	19		21			
other	51		72			
Total deaths	784	152.4	964	187.8	20% (27% to 12%)	<0.001

Mean follow-up was 5.2 years.
Adapted with permission from ref. 35.

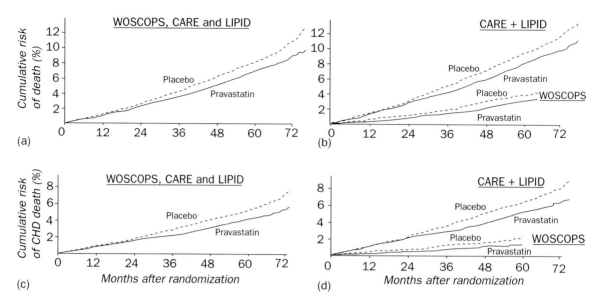

Fig. 11.1 Mortality by treatment group: pravastatin versus placebo (Prospective Pravastatin Pooling Project). (Adapted with permission from ref. 35.)

per 10 000 participants per year) compared with 964 deaths among the 9873 patients randomized to placebo (= 188 deaths per 10 000 per year). This was a 20% reduction (95% confidence interval (CI) 27–12%) in all-cause mortality ($p < 0.001$). If the trials are split between primary and secondary prevention, there is a 19% reduction in all-cause mortality in the combined CARE/LIPID population, which is comparable to the 22% reduction in WOSCOPS, although the mortality rates in WOSCOPS are much smaller.[35] (Data not shown.)

There was a 24% reduction in both fatal CHD mortality ($p < 0.001$) and total CVD mortality ($p < 0.001$). Within total CVD, there was an overall, non-significant 17% reduction in 'Other Fatal CVD'. There was also an overall, non-significant 12% reduction in 'Total Non-CVD Mortality'.

Treatment group-specific lifetable curves for all-cause and CHD mortality are presented in Fig. 11.1, which also presents data stratified by primary and secondary prevention.[35] Whereas the curves for either outcome are lower for WOSCOPS, participants in the pravastatin group consistently had lower event rates in all three trials. Also, the curves in (a) and (c)

appear to begin to diverge after six months of treatment, although the divergence clearly accelerates after two years of treatment.

In the overall PPP database, the beneficial effects of pravastatin on all-cause and CHD mortalities were evident across a wide range of population sub-groups.[35] When the population was stratified by age, gender and qualifying event (data not shown here), the relative benefit of pravastatin was similar for either outcome. For example, although there was an observed 17% ($p = 0.006$) and a 22% ($p < 0.001$) reduction in all-cause mortality in participants less than 65 years and 65–75 years, respectively, there was no evidence that these two relative reductions were different (i.e. there is no evidence of a statistical interaction).

With respect to CHD mortality, the following sub-groups had reductions in events attributable to pravastatin at p-values less than 0.05: age <65 years (21% reduction), age 65–75 years (28% reduction), men (25% reduction), patients with a prior MI (22% reduction), patients with no prior MI but with a history of unstable angina (26% reduction) and patients with no history of clinical CHD (34% reduction).[35] Women, who comprised 11% of the PPP database, had a 20% reduction in CHD mortality, although this difference was not statistically significant ($p = 0.23$).

PPP: effect of pravastatin on coronary incidence

The effect of pravastatin on coronary incidence (defined as the first post-randomization occurrence of a non-fatal MI or fatal CHD event) was also examined in a wide range of population subgroups.[36,37] Table 11.3 presents the highlights of these analyses for the overall pooled database of WOSCOPS, CARE and LIPID data. Overall, there were 947 pravastatin group participants who experienced a coronary event (= 184 events per 10 000 participants per year) compared with 1247 placebo group participants (= 243 events per 10 000 per year). This corresponds to a 26% reduction (95% CI 32–19%) in coronary incidence attributable to pravastatin ($p < 0.001$).

Examination of the interaction p-values in Table 11.3 indicates that there is no evidence for a different relative benefit of pravastatin according to baseline age, gender, smoking status, diabetes status or CHD presence.[36] Among the 25 sub-groups presented in Table 11.3, there was at least a 14% reduction in coronary incidence attributable to the drug. In fact, the sub-group experiencing the 14% reduction (patients with a history of hypertension) still had a statistically significant reduction in events (95% CI 24–2%, $p = 0.03$), although this reduction itself appeared to be statistically lower that the 33% reduction noted among participants without a history of hypertension (95% CI 40–25%, interaction $p = 0.003$). Only two sub-groups (patients with a history of diabetes, who comprised 7% of the database, and patients with a triglyceride level of at least 220 mg/dl or 2.5 mmol/l) had sub-group-specific p-values greater than 0.05, and both of these were only slightly greater (0.08 and 0.06, respectively). Also, examination of the interaction p-values suggests that the relative benefit of pravastatin may be less among patients who begin therapy with lower LDL-C (interaction $p = 0.07$).[36,37]

Figure 11.2 presents the treatment group-specific coronary incidence lifetable curves for both the total PPP population (a) and the secondary prevention trials only (b).[36] In both graphs, there is a similar reduction in coronary events attributable to pravastatin and the event curves appear to begin to diverge within one year of follow-up.

When this protocol-specified outcome measure was expanded to include coronary artery bypass grafts (CABG) and percutaneous transluminal coronary angioplasty (PTCA) (which added 1523 or 69% additional events), all sub-groups had statistically significant reductions in coronary events or procedures.[36] (Data not shown.) However, there was still a statistically significant interaction (interaction $p = 0.01$) in relative event reductions observed between participants with a history of hypertension (16% reduction) and those without (29% reduction). This *post-hoc* analysis also provided additional evidence that the relative benefit of pravastatin may be less among patients who begin therapy with lower LDL-C (interaction $p = 0.02$).

THE HEART PROTECTION STUDY

Background to the study

The HPS was established in the early 1990s to assess in a factorially designed trial the effects of cholesterol-lowering therapy and anti-oxidant vitamin supplementation on mortality and major cardiovascular events among patients at high risk of CHD events, regardless of their pre-treatment lipid levels.[27,38–41] The trial was designed to be extremely large to provide reliable estimates of overall and sub-group treatment effects and to avoid problems with interpretation. Ultimately, 20 536 high-risk individuals were randomized.

As with the trials that comprised the PPP, the rationale for the cholesterol portion of HPS was based on the observations made from longitudinal studies that the risk of CHD events increased with increasing cholesterol levels and from the results of the early (non-statin) lipid-lowering trials. The HPS investigators were specifically intrigued by observations from the

Table 11.3 Coronary incidence by treatment group and patient sub-group in PPP: all three trials combined

Baseline sub-group	Pravastatin group			Placebo group			Percent reduction in relative risk (95% CI)	Sub-group p-value	Interaction p-value
	No. of patients	No. of events	Rate/10 000/yr	No. of patients	No. of events	Rate/10 000/yr			
Overall coronary incidence	9895	947	184.0	9873	1247	242.9	26% (32% to 19%)	<0.001	–
Age group									
<55 y	3311	213	123.7	3326	306	176.9	32% (43% to 19%)	<0.001	0.31
55–64 y	4180	388	178.5	4108	479	224.2	21% (31% to 10%)	<0.001	
65–75 y	2404	346	276.8	2439	462	364.3	26% (35% to 14%)	<0.001	
Gender									
men	8853	834	181.2	8823	1104	240.6	26% (33% to 19%)	<0.001	0.08
women	1042	113	208.5	1050	143	261.9	20% (38% to – 2%)	0.07	
Current smoker									
yes	1916	193	193.7	1944	290	286.9	35% (45% to 22%)	<0.001	0.13
no	7979	754	181.7	7929	957	232.1	23% (30% to 15%)	<0.001	
History of diabetes									
yes	719	131	350.4	725	157	416.4	19% (36% to – 2%)	0.08	0.43
no	9176	816	171.0	9148	1090	229.1	27% (33% to 20%)	<0.001	
History of hypertension									
yes	3273	424	249.1	3295	488	284.8	14% (24% to 2%)	0.03	0.003
no	6622	523	151.9	6578	759	221.9	33% (40% to 25%)	<0.001	
CHD presence									
MI	4960	610	236.5	4953	772	299.7	22% (30% to 14%)	<0.001	0.42
Unstable angina (no MI)	1633	159	187.2	1627	216	255.3	29% (42% to 12%)	0.001	
none	3302	178	103.7	3293	259	151.3	33% (44% to 18%)	<0.001	
Total cholesterol (mg/dl)									
<213	3160	353	214.8	3116	414	255.5	17% (28% to 5%)	0.009	0.24
213–249	3227	345	205.6	3267	494	290.8	30% (39% to 20%)	<0.001	
≥250	3508	249	136.5	3490	339	186.8	30% (40% to 17%)	<0.001	

Table 11.3 *Continued*

Baseline sub-group	Pravastatin group			Placebo group			Percent reduction in relative risk (95% CI)	Sub-group p-value	Interaction p-value
	No. of patients	No. of events	Rate/10 000/yr	No. of patients	No. of events	Rate/10 000/yr			
LDL-C (mg/dl)									
<135	2298	249	208.4	2220	304	263.3	22% (34% to 7%)	0.005	0.07
135–174	3992	426	205.2	3994	552	265.8	23% (32% to 13%)	<0.001	
≥175	3605	272	145.1	3658	391	205.6	32% (42% to 21%)	<0.001	
HDL-C (mg/dl)									
<39	5146	603	225.3	5158	789	294.2	24% (32% to 16%)	<0.001	0.48
≥39	4749	344	139.3	4714	458	186.8	28% (37% to 17%)	<0.001	
Triglycerides (mg/dl)									
<133	4198	373	170.9	4312	531	236.8	29% (38% to 19%)	<0.001	0.42
133–219	4006	378	181.5	3927	498	243.9	26% (35% to 16%)	<0.001	
≥220	1691	196	222.9	1634	218	256.6	17% (32% to – 1%)	0.06	

Mean follow-up was 5.2 years.
Coronary incidence defined as the first post-randomization occurrence of a non-fatal MI or fatal CHD.
Adapted with permission from ref. 36.

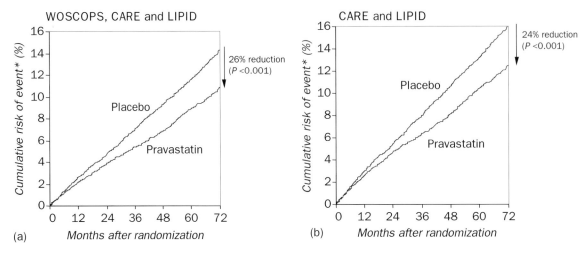

Fig. 11.2 Coronary incidence by treatment group: pravastatin versus placebo (Prospective Pravastatin Pooling Project). *Coronary incidence defined as first post-randomization occurrence of a non-fatal MI or CHD death.

prospective studies that the relationship between cholesterol level and CHD risk was linear when the risk was plotted on a doubling scale. This implied that an absolute reduction in cholesterol would be associated with a proportional reduction in CHD events across the entire range of cholesterol values in the general population. Thus, in contrast to early lipid-lowering trials in which participants with high cholesterol were treated, HPS would study participants with a wider range of lipid values. (As noted above, the CARE and LIPID investigators had similar thoughts.)

The HPS investigators were also concerned about risk versus benefit, specifically because of observations noted in the early trials and in prospective studies that suggested that there may be danger in lowering cholesterol levels too far.[42] It was unclear whether these purported inverse relationships were real or due to chance or confounding. Even the early trials, which were powered to detect treatment effects on major coronary events or deaths, were too small to detect adverse treatment effects on other outcomes, or to detect any effect on all-cause mortality. Thus, the HPS investigators wanted to have a large enough trial to address and preferably resolve the issues related to the risks and benefits of cholesterol therapy across a wide range of patient sub-groups.

The rationale for the antioxidant portion of the trial was partly based upon animal studies suggesting that antioxidants may slow atherosclerotic progression[43,44] and partly upon suggestions from some observational studies that a lower risk of CHD events may be moderately associated with increased dietary intake of antioxidant vitamins.[45,46] During the design phase of their trial, the HPS investigators recognized that if the effect of an antioxidant on coronary events was only moderate, then a very large trial would be required to test the hypothesis reliably.

HPS design

The HPS, conducted in the UK, was designed as an extremely large factorial trial, with 20 536 randomized participants. Men and women, 40–80 years of age, with a cholesterol level of at least 135 mg/dl (3.5 mmol/l) and at high risk of a coronary event were randomized to one of four treatment groups: simvastatin + vitamin supplementation; simvastatin + vitamin placebo; simvastatin placebo + vitamin supplementation; and double placebo. 'High risk' was defined as being at increased risk of dying within five years from a CHD event because of a history of coronary disease, occlusive disease, diabetes or treated hypertension (if also a male 65+ years of

Table 11.4 Baseline description of HPS participants	
Baseline characteristic	*%*
Age	
<65 years	47.9
65–69 years	23.8
70–74 years	22.1
>74 years	6.2
	100.0
Female	24.7
Prior disease status	
myocardial infarction	41.4
other CHD	23.7
no CHD	34.9
	100.0
Cholesterol level	
<193 mg/dl (5.0 mmol/l)	19.8
≥193 to <232 mg/dl	38.4
≥232 mg/dl (6.0 mmol/l)	41.8
	100.0
LDL-C level	
<116 mg/dl (3.0 mmol/l)	33.1
≥116 to <135 mg/dl	24.7
≥135 mg/dl (3.5 mmol/l)	42.3
	100.0
History of cerebrovascular disease	16.0
History of PVD	32.9
History of diabetes	29.0
Treated for hypertension	41.2
On aspirin/other anti-platelet	63.0

Total sample size = 20 536
MI, myocardial infarction; CHD, coronary heart disease; LDL-C, low-density lipoprotein cholesterol; PVD, peripheral vascular disease.
Adapted with permission from refs 27 and 47.

be summarized that vitamin use had no observed effect on the five-year event rates of any fatal/non-fatal vascular, cancer or other outcome.[40,41]

The primary HPS outcome was all-cause mortality. Other outcomes included CHD mortality, other causes of death, 'major coronary events' (defined as non-fatal MI or CHD death), and 'major vascular events' (defined as major coronary events, fatal/non-fatal stroke or any coronary/non-coronary revascularization). Randomized participants were followed for an average of 5 years (providing over 100 000 patient years of experience).

HPS: baseline characteristics and comparison with PPP

Table 11.4 describes the HPS population at baseline.[27,39,47] HPS had an older population compared with PPP: 52% of the HPS participants were 65 years or older, compared with 25% of the PPP participants. More of the HPS participants were female: 25% compared with the 11% noted in PPP. However, like PPP, almost two-thirds of the HPS participants were secondary prevention. With respect to the baseline lipids, PPP had higher values: 42% of the HPS participants had an LDL-C of 135 mg/dl (3.5 mmol/l) or greater, compared with 77% of the PPP participants. HPS had a higher proportion of patients with diabetes (29%) compared with PPP (7%). The prevalence of aspirin use was roughly comparable between the two studies (63% HPS vs 56% PPP).

HPS: adherence to study medications and effect of simvastatin on lipids

Four percent of the HPS placebo group participants were on an open-labeled statin at one year post randomization, although 32% were on a statin at five years.[27] Conversely, 11% of the HPS participants assigned to simvastatin were off their masked study medication at one year, and this only rose to 18% at five years post randomization.[27]

Although the effects of simvastatin on lipid levels across time[27] were greater than those

age). Participants received either 40 mg/day simvastatin or matching placebo tablet, and either antioxidant vitamins (600 mg vitamin E, 250 mg vitamin C, and 20 mg beta-carotene daily) or matching placebo capsules.

Because the focus of this book is the use of statins, the HPS antioxidant results will not be presented in detail; only the marginal simvastatin results will be presented. However, it can observed with the non-statins in the first generation of lipid trials, the effects were slightly less than those observed in PPP with pravastatin. Using an intention-to-treat analysis and compared with placebo participants, in HPS there was a 31 mg/dl (0.8 mmol/l) greater mean reduction in total cholesterol levels among the simvastatin participants over five years of follow-up. Among these simvastatin participants, there was also a 27 mg/dl (0.7 mmol/l) greater decrease in LDL-C, a 0.8 mg/dl (0.02 mmol/l) greater increase in HDL-C and an 18 mg/dl (0.2 mmol/l) greater decrease in triglycerides.

HPS: effect of simvastatin on mortality

The HPS mortality results are presented in Table 11.5.[27,41,47] Comparable to PPP, 61% of the deaths in HPS were vascular in nature. For the primary outcome measure, all-cause mortality, participants assigned to the simvastatin group had a 13% lower death rate (95% CI 19–6%; $p < 0.001$). There were 1328 deaths among the 10 269 participants randomized to the simvastatin group (= 259 deaths per 10 000 participants per year) compared with 1507 deaths among the 10 267 participants randomized to the placebo group (= 294 deaths per 10 000 participants per year).

HPS also reported a 17% reduction in vascular deaths among simvastatin participants (95% CI 25–9%, $p < 0.001$), with fewer coronary, stroke and other vascular deaths in the simvastatin group. There was a comparable number of non-vascular deaths between the simvastatin and placebo groups ($p = 0.4$).

HPS: effect of simvastatin on major coronary and vascular events

The effect of simvastatin on major coronary events (defined, as in PPP, as non-fatal MI or CHD death) was examined (Table 11.6).[27,48] Overall, there were 898 simvastatin group participants who experienced a coronary event (= 175 events per 10 000 participants per year) compared with 1212 placebo group participants (= 236 events per 10 000 per year). This is a 26%

reduction in coronary incidence attributable to simvastatin ($p < 0.001$).

This beneficial effect of simvastatin was observed in all reported patient sub-groups (Table 11.6).[49] Examination of the interaction p-values in the table indicates that there is no evidence for a different relative effect of simvastatin according to any reported baseline characteristic, including age, gender, smoking status, diabetes status, CHD presence or lipid level. Among the 22 sub-groups presented in Table 11.6, there was at least an 18% reduction in major coronary events attributable to the drug and all sub-groups had statistically significant p-values.

When this outcome is expanded to include fatal or non-fatal strokes and revascularizations, this new outcome ('major vascular events') added 2508 (or 118%) more events (80% of which were revascularizations).[27] Simvastatin was associated with a 24% reduction in these events (95% CI 28–19%, $p < 0.001$). Figure 11.3 presents the treatment group-specific lifetable curves for this outcome measure.[27] It is noted that the curves begin to diverge after 12 months of treatment.

COMPARISON OF THE MAIN RESULTS FROM PPP AND HPS

It is noted in Table 11.5 that the overall, annualized placebo group all-cause mortality rate in HPS (294 deaths per 10 000 participants per year) is 56% higher than the comparable statistic for PPP reported in Table 11.2 (188 deaths per 10 000 participants per year). This difference in all-cause mortality is mirrored by higher placebo-group mortality rates in HPS for both vascular deaths (183 deaths per 10 000 per year in HPS vs 124 CVD deaths per 10 000 per year in PPP) and non-vascular deaths (111 deaths per 10 000 per year vs 64 non-CVD deaths per 10 000 per year in PPP).

Comparing the baseline characteristics between the trials provides two possible contributors for these differentials: the HPS population was older than PPP and HPS had a higher proportion of patients with diabetes (29%) compared with PPP (7%). On the other hand, PPP

Table 11.5   Mortality rates by treatment group in HPS simvastatin trial

Cause of death	Simvastatin group (n = 10 269)		Placebo group (n = 10 267)		Percent reduction in relative risk (95% CI)	p-value
	No. of deaths	Rate/10 000/yr	No. of deaths	Rate/10 000/yr		
Vascular causes	781	152.1	937	182.5	17% (25% to 9%)	<0.001
coronary	587		707			
stroke	96		119			
other vascular	98		111			
Non-vascular	547	106.5	570	111.0	5% (15% to −7%)	0.4
cancer	359		345			
respiratory	90		114			
other medical	82		90			
non-medical	16		21			
Total deaths	1328	258.6	1507	293.6	13% (19% to 6%)	<0.001

Mean follow-up was 5.0 years.
Adapted with permission from ref. 27.

Table 11.6 Effect of simvastatin on first major coronary event by patient sub-group in HPS

Baseline sub-group	Simvastatin group			Placebo group			Percent reduction in relative risk	Sub-group p-value	Interaction p-value
	No. of patients	No. of events	Rate/10 000/yr	No. of patients	No. of events	Rate/10 000/yr			
First major coronary event	10 269	898	174.9	10 267	1212	236.1	26%	<0.001	–
Age group									
<65 y	4903	304	124.0	4936	453	183.5	32%	<0.001	0.19
65–69 y	2447	232	189.6	2444	320	261.9	28%	<0.001	
70+ y	2919	362	248.0	2887	439	304.1	18%	0.002	
Gender									
men	7727	767	198.5	7727	1015	262.7	24%	<0.001	0.35
women	2542	131	103.1	2540	197	155.1	34%	<0.001	
Current smoker									
yes	1446	127	175.7	1467	207	282.2	38%	<0.001	0.16
no	8823	771	174.8	8800	1005	228.4	23%	<0.001	
Prior disease									
MI	4257	539	253.2	4253	681	320.2	21%	<0.001	0.14
other CHD	2437	178	146.1	2439	246	201.7	28%	0.001	
no prior CHD	3575	181	101.3	3575	285	159.4	36%	<0.001	
Cholesterol level									
<193 mg/dl (<5.0 mmol/l)	2030	164	161.6	2042	220	215.5	25%	0.003	0.71
≥193 to <232 mg/dl (<6.0 mmol/l)	3942	315	159.8	3941	464	235.5	32%	<0.001	
≥232 mg/dl (≥6.0 mmol/l)	4297	419	195.0	4284	528	246.5	21%	<0.001	
LDL-C level									
<116 mg/dl (<3.0 mmol/l)	3389	268	158.2	3404	356	209.2	24%	<0.001	0.96
≥116 to <135 mg/dl (≥3.5 mmol/l)	2549	199	156.1	2514	293	233.1	33%	<0.001	
≥135 mg/dl (≥3.5 mmol/l)	4331	431	199.0	4349	563	258.9	23%	<0.001	

Table 11.6 *Continued*

Baseline sub-group	Simvastatin group			Placebo group			Percent reduction in relative risk	Sub-group p-value	Interaction p-value
	No. of patients	No. of events	Rate/10 000/yr	No. of patients	No. of events	Rate/10 000/yr			
HDL-C level									
<35 mg/dl (<0.9 mmol/l)	3617	368	203.5	3559	514	288.8	30%	<0.001	0.59
≥35 to <43 mg/dl	2795	249	178.2	2871	337	234.8	24%	<0.001	
≥43 mg/dl (≥1.1 mmol/l)	3857	281	145.7	3837	361	188.2	23%	0.001	
Triglyceride level									
<177 mg/dl (<2.0 mmol/l)	6011	493	164.0	6034	679	225.1	27%	<0.001	0.99
≥177 to <354 mg/dl	3445	335	194.5	3443	427	248.0	22%	<0.001	
≥354 mg/dl (≥4.0 mmol/l)	813	70	172.2	790	106	268.4	36%	0.002	

Mean follow-up was 5.0 years.
Adapted with permission from refs 27 and 49.

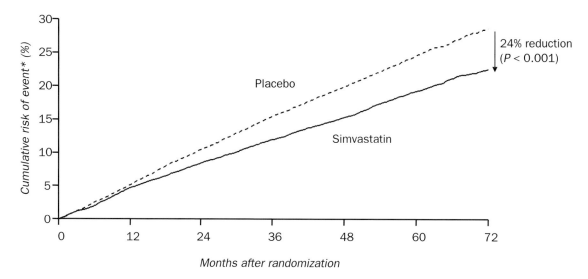

Fig. 11.3 Occurrence of major vascular events by treatment group: simvastatin versus placebo (Heart Protection Study). *Major vascular event defined as the first occurrence of a fatal or non-fatal coronary event, fatal or non-fetal stroke or any coronary or non-coronary revascularization. (Adapted with permission from ref. 27.)

and HPS had a similar prevalence of secondary prevention and PPP had higher prevalence of an LDL-C of 135 mg/dl (3.5 mmol/l) or greater: 77% PPP vs 42% HPS. The prevalence of aspirin use was roughly comparable between the two studies (63% HPS vs 56% PPP).

Regarding the effects of the statins on events, both trials provide evidence that statins reduce all-cause and some cause-specific mortality rates. Pravastatin in PPP was associated with a 20% reduction in all-cause mortality (Table 11.2) and simvastatin in HPS was associated with a 13% reduction (Table 11.5), with some overlap in the 95% confidence intervals. Pravastatin was also associated with 24% reduction in total fatal CVD events and simvastatin with a relatively comparable 17% reduction in deaths from vascular causes. Both trials also had non-statistically significant reductions in non-CVD/non-vascular deaths: 12% in PPP and 5% in HPS.

Although there were differences between the trials in mortality rates, PPP and HPS had nearly identical placebo group rates for fatal/non-fatal coronary events: 243 events per 10 000 per year in PPP versus 236 in HPS. Both trials also provided strong evidence that these statins reduce this rate of coronary incidence:

both had a 26% reduction in these events associated with a statin (Tables 11.3 and 11.6). Furthermore, this benefit was apparent among a wide range of patient characteristics.

COMPARISON OF THE EFFECTS OF PRAVASTATIN AND SIMVASTATIN ON STROKE

Both the constituent trials of PPP and HPS itself were designed to answer the broad questions of the effects of a statin on coronary events and/or mortality. However, both PPP and HPS did specify *a priori* that a question of interest would be the effect of a statin on risk of stroke.[27,28]

For decades, there was skepticism that strokes were related to increased levels of cholesterol and that therefore a reduction of lipids would not translate into a reduction in strokes. This skepticism was fueled by the results of large observational studies in which there was little, if any, relationship between stroke incidence (in which haemorrhagic and non-haemorrhagic strokes were combined) and increased lipid levels.[50] As late as 1995, a meta-analysis of 11 clinical trials (none of which used a statin) was published reporting that total stroke was not reduced by lipid therapy.[51] However, in that same 4S trial reported that simvastatin use was associated with a reduction in cerebrovascular events.[23] Subsequently, CARE and LIPID independently reported that pravastatin was also associated with a reduction in stroke events.[25,26]

Both HPS and PPP (for which CARE and LIPID had the most data) reported benefit of statin therapy in reducing stroke events, specifically on non-haemorrhagic or ischaemic strokes and on non-fatal strokes (Table 11.7).[27,52] In this table it is noted that most strokes in these study populations were non-fatal and that most were non-haemorrhagic or ischaemic. Pravastatin in PPP was associated with a 22% reduction in total fatal or non-fatal stroke (95% CI 35–7%, $p = 0.01$) (Fig. 11.4), and simvastatin in HPS was associated with a nearly identical 25% reduction (95% CI 34–15%, $p < 0.001$). Most of this effect was because of a reduction in non-haemorrhagic or ischaemic stroke; there was essentially no effect of a statin on haemorrhagic stroke. Also, most of this effect was related to a reduction in non-fatal stroke (25% reduction in PPP and 27% reduction in HPS); the effect, if any, of statins on fatal stroke was minimal in both trials.

COMPARISON OF THE SAFETY PROFILES OF PRAVASTATIN AND SIMVASTATIN

Both PPP and HPS had as a major objective the long-term confirmation of statin safety.[27,28] The periodic measurement of liver and muscle enzymes was performed in both trials and the incidence of cancer monitored.

PPP reported that 8.8% of pravastatin and 8.2% of placebo participants ever had an alanine aminotransferase (ALT) more than 50% greater than the upper limit of normal (ULN) for the laboratory ($p = $ not significant).[53] HPS reported that 1.8% of simvastatin and 1.6% of the placebo participants had an ALT that was more than 100% greater than the ULN ($p = $ not significant).[27] PPP also reported that 2.1% of pravastatin and 1.9% of placebo participants ever had a creatine kinase (CK) more than three times greater than ULN ($p = $ not significant). HPS reported that 0.3% of simvastatin and 0.2% of the placebo participants had a CK that was more than four times

greater than the ULN ($p = $ not significant). PPP also reported that there were no cases of myopathy or rhabdomyolysis noted in either treatment group. HPS reported that there were ten cases of myopathy in the simvastatin group and four in the placebo group ($p = $ not significant), and that there were five cases of rhabdomyolysis in the simvastatin group and three in the placebo group. Both groups reported that the drugs appeared to be safe with respect to possible liver and muscle problems.

Table 11.8 presents the comparison of treatment group-specific rates of cancer for the two trials.[27,53] PPP and HPS had similar overall placebo group rates of any cancer: 18 per 1000 per year in PPP versus 16 per 1000 per year in HPS. Regarding any possible effect of a statin on cancer, there was no treatment group difference in either mega-trial in cancer rates for any grouping of cancers.

The CARE trial had previously reported an excess of breast cancer in the statin group[25] but neither LIPID nor HPS confirmed this. In LIPID, 1.3% of the pravastatin women developed breast cancer compared with 1.1% of the placebo women; two men in the placebo group also developed breast cancer.[26] In HPS, 1.5% of the simvastatin women developed breast cancer compared with 2.0% of the placebo women.[27]

CONCLUSION

The PPP Project and the HPS have both provided strong evidence that pravastatin and simvastatin safely reduce cardiovascular mortality and morbidity in patients with a wide range of baseline characteristics. Both simvastatin and pravastatin were associated with similar reductions in fatal and non-fatal coronary events. The extremely large sample sizes for these mega-trials have provided reliable estimates of these effects and confirm their benefit in every examined sub-group. The reduction of all-cause mortality in both trials is particularly striking in that it addresses the earlier concern of a possible increase in non-vascular deaths, thus demonstrating an extremely favourable balance between benefit and risk.

Table 11.7 Effect of statin on stroke in PPP and HPS

i. Pravastatin in the PPP (CARE/LIPID only: 5.4 years' mean follow-up)

Event/stroke type	Pravastatin group (n = 6593)		Placebo group (n = 6580)		Percent reduction in relative risk (95% CI)	p-value
	No. of strokes	Rate/1000/yr	No. of strokes	Rate/1000/yr		
Total stroke (fatal/non-fatal)	221	6.2	280	7.9	22% (35% to 7%)	0.01
non-haemorrhagic	171	4.8	218	6.1	23%	
haemorrhagic	19	0.5	15	0.4	−25%	
unknown type	31	0.9	47	1.3	35%	
Non-fatal stroke	194	5.4	255	7.2	25% (38% to 10%)	
Fatal stroke	31	0.9	32	0.9	4% (42% to −57%)	

ii. Simvastatin in the HPS (5.0 years mean follow-up)

Event/stroke type	Simvastatin group (n = 10 269)		Placebo group (n = 10 267)		Percent reduction in relative risk (95% CI)	p-value
	No. of strokes	Rate/1000/yr	No. of strokes	Rate/1000/yr		
Total stroke (fatal/non-fatal)	444	8.6	585	11.4	25% (34% to 15%)	<0.001
ischaemic	290	5.6	409	8.0	29%	
haemorrhagic	51	1.0	53	1.0	4%	
unknown type	103	2.0	134	2.6	23%	
Non-fatal stroke	366	7.1	499	9.7	27% (35% to 17%)	
Fatal stroke	96	1.9	119	2.3	19% (38% to −5%)	

Adapted with permission from refs 27 and 52.

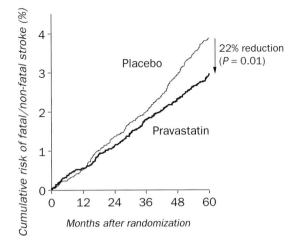

Fig. 11.4 Occurrence of any fatal/non-fatal stroke by treatment group: pravastatin versus placebo (Prospective Pravastatin Pooling Project). (Adapted with permission from ref. 52.)

REFERENCES

1. Coronary Drug Project Research Group. The Coronary Drug Project: Design, methods, and baseline results. American Heart Association Monograph Number 38. *Circulation* 1973; **47** (Suppl I): I1–I79.
2. Coronary Drug Project Research Group. Clofibrate and niacin in coronary heart disease. *JAMA* 1975; **231**: 360–81.
3. Canner PL, Berge KG, Wenger NK et al., for the Coronary Drug Project Research Group. Fifteen-year mortality in Coronary Drug Project patients: long-term benefit with niacin. *J Am Coll Cardiol* 1986; **8**: 1245–55.
4. Committee of Principal Investigators. A cooperative trial in the prevention of ischaemic heart disease using clofibrate. *Br Heart J* 1978; **40**: 1069–118.
5. Committee of Principal Investigators. WHO cooperative trial on primary prevention of

Table 11.8   Effect of statin on incidence of site-specific primary cancers in PPP and HPS

Body system/study		Statin group No. of cancers	Rate/1000/yr	Placebo group No. of cancers	Rate/1000/yr	Percent reduction in relative risk	p-value*
Any cancer							
	PPP	946	19.0	914	17.8	–6%	0.48
	HPS	814	15.9	803	15.6	–1%	0.78
Genitourinary							
	PPP	266	5.3	247	4.8	–11%	0.42
	HPS	259	5.0	272	5.3	5%	0.57
Gastrointestinal							
	PPP	137	2.7	149	2.9	5%	0.48
	HPS	228	4.4	223	4.3	–2%	0.81
Respiratory							
	PPP	122	2.4	133	2.6	6%	0.49
	HPS	179	3.5	167	3.3	–7%	0.52
Haematological							
	PPP	38	0.8	52	1.0	25%	0.14
	HPS	64	1.2	52	1.0	–23%	0.26
Nervous system							
	PPP	16	0.3	12	0.2	–37%	0.57
	HPS	12	0.2	6	0.1	–100%	0.16

* Difference between incidence rates.
PPP followed 9895 pravastatin and 9873 placebo participants for a mean of 5.2 years.
HPS followed 10 269 simvastatin and 10 267 placebo participants for a mean of 5.0 years.
Adapted with permission from refs 27 and 53.

ischaemic heart disease using clofibrate to lower serum cholesterol: mortality follow-up. *Lancet* 1980; **ii**: 379–85.

6. Committee of Principal Investigators. WHO cooperative trial on primary prevention of ischaemic heart disease using clofibrate to lower serum cholesterol: final mortality follow-up. *Lancet* 1984; **ii**: 600–4.

7. Lipid Research Clinics Program. The Coronary Primary Prevention Trial: design and implementation. *J Chron Dis* 1979; **32**: 609–31.

8. Lipid Research Clinics Program. The Lipid Research Clinics Coronary Primary Prevention Trial results. I. Reduction in incidence of coronary heart disease. *JAMA* 1984; **251**: 351–64.

9. Lipid Research Clinics Program. The Lipid Research Clinics Coronary Primary Prevention Trial results. II. The relationship of reduction in incidence of coronary heart disease to cholesterol lowering. *JAMA* 1984; **251**: 365–74.

10. Frick MH, Elo O, Haapa K et al. Helsinki Heart Study: primary prevention trial with gemfibrozil in middle-aged men with dyslipidemia. Safety of treatment, changes in risk factors, and incidence of coronary heart disease. *N Engl J Med* 1987; **317**: 1237–45.

11. Gould AL, Rossouw JE, Santanello NC et al. Cholesterol reduction yields clinical benefit. A new look at old data. *Circulation* 1995; **91**: 2274–82.

12. Gordon DJ. Cholesterol lowering and total mortality. In: Rifkind BM, ed. *Lowering Cholesterol in High-Risk Individuals and Populations*. New York: Marcel Dekker, 1995.

13. Coronary Drug Project Research Group. Findings leading to discontinuation of the 2.5 mg/day estrogen group. *JAMA* 1973; **226**: 652–7.

14. Coronary Drug Project Research Group. Findings leading to further modifications of its protocol with respect to dextrothyroxine. *JAMA* 1972; **220**: 886–1008.

15. Blankenhorn DH, Nessim SA, Johnson RL et al. Beneficial effects of combined colestipol–niacin therapy on coronary atherosclerosis and coronary venous bypass grafts. *JAMA* 1987; **257**: 3233–40.

16. Blankenhorn DH, Azen SP, Kramsch DM et al. Coronary angiographic changes with lovastatin therapy: the Monitored Atherosclerosis Regression Study (MARS). *Ann Intern Med* 1993; **119**: 969–76.

17. Waters D, Higginson L, Gladstone P et al. Effects of monotherapy with an HMG-CoA reductase inhibitor on the progression of coronary atherosclerosis as assessed by serial quantitative angiography: the Canadian Coronary Atherosclerosis Intervention Trial. *Circulation* 1994; **89**: 959–68.

18. Pitt B, Mancini GBJ, Ellis S et al. for the PLAC I Investigators. Pravastatin Limitation of Atherosclerosis in the Coronary Arteries (PLAC I): reduction in atherosclerosis progression and clinical events. *J Am Coll Cardiol* 1995; **26**: 1133–9.

19. Jukema JW, Bruschke AVG, van Boven AJ et al. Effects of lipid lowering by pravastatin on progression and regression of coronary artery disease in symptomatic men with normal to moderately elevated serum cholesterol levels. The Regression Growth Evaluation Statin Study (REGRESS). *Circulation* 1995; **91**: 2528–40.

20. Furberg CD, Adams HP, Applegate WB et al. for the Asymptomatic Carotid Artery Progression Study (ACAPS) Research Group. Effect of lovastatin on early carotid atherosclerosis and cardiovascular events. *Circulation* 1994; **90**: 1679–87.

21. Crouse JR, Byington RP, Bond MG et al. Pravastatin, Lipids, and Atherosclerosis in the Carotid Arteries (PLAC-II). *Am J Cardiol* 1995; **75**: 455–9.

22. Mercuri M, Bond MG, Sirtori CR et al. Pravastatin reduces carotid intima-media thickness progression in an asymptomatic hypercholesterolemic Mediterranean population: the Carotid Atherosclerosis Italian Ultrasound Study. *Am J Med* 1996; **101**: 627–34.

23. Scandinavian Simvastatin Survival Study Group. Randomised trial of cholesterol lowering in 4444 patients with coronary heart disease: the Scandinavian Simvastatin Survival Study (4S). *Lancet* 1994; **344**: 1383–9.

24. Shepherd J, Cobbe SM, Ford I et al. for the West of Scotland Coronary Prevention Study Group. Prevention of coronary disease with pravastatin in men with hypercholesterolemia. *N Eng J Med* 1995; **333**: 1301–7.

25. Sacks FM, Pfeffer MA, Moye LA et al. for the Cholesterol and Recurrent Events Trial Investigators. The effect of pravastatin on coronary events after myocardial infarction in patients with average cholesterol levels. *N Engl J Med* 1996; **335**: 1001–9.

26. Long-term Intervention with Pravastatin in Ischaemic Disease (LIPID) Study Group. Prevention of cardiovascular events and death with pravastatin in patients with coronary heart

disease and a broad range of initial cholesterol levels. *N Engl J Med* 1998; **339**: 1349–57.

27. Heart Protection Study Collaborative Group. MRC/BHF Heart Protection Study of cholesterol lowering with simvastatin in 20,536 high-risk individuals: a randomised placebo-controlled trial. *Lancet* 2002; **360**: 7–22.

28. PPP Project Investigators. Design, rationale, and baseline characteristics of the Prospective Pravastatin Pooling (PPP) Project – a combined analysis of three large-scale randomized trials: Long-term Intervention with Pravastatin in Ischemic Disease (LIPID), Cholesterol and Recurrent Events (CARE), and West of Scotland Coronary Prevention Study (WOSCOPS). *Am J Cardiol* 1995; **76**: 899–905.

29. Muldoon MF, Manuck SB, Matthews KA. Lowering cholesterol concentrations and mortality: a quantitative review of primary prevention trials. *BMJ* 1990; **301**: 309–14.

30. Davey-Smith G, Pekkanen J. Should there be a moratorium on the use of cholesterol-lowering drugs? *BMJ* 1992; **304**: 431–4.

31. Collins R, Keech A, Peto R, Sleight P (ISIS), Kjekshus J, Wilhelmsen L (4S), MacMahon S, Shaw J, Simes J (LIPID), Braunwald E, Buring J, Hennekens C et al. (CARE, Women's Health Study, Physicians' Health Study, SAVE), Probstfield J, Yusuf S (Post-CABG Study), Downs JR, Gotto A (AFCAPS/TexCAPS), Cobbe S, Ford I, Shepherd J (WOSCOPS). Cholesterol and total mortality: need for larger trials (Letter). *BMJ* 1992; **304**: 1689.

32. West of Scotland Coronary Primary Prevention Study Group. A coronary primary prevention study of Scottish men age 45–64 years: trial design. *J Clin Epidemiol* 1992; **45**: 849–60.

33. Sacks FM, Pfeffer MA, Moye L et al. Rationale and design of a secondary prevention trial of lowering normal plasma cholesterol levels after acute myocardial infarction: the Cholesterol and Recurrent Events trial (CARE). *Am J Cardiol* 1991; **68**: 1436–46.

34. Lipid Study Group. Design features and baseline characteristics of the LIPID (Long-term Intervention with Pravastatin in Ischaemic Disease) Study: a randomized trial in patients with previous acute myocardial infarction and/or unstable angina pectoris. *Am J Cardiol* 1995; **76**: 474–9.

35. Simes J, Furberg CD, Braunwald E et al. Effects of pravastatin on mortality in patients with and without coronary heart disease across a broad range of cholesterol levels. Prospective Pravastatin Pooling Project. *Eur Heart J* 2001; **23**: 207–15.

36. Sacks FM, Tonkin AM, Shepherd J et al., for the Prospective Pravastatin Pooling Project. Effect of pravastatin on coronary disease events in subgroups defined by coronary risk factor. The Prospective Pravastatin Pooling Project. *Circulation* 2000; **102**: 1893–900.

37. Sacks FM, Tonkin AM, Craven T et al. Coronary heart disease in patients with low LDL-cholesterol. Benefit of pravastatin in diabetics and enhanced role for HDL-cholesterol and triglycerides as risk factors. *Circulation* 2002; **105**: 1424–8.

38. Armitage J, Collins R. Need for large-scale randomised evidence about lowering LDL cholesterol in people with diabetes mellitus. MRC/BHF heart protection study and other major trials. *Heart* 2000; **84**: 357–60.

39. MRC/BHF Heart Protection Study Collaborative Group. MRC/BHF Heart Protection Study of cholesterol-lowering therapy and of antioxidant vitamin supplementation in a wide range of patients at increased risk of coronary heart disease death: early safety and efficacy experience. *Eur Heart J* 1999; **20**: 725–41.

40. Heart Protection Study Collaborative Group. MRC/BHF Heart Protection Study of antioxidant vitamin supplementation in 20,536 high-risk individuals: a randomised placebo-controlled trial. *Lancet* 2002; **360**: 23–33.

41. Heart Protection Study Collaborative Group. Heart Protection Study Homepage. http://www.ctsu.ox.ac.uk/~hps/. (Accessed 4 March 2003.)

42. Jacobs D, Blackburn H, Higgins M et al. Report of the conference on low blood cholesterol: mortality associations. *Circulation* 1992; **86**: 1046–60.

43. Carew TE, Schwenke DC, Steinberg D. Antiatherogenic effects of probucol unrelated to its hypercholesterolemic effect: evidence that antioxidants *in vivo* can selectively inhibit LDL degradation in macrophage-rich fatty streaks and slow the progression of atherosclerosis in WHHL rabbit. *Proc Natl Acad Sci USA* 1987; **84**: 7725–9.

44. Williams RJ, Motteram JM, Sharp CH et al. Dietary vitamin E and the attenuation of early lesion development in modified Watanabe rabbits. *Atherosclerosis* 1992; **94**: 153–9.

45. Stampfer MJ, Hennekens CH, Manson JE et al. Vitamin E consumption and the risk of coronary

disease in women. *N Engl J Med* 1993; **328**: 1444–9.

46. Gey KF, Puska P, Jordan P, Moser UK. Inverse correlation between plasma vitamin E and mortality from ischemic heart disease in cross-cultural epidemiology. *Am J Clin Nutr* 1991; **53** (Suppl 1): 326S–334S.

47. Heart Protection Study Collaborative Group. HPS info – slideshow presentation. http://www.ctsu.ox.ac.uk/~hps/hps_slides.shtml. (Accessed 4 March 2003.)

48. Heart Protection Study Collaborative Group. Webfigure1: Effects of simvastatin allocation on first major coronary event in different prior disease categories. *Lancet* 2002; **360**: http://image.thelancet.com/extras/02art5389webfigure1.pdf. (Accessed 4 March 2003.)

49. Heart Protection Study Collaborative Group. Webfigure2: Effects of simvastatin allocation on first major coronary event in different categories of participant. *Lancet* 2002; **360**: http://image.thelancet.com/extras/02art5389webfigure2.pdf. (Accessed 4 March 2003.)

50. Prospective Studies Collaboration. Cholesterol diastolic blood pressure, and stroke: 13,000 strokes in 450,000 people in 45 prospective cohorts. *Lancet* 1995; **346**: 1647–53.

51. Hebert PR, Gaziano JM, Hennekens CH. An overview of trials of cholesterol lowering and risk of stroke. *Arch Intern Med* 1995; **155**: 50–5.

52. Byington RP, Davis BR, Plehn JF et al. Reduction of stroke events with pravastatin – the Prospective Pravastatin Pooling (PPP) Project. *Circulation* 2001; **103**: 387–92.

53. Pfeffer MA, Keech A, Sacks FM et al. Safety and tolerability of pravastatin in long-term clinical trials. Prospective Pravastatin Pooling (PPP) Project. *Circulation* 2002; **105**: 2341–6.

12

The Prospective Study of Pravastatin in the Elderly at Risk (PROSPER)

James Shepherd, Gerard Jan Blauw, Michael B Murphy and Allan Gaw

INTRODUCTION

Circulatory diseases account for approximately 30% of the 55 million deaths that occur in the world each year, and represent the major cause of mortality in industrialized nations. In the Western world, vascular disease claims two-fifths of all lives lost, the vast majority of these coming from stroke and heart attack. While atherosclerotic coronary occlusion is the most important cause of premature death (especially among men) in Western society, its main impact overall falls on the elderly, and in particular on elderly women (Fig. 12.1).[1–3] In fact, more than 80% of those who die from coronary heart disease (CHD) are older than 65. Similarly, strokes affect primarily the elderly and women (see Fig. 12.1). In parallel with this cumulative degenerative pathology in the elderly population come the spectres of physical and mental disability, both of which will increasingly stress the healthcare and social services of industrialized countries. Particular weight needs to be given to the management of cerebral degeneration associated with Alzheimer's and ischaemic brain disease, and to the maintenance of blood flow through the coronary and peripheral arterial beds. Unfortunately, the extent of these problems, uncertainties over appropriate management strategies, and constraints on healthcare budgets all conspire to limit strategic development and the implementation of workable and affordable policies. This chapter reviews our understanding of coronary and cerebral well-being in the elderly.

CORONARY ARTERY DISEASE IN THE ELDERLY

Despite the high prevalence of coronary artery disease in elderly populations, it is still unclear whether predictors of vascular disease among the middle-aged remain clinically apt as age increases. Cholesterol, for example, which is a clear marker for premature death in the middle-aged, apparently does not carry the same predictive power in older people.[4] Initial studies,[5,6] although not entirely consistent,[7–10] suggested that while significant elevations of plasma cholesterol predicted earlier death, very low cholesterol values were similarly predictive in contrast to intermediate levels. Some interpreted these findings at face value and raised concerns over lowering plasma cholesterol too enthusiastically. Closer inspection of the data, however, led many to conclude that the low cholesterol values which ultimately were associated with premature death in fact reflected pre-existing subclinical pathology. This controversy has been revisited in the Marshfield Epidemiologic Study Area,[4] using a prospective approach which began with the registration and risk-factor assessment of 989 subjects within an observational programme – the ultimate outcome was total mortality. Ten years later they reported that in regard to plasma lipids and lipoproteins, survival among men was associated with higher baseline values of high-density lipoprotein cholesterol (HDL-C) and lower initial total cholesterol/HDL-C ratios. Individuals with HDL-C values greater than 50 mg/dl (1.3 mmol/l) had a

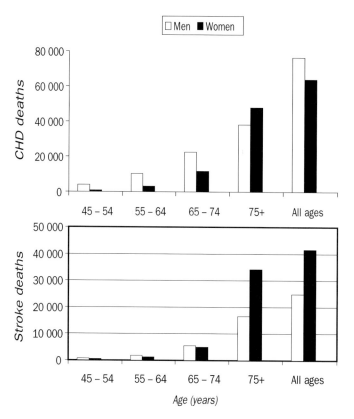

Fig. 12.1 Coronary heart disease and stroke deaths in the United Kingdom in 1997 by age.

relative risk of death of 52% that of men whose HDL-C level was below 35 mg/dl (0.9 mmol/l), and these findings were independent of age or the potentially confounding influences of CHD, stroke or cancer prevalence on all-cause mortality. Although challenged in some quarters,[10] this is consistent with earlier publications[5,11] and essentially exonerates low cholesterol as a risk factor. Interestingly, the protective effect of HDL-C appeared to act in synergy with age. Younger participants with high HDL-C had a risk of death which was 84% lower than that of older men with the lowest HDL-C. In light of these findings, it is gratifying to note that the recently published National Cholesterol Education Program guidelines[12] place greater emphasis than previously on the role of the metabolic syndrome and the cardiovascular risk associated with low HDL-C.

In contrast to the findings in men, epidemiological studies have suggested that there is no association between lipid and lipoprotein values and all-cause mortality in women older than 65,[4] despite the fact that two previous studies[5,6] that had reported positively for men had also done so for women. Whether this related to non-randomness in sample selection, to the limited number of females in the cohort, or to some more subtle metabolic phenomenon which selectively targets women and might have influenced plasma HDL-C values like the menopause[13] or the presence of sub-clinical hypothyroidism[14] is not clear at this time. Although therapeutic interventions (HRT and thyroxine replacement therapy) against both of the above independently improve the atherogenicity of the lipid risk profile, neither has been shown to alter life expectancy or improve cardiovascular risk.[15,16]

LIPID LOWERING FOR VASCULAR RISK MANAGEMENT IN THE ELDERLY

Over the last 40 years, a substantial body of research has established the importance of lipids and lipoproteins as risk factors for developing cardiovascular disease. Elevated plasma levels of total and low-density lipoprotein cholesterol (LDL-C) are associated with increased risk[17,18] while the plasma HDL-C level is inversely related to CHD risk.[19] Despite these epidemiological associations between cholesterol and risk of vascular disease, it was not until the formal testing of the lipid hypothesis that most of the clinical community took real notice of this field.

The lipid hypothesis states that an elevated plasma cholesterol level is causally associated with cardiovascular disease and that lowering it will, in turn, reduce the patient's risk of disease. This hypothesis was put to the test in a series of early trials, mainly using the bile acid sequestrant resin cholestyramine, or the fibric acid derivatives clofibrate or gemfibrozil.[20–22] Although the results of these studies in part supported the notion that cholesterol lowering was beneficial in terms of reducing cardiovascular risk, there were a number of significant concerns about the overall safety of lipid-lowering therapy. Apparent increases in non-vascular events in these trials prompted some to question the overall safety of lipid-lowering drugs[23] and others to go further and call for a halt to their prescription altogether.[24] However, such concerns were put to rest when a new generation of lipid-lowering drugs was developed and tested. The HMG-CoA reductase inhibitors, or statins, were introduced in the 1980s and used to test the lipid hypothesis in a series of landmark trials that have changed the face of preventive cardiology around the globe.[25–31]

These trials were primarily designed to answer the big questions of the day – were the statins safe and effective in moderate- or high-risk populations? At the time, the main patient group that was of concern to clinicians was middle-aged males and these were the patients who overwhelmingly constituted the study populations and who gained benefit from the statin interventions. A relatively small number of women were included in the trials and relatively few young or old patients were studied. Despite the apparent cardiovascular utility of statins in these elderly sub-groups,[28,32,33] criticisms have been levelled at the wisdom of applying the

results in these small sub-groups to the elderly population as a whole. Recent studies have significantly expanded the size of our female and elderly database;[30] and the results of PROSPER,[34] a trial specifically dedicated to examination of the value of statins in the elderly, have recently appeared in print. Prior to the availability of this information, it is useful to look at what evidence already existed to support the use of lipid-lowering drug therapy in the elderly.

In the Scandinavian Simvastatin Survival Study (4S), a sub-group analysis was performed in individuals aged 65 years or over and it was clear that this group, although relatively small in number in the study, enjoyed similar event reduction to that of their younger counterparts.[32,33] In the second major secondary prevention trial with a statin – the Cholesterol and Recurrent Events (CARE) trial – a similar analysis was performed on individuals from 60 to 80 years of age, and again the same result was found: older individuals appeared to benefit from statin therapy in much the same way as younger trial participants.[28]

Figure 12.2 shows the cardiovascular event reduction in age-specific sub-groups from the Long-term Intervention with Pravastatin in Ischaemic Disease (LIPID) study. Perhaps best of all, this demonstrates the difficulty in relying on sub-group analyses and the reasons behind the recent controversy over the use of lipid-lowering drugs in the elderly. In the LIPID study, which was a large trial performed in Australia and New Zealand involving more than 9000 subjects, the benefits of prescribing pravastatin to high-risk individuals were tested.[27] Overall, the group showed highly significant reductions in total and CHD mortality. In common with the 4S and CARE investigators, the LIPID investigators also examined the effect of age on event reduction. Younger and middle-aged groups appeared to do well, as did those up to the age of 69 years, but in the 70 and older group there was no significant change in the risk of cardiovascular events. Does this mean that those aged over 69 years do not benefit or is this simply a function of the relatively small numbers of individuals in this age group recruited into the LIPID trial, which

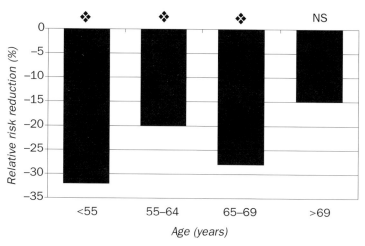

Fig. 12.2 Relative risk reductions in coronary events (CHD death and non-fatal MI) compared with placebo in high-risk patients with ischaemic heart disease receiving pravastatin: an age-dependent analysis of the Long-term Intervention with Pravastatin in Ischaemic Disease (LIPID) study.[27] (NS, non-significant; ❖, $p < 0.05$ versus placebo.)

after all was not primarily a study of the elderly? Almost certainly it is the latter, since recently published findings from PROSPER[34] and the Heart Protection Study,[30] both of which recruited more than 5000 individuals aged over 70 years, indicate that the cardiovascular benefits from statin administration are as strong in that age group as in younger individuals.

Thus far, we have looked exclusively at the evidence for using statins in the elderly to prevent CHD. However, we should not forget that one of the principal manifestations of atherosclerotic disease in the elderly is cerebrovascular disease. Stroke rates are mercifully very low in younger populations but increase exponentially as we age, with the highest rates in the over-70s. Is there any evidence that stroke rates can be affected by lipid-lowering therapy?

The first concrete evidence that manipulation of the lipid profile using a statin would reduce the risk of stroke came from a *post-hoc* analysis of the 4S study.[25,35] In this study hypercholesterolaemic patients with clinical CHD were randomized to simvastatin 20–40 mg/day or placebo and followed for approximately five years. The 4S investigators conducted a follow-up analysis of their data to determine whether simvastatin reduces cerebrovascular risk in patients with established coronary disease and raised total cholesterol levels. They observed a 28% reduction ($p = 0.03$) in the relative risk of total cerebrovascular events (stroke plus transient ischaemic attack (TIA)).

Definitive evidence that stroke rates could be reduced in high-risk individuals came from two further major statin trials: the CARE trial and the LIPID study. Importantly, in both of these studies stroke was a pre-specified end-point. In the CARE trial over 4000 survivors of myocardial infarction (MI) with average total cholesterol levels were examined. Using a fixed dose of pravastatin (40 mg/day), the investigators obtained significant reductions in the relative risk of cardiovascular events and a 32% decrease ($p = 0.03$) in the risk of stroke.[36]

The LIPID study, which is one of the larger statin intervention trials to date, used the same dose of pravastatin as in CARE and again demonstrated significant risk reduction for stroke, which was also a pre-specified end-point. In patients who had experienced either MI or unstable angina there was a 19% reduction ($p < 0.05$) in the relative risk of stroke.[27]

These clinical trials offer compelling evidence that statin therapy will reduce the risk of stroke as well as CHD in high-risk patients, but does this equally apply to the elderly? Because the majority of patients in the 4S, CARE and LIPID studies were middle-aged, some clinicians remained unconvinced about the use of statins to prevent the clinical consequences of cerebrovascular disease in the elderly. What was required was trial evidence for the prevention of both coronary and cerebrovascular disease in large, elderly cohorts. Two studies have now addressed this deficiency in our evidence portfolio.

The Heart Protection Study (HPS) has recently presented data on the effect of simvastatin in a large patient group that included over 5000 patients aged between approximately 70 and 75 years. The clear message was that this patient group benefited significantly from statin therapy.[30]

To gain insight into the value of statin therapy in a wider elderly cohort, we need to turn to the Prospective Study of Pravastatin in the Elderly at Risk (PROSPER), a project dedicated to the treatment of 70- to 82-year-old men and women at very high risk of a first or recurrent vascular event.[34]

PROSPER: PRAVASTATIN TREATMENT OF THE ELDERLY

PROSPER is a double-blind, randomized, placebo-controlled trial designed to examine the hypothesis that pravastatin at a dose of 40 mg/day will reduce the risk of cardiovascular and cerebrovascular events in elderly subjects with vascular disease or at high risk of developing vascular disease.[37] Three European co-ordinating centers – Glasgow, Scotland, Cork, Ireland and Leiden in The Netherlands – collaborated in the project, which was based in primary care (general practice), in trial centres in close proximity to each of the three co-ordinating centres.

Into this study were enrolled 5804 elderly men and women (2804 men and 3000 women), 70–82 years of age, with plasma total cholesterol of 4.0–9.0 mmol/l (155–350 mg/dl), triglycerides ≤6.0 mmol/l (530 mg/dl) and good cognitive function (Mini-Mental Score >24 at baseline),[38] using the eligibility criteria outlined in Table 12.1. Forty-four percent of the study population had evidence of vascular disease at enrolment, and the other 56% were at high risk for vascular disease because they had at least one major vascular risk factor (e.g. hypertension, cigarette smoking or diabetes mellitus).

Individuals were identified in the primary care setting during a ten-week screening and enrolment programme which ran from December 1997 to May 1999 and which, for eligible candidates, was followed by a double-blind treatment period. After two initial screening visits conducted by a study nurse, eligible subjects entered a four-week single-blind placebo lead-in period (Fig. 12.3). At the end of the placebo lead-in, the 5804 subjects who continued to satisfy the enrolment criteria (as assessed by a physician) and were ≥75% compliant with placebo medication (by tablet count) were randomized on a double-blind basis and in a 1:1 ratio to receive pravastatin 40 mg or placebo once daily for 3.2 years (see Fig. 12.3). Throughout the project, all subjects received nutritional advice and health counselling, and were exhorted to follow the National Cholesterol Education Program Step 1 diet or a local equivalent that provides <30% of total calories from fat (<10% as saturated fat) and a cholesterol intake of <300 mg/day. During the double-blind phase, subjects were seen at clinic visits in the trial centres every three months.

To assess changing cognitive function, the Mini-Mental State Examination (MMSE) and a series of psychometric tests (picture-word learning test, Stroop colour word test and letter digit coding test) were administered at each of two baseline visits, and disability questionnaires (20-point Barthel and instrumental activities of daily living) were completed.[37,39,40] We excluded individuals with poor cognitive function (MMSE score <24). The institutional ethics review boards of all centres approved the protocol, and all participants gave written informed consent. The protocol was consistent with the Declaration of Helsinki. Lipoprotein profiles were measured at baseline and then subsequently at 3, 6, 12, 24 and 36 months at the Centre for Disease Control certified central lipoprotein laboratory in Glasgow. A 12-lead electrocardiogram was recorded annually and transmitted electronically to the electrocardiogram core laboratory at Glasgow Royal Infirmary, where all computer interpretations were reviewed and automated Minnesota coding carried out.[41] The cognitive function tests and disability assessments were repeated annually. All the data were processed and analysed at the study data centre in The Robertson Centre for Biostatistics, Glasgow.

Table 12.1   Inclusion and exclusion criteria in PROSPER[37]

Inclusion criteria
- Men or women aged 70–82 years
- Total cholesterol 4.0–9.0 mmol/l
- Physician-diagnosed stable angina or intermittent claudication
- Stroke, transient ischaemic attack, myocardial infarction, arterial surgery or amputation for vascular disease >6 months prior to study entry
- One or more of the following risk factors for vascular disease:
  current smoker
  hypertension, currently receiving drug treatment
  known diabetes mellitus or fasting blood glucose >7 mmol/l

Exclusion criteria
- Recent stroke, transient ischaemic attack, myocardial infarction, arterial surgery or amputation for vascular disease ≤6 months prior to study entry
- Any surgery requiring overnight hospitalization for a medical reason (including angioplasty) ≤6 months prior to study entry
- Poor cognitive function at baseline (Mini-Mental Score Examination <24)
- Physically or mentally unable to attend the clinic for the screening visit
- Total cholesterol <4.0 mmol/l or >9.0 mmol/l
- Total triglyceride >6.0 mmol/l
- History of malignancy within the past five years except localized basal cell carcinoma of the skin
- Congestive heart failure (New York Heart Association Functional Class III or IV)
- Electrocardiographic evidence of atrial fibrillation or other significant arrhythmia or Wolff–Parkinson–White syndrome
- Implanted cardiac pacemakers with the capacity for ventricular pacing
- Organ transplant recipient
- Current lipid-lowering drug treatment
- Cyclosporin treatment
- Previous participation in a clinical trial using an HMG-CoA reductase inhibitor
- Inability to give informed consent
- Planned long-term travel or emigration within next three years
- Current alcohol or drug abuse
- Co-habitation with another trial participant
- <75% or >120% compliance with placebo lead-in medication
- Receipt of any investigational drugs (including placebo) within 30 days of enrolment
- Inability to tolerate oral medication or a history of significant malabsorption
- Any other medical condition which renders the patient unable to complete the study or which would interfere with optimal participation in the study or produce significant risk to the patient
- Abnormal laboratory findings, including:
  haemoglobin <11 g/dl and haematocrit <33%
  thyroid stimulating hormone >20 u/l or >10 u/l with an abnormal free thyroxine
  glucose >15 mmol/l
  platelet count <100 000/mm^3
  white blood cell count <3500/mm^3 or >15 000/mm^3
  serum creatinine >200 μmol/l
  aspartate aminotransferase or alanine aminotransferase >3.0 times upper limit of normal for the laboratory
  creatine kinase >3 times upper limit of normal for the laboratory

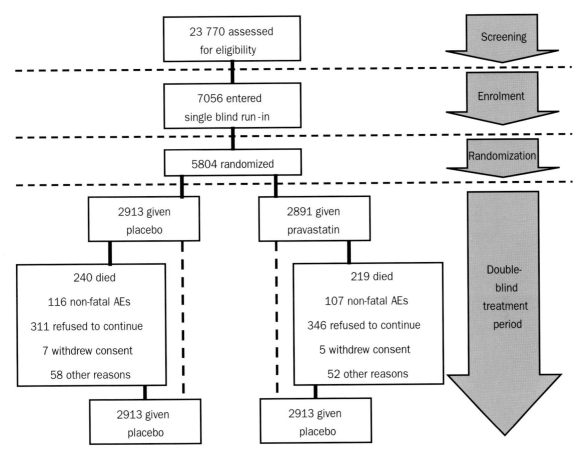

Fig. 12.3 Flow chart of PROSPER outlining major milestones and events in the conduct of the study.

Our primary outcome was the combined end-point of definite or suspect death from CHD, non-fatal MI, and fatal or non-fatal stroke, assessed in the entire cohort. Secondary outcomes included examination of the coronary and cerebrovascular components separately. Additionally, we assessed the primary outcome separately for men and women and for those with and without pre-existing disease. Tertiary end-points included an assessment of TIA, disability and cognitive function. We also planned to examine the magnitude of benefit in relation to baseline risk factors (including smoking status, history of hypertension, sex, diabetes, and LDL-C and HDL-C concentrations).[37] At baseline, the two treatment groups were balanced with respect to all relevant characteristics,[34] and compliance with the prescribed treatments was good. The proportion of potential visits to trial centres actually attended, and at which study medication was issued, was 86% in both the placebo and pravastatin groups. For participants given study medication, the average adherence, calculated as the number of pills received less the number returned at the next visit, divided by the days between these two visits, was 94% in both the placebo and pravastatin groups; 277 (10%) and 131 (5%) individuals in these respective groups initiated non-study statin therapy.

At three months' follow-up (Fig. 12.4), mean LDL-C in the pravastatin group was 2.5 mmol/l, 34% lower than the value in the placebo group, HDL-C was 5% higher, and plasma triglyceride concentrations 13% lower in compliant individuals (LDL-C 32% lower, HDL-C 5% higher and triglyceride 12% lower for the entire cohort). The

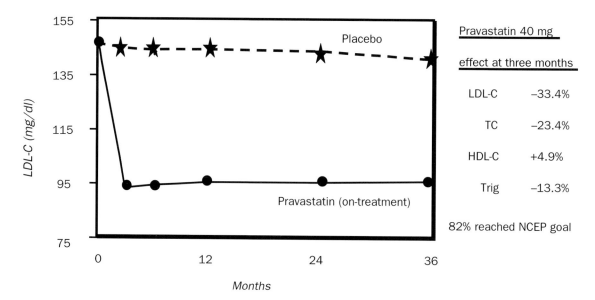

Fig. 12.4 The effects of placebo and pravastatin treatment (40 mg/day) on lipids and lipoproteins in PROSPER throughout the 3.2 years of the study; 82% of those taking pravastatin achieved the NCEP goals consistent with their risk (LDL-C = 100 mg/dl for individuals with diabetes or existing vascular disease and 130 mg/dl for others at high risk of disease because of their risk factor profile).

LDL-C reduction was sustained (see Fig. 12.4) in those who continued to take pravastatin, and at the second annual visit post randomization the pravastatin-induced decrease in LDL-C was 33% in compliant individuals and 27% in the entire cohort.

Treatment with pravastatin reduced (Fig. 12.5a) the risk of a primary end-point (CHD death, non-fatal MI or fatal or non-fatal stroke) over the 3.2 years of the study by 15% ($p = 0.014$); and when this was separated into its coronary and cerebrovascular components (Fig. 12.5b–d) it was clear that the coronary circulation fared better than the cerebrovascular tree. Coronary deaths were reduced by 24% ($p = 0.043$) and combined coronary deaths and non-fatal infarcts by 19% ($p = 0.006$). Conversely, there was no discernible effect of pravastatin treatment on cerebrovascular events (see Fig. 12.5c) although TIAs fell 25% to borderline significance ($p = 0.051$).

In order to gauge whether the benefits of pravastatin therapy were measurably different in middle-aged individuals versus the elderly PROSPER cohort, we amalgamated the results of the CARE[28] and LIPID[27] trials and truncated

the composite findings of these to the same 3.2-year treatment period as used in PROSPER. As far as the coronary circulation is concerned (Fig. 12.6), it is clear that treatment of high-risk middle-aged individuals (in CARE and LIPID) not only reduces their risk of CHD death and non-fatal MI by 24% over 5–6 years but also achieves the same effect in as little as 3.2 years. So, the response of the coronary tree in the elderly in PROSPER (a 19% reduction in composite coronary events) is the same as that seen in the middle-aged CARE and LIPID cohorts. Not surprisingly then, the number needed to treat for 3.2 years to avoid a fatal or non-fatal MI in the high-risk elderly PROSPER cohort matches closely the same variables in CARE and LIPID (Table 12.2).

But why did pravastatin (40 mg/day) not prevent strokes in PROSPER over 3.2 years whereas it had done so in the middle-aged cohorts in CARE and LIPID over five and six years' treatment respectively? To explore this issue, let us again examine the influence of the statin on stroke events[42] in the middle-aged individuals in CARE and LIPID over the same 3.2 year time frame as PROSPER (Fig. 12.7).

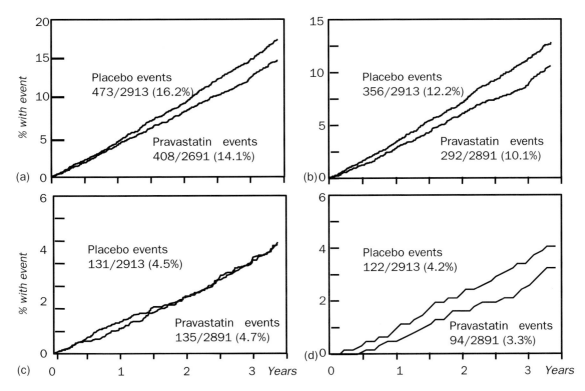

Fig. 12.5 Effects of pravastatin on major end-points in PROSPER (Kaplan–Meier analysis). (a) Primary end-point (CHD death + non-fatal MI and fatal + non-fatal stroke). Treatment reduced risk of the primary end-point by 15% (p = 0.014). (b) CHD death + non-fatal MI was reduced by 19% (p = 0.006) as a result of pravastatin. (c) Fatal + non-fatal stroke. No effect of statin therapy was evident over the 3.2 years of the study. (d) CHD death fell by 24% (p = 0.043) as a consequence of pravastatin treatment.

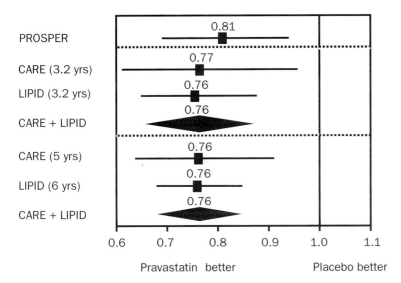

Fig. 12.6 Comparison of the coronary benefits of pravastatin (40 mg/day) in middle-aged individuals in CARE and LIPID and in the elderly PROSPER cohort. The significance of the effects of the statin is depicted in the solid symbols and the 95% confidence intervals associated with them.

Table 12.2   Comparative benefits of pravastatin 40 mg/day in preventing CHD death/non-fatal MI over 3.2 years in high-risk middle-aged or elderly patients

	RRR*	NNT**
PROSPER	19	48
LIPID	24	49
CARE	23	52
WOSCOPS	34	59
PROSPER***	22	25

* Relative risk reduction.
** Number needed to treat to prevent one CHD death or non-fatal MI.
*** Secondary prevention.

Table 12.3   Categorization of the recorded stroke events in PROSPER

	Placebo (n = 2913)	Pravastatin (n = 2891)
Ischaemic stroke	91 (3.1%)	88 (3.0%)
Intracerebral haemorrhage	8 (0/3%)	9 (0.3%)
Unspecified	32 (1.1%)	38 (1.3%)
None	2782	2756

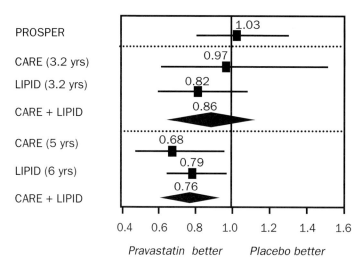

PROSPER 1.03
CARE (3.2 yrs) 0.97
LIPID (3.2 yrs) 0.82
CARE + LIPID 0.86
CARE (5 yrs) 0.68
LIPID (6 yrs) 0.79
CARE + LIPID 0.76

0.4 0.6 0.8 1.0 1.2 1.4 1.6

Pravastatin better   Placebo better

Fig. 12.7 Comparison of the stroke benefits of pravastatin (40 mg/day) over 3.2 and 5–6 years in middle-aged and elderly individuals at high risk of vascular disease. The treatment benefit seen over 5–6 years in middle-aged individuals in CARE and LIPID was not evident over a 3.2-year truncated treatment period in these studies. Consequently, the findings in CARE, LIPID and PROSPER are entirely consistent.

Clearly, five or six years of pravastatin therapy in CARE and LIPID reduced stroke risk in middle-aged individuals by 32% and 21% respectively.

However, truncation of the treatment period to 3.2 years eliminated this benefit in both trials, although the LIPID cohort, presumably because of its larger size (*n* = 9014), showed a trend towards benefit. Hence the lower stroke event rate in 9014 middle-aged individuals or in the 5804 elderly subjects in PROSPER failed to generate enough power to reveal cerebrovascular benefit after 3.2 years of pravastatin therapy.

That said, it is important to note that there was a marginal improvement in TIAs and that the failure to show stroke benefit did not derive from an increased number of haemorrhagic strokes in the pravastatin-treated cohort in PROSPER. The subjects in both treatment categories experienced the same number of intracerebral haemorrhagic events over the 3.2 years of the trial (Table 12.3).

Cursory examination of the benefits of pravastatin in the various pre-defined subgroups in PROSPER might lead one to surmise that men, especially those with pre-existing

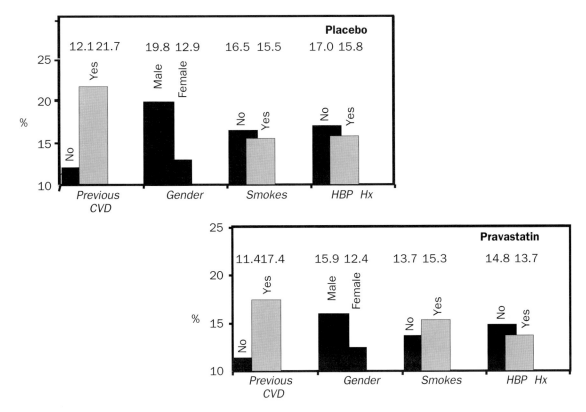

Fig. 12.8 Sub-group analysis of the benefits of pravastatin in PROSPER. CVD, cardiovascular disease; HBP Hx, history of high blood pressure.

vascular disease, gained more benefit than women. However, a more careful inspection of the data (Fig. 12.8) shows that while those at highest risk gained more absolute benefit from intervention, there was no significant difference in the response of these sub-groups to intervention. It is therefore unjustifiable to conclude that primary vascular disease prevention or statin prescriptions for women are of doubtful clinical validity among the elderly. Epidemiological studies in the elderly have suggested that LDL-C does not predict risk of either heart attack or stroke,[43,44] while HDL-C is strongly cardioprotective.[4,5,11] The PROSPER findings substantiate these proposals.[34] Variation in baseline LDL-C related neither to the risk of a coronary event nor to the efficacy of pravastatin in preventing one. Conversely, the greatest vascular risk was found among those with the lowest baseline HDL-C and these individuals gained the most from treatment.

The increased risk of incident cancer was a surprising and unexpected finding in PROSPER,[34] refuelling the controversy which arose from the finding of an inverse association between plasma cholesterol and cancer rates, especially in older persons,[45] and from the results of early trials.[23,24] More recent experience with statins in long-term trials[46] allayed concerns that there was a cause-and-effect relation, and formal meta-analyses indicate no effect of these drugs on cancer incidence.[46] The finding in PROSPER of more diagnosed cancers in those allocated to pravastatin should be interpreted in the context of this body of evidence. A meta-analysis of pravastatin trials, including PROSPER, revealed no significant effect of the drug on cancer rates.[34] Inclusion of other statin trials in this analysis lends support to this contention. Furthermore, the HPS,[30] to which large numbers of women and elderly individuals were recruited, showed no effect of

Table 12.4 Unique features of the PROSPER design

PROSPER baseline data

Characteristic	Value	Comments
Mean age (years)	75.3	First dedicated statin study at this age
% male	48	More than 50% female
History of CVD (%)	44	Equally balanced primary/secondary prevention
Total cholesterol (mg/dl)	221	Virtually unrestricted lipids
SBP/DBP (mmHg)	155/84	Higher BP than previously
Concomitant drugs	≤16	Significant polypharmacy

the drugs on cancer. That said, the PROSPER population differed in age from the other trials used in the meta-analyses, and cancer risk in all statins trials that recruit elderly individuals should be assessed. In view of the available evidence, the most likely explanation is that the imbalance in cancer rates in PROSPER was a chance finding, which could in part have been driven by the recruitment of individuals with occult disease. This proposal is currently under investigation by detailed analysis of the PROSPER database.

Finally, what should the busy primary care physician make of PROSPER? First, the uniqueness of its features should be recognised (Table 12.4). It is the first study exclusively dedicated to the elderly, and it speaks loudly in favour of managing their vascular risk with lipid-lowering statin therapy. More than half of the individuals recruited to the project were women, and they gained as much benefit as did the men. Forty-four percent of recruits came to the trial with clinically evident vascular disease and the remainder were at high risk of a first vascular event. Despite this high risk (greater on average – 5.1% per annum risk of a primary end-point – than any of the other statin trials), tangible benefit was apparent within the short space of 3.2 years of statin treatment. Baseline total cholesterol or LDL-C did not predict who were at greatest risk or would gain most from therapy. However, low HDL-C was a strong indicator of both. Consequently, targeting statins at elderly individuals with low HDL-C and high vascular

risk, irrespective of their total plasma cholesterol value, makes good clinical sense. And finally, despite the presence of significant polypharmacy in PROSPER (average drug consumption was four different medications per day), this proved not to be a barrier to statin therapy. Liver dysfunction and myopathy were conspicuously absent over the 3.2-year trial period. The findings of PROSPER therefore suggest that the vascular risk management strategy currently applied to the middle-aged would offer similar cardiovascular benefits to the elderly.

REFERENCES

1. Office for National Statistics, London.
2. General Register Office, Edinburgh.
3. Statistics and Research Agency, Belfast, Northern Ireland.
4. Chyou P-H, Eaker ED. Serum cholesterol concentrations and all-cause mortality in older people. *Age Ageing* 2000; **29**: 69–74.
5. Nikkila M, Heikkinen J. Serum cholesterol, high-density lipoprotein cholesterol and five-year survival in elderly people. *Age Ageing* 1990; **19**: 403–8.
6. White AD, Haines CG, Tyroler HA. Serum cholesterol and 20-year mortality in black and white men and women aged 65 and older in the Evans County Heart Study. *Ann Epidemiol* 1992; **2**: 85–91.
7. Paterson TC, Armstrong R, Armstrong EC. Serum lipid levels and the severity of coronary and cerebral atherosclerosis in adequately nourished men 60–69 years of age. *Circulation* 1963; **27**: 229–36.
8. Agner E. Some cardiovascular risk markers are also important in old age. *Acta Med Scand* 1984; **696** (Suppl): 1–50.

9. Anderson KM, Castelli WP, Levy D. Cholesterol and mortality. 30 years of follow-up from the Framingham Study. *JAMA* 1987; **257**: 2176–80.

10. Krumholz HM, Seeman TE, Merrill SS et al. Lack of association between cholesterol and coronary heart disease mortality and morbidity and all-cause mortality in persons older than 70 years. *JAMA* 1994; **272**: 1335–40.

11. Zimetbaum P, Fuchman WH, Ooi WL et al. Plasma lipids and lipoproteins and the incidence of cardiovascular disease in the very elderly. *Atheroscler Thromb* 1992; **12**: 416–23.

12. Executive Summary of the Third Report of the National Cholesterol Education Program (NCEP) Expert Panel on Detection, Evaluation and Treatment of High Blood Cholesterol in Adults (Adults Treatment Panel III). *JAMA* 2001; **285**: 2486–97.

13. Binder EF, Williams DB, Schechtman KB et al. Effects of hormone replacement therapy on serum lipids in elderly women. *Ann Intern Med* 2001; **134**: 754–60.

14. Kahaly GJ. Cardiovascular and atherogenic aspects of subclinical hypothyroidism. *Thyroid* 2000; **10**: 665–79.

15. Sawin CT, Geller A, Hershman JM et al. The aging thyroid. The use of thyroid hormone in older persons. *JAMA* 1989; **261**: 2653–5.

16. Poulter N. Oestrogen and protection against cardiovascular disease potential versus reality. *Br J Cardiol* 2001; **7**: 383–90.

17. Castelli WP. Epidemiology of coronary heart disease: the Framingham study. *Am J Med* 1984; **76**: 4–12.

18. Stamler J, Wentworth D, Neaton JD. Is the relationship between serum cholesterol and risk of premature death from coronary heart disease continuous and graded? Findings in 356,222 primary screenees of the Multiple Risk Factor Intervention Trial (MRFIT). *JAMA* 1986; **256**: 2823–8.

19. Assmann G, Schulte H. Relation of high-density lipoprotein cholesterol and triglyceride to incidence of atherosclerosis coronary artery disease (the PROCAM experience). *Am J Cardiol* 1992; **70**: 733–7.

20. Lipid Research Clinics Program. The Lipid Research Clinics Coronary Primary Prevention Trial results. I. Reduction in incidence of coronary heart disease. *JAMA* 1984; **251**: 351–64.

21. Frick MH, Elo O, Haapa K et al. Helsinki Heart Study: primary prevention trial with gemfibrozil in middle-aged men with dyslipidemia: safety of treatment, changes in risk factors, and incidence of coronary heart disease. *N Engl J Med* 1987; **317**: 1237–45.

22. Report from the committee of principal investigators. A co-operative trial in the primary prevention of ischaemic heart disease using clofibrate. *Br Heart J* 1978; **40**: 1069–118.

23. Keech AC. Does cholesterol lowering reduce total mortality? *Postgrad Med J* 1992: **68**: 870–1.

24. Davey Smith G, Pekkanen J. Should there be a moratorium on the use of cholesterol lowering drugs? *BMJ* 1992; **304**: 431–4.

25. Scandinavian Simvastatin Survival Study Group. Randomised trial of cholesterol lowering in 4444 patients with coronary heart disease: the Scandinavian Simvastatin Survival Study (4S). *Lancet* 1994; **344**: 1383–9.

26. Shepherd J, Cobbe SM, Ford I et al. Prevention of coronary heart disease with pravastatin in men with hypercholesterolemia. *N Engl J Med* 1995; **333**: 1301–7.

27. Long-term Intervention with Pravastatin in Ischemic Disease (LIPID) Study Group. Prevention of cardiovascular events and death with pravastatin in patients with coronary heart disease and a broad range of initial cholesterol levels. *N Engl J Med* 1998; **339**: 1349–57.

28. Sacks FM, Pfeffer MA, Moye LA et al. for the Cholesterol and Recurrent Events Trial Investigators. The effect of pravastatin on coronary events after myocardial infarction in patients with average cholesterol levels. *N Engl J Med* 1996; **335**: 1001–9.

29. Downs JR, Clearfield M, Weis S et al. Primary prevention of acute coronary events with lovastatin in men and women with average cholesterol levels: results of AFCAPS/TexCAPS Research Group. *JAMA* 1998; **279**: 1615–22.

30. Heart Protection Study Collaborative Group. MRC/BHF Heart Protection Study of cholesterol lowering with simvastatin in 20,536 high-risk individuals: a randomised placebo-controlled trial. *Lancet* 2002; **360**: 7–22.

31. Sever PS, Dahlof B, Poulter NR et al. Prevention of coronary and stroke events with atorvastatin in hypertensive patients who have average or lower-than-average cholesterol concentrations, in the Anglo-Scandinavian Cardiac Outcomes Trial – Lipid-Lowering Arm (ASCOT-LLA): a multicentre randomised controlled trial. *Lancet* 2003; **361**: 1149–58.

32. Miettinen TA, Pyörälä K, Olsson AG et al. Cholesterol-lowering therapy in women and

elderly patients with myocardial infarction or angina pectoris. *Circulation* 1997; **96**: 4211–18.

33. Pedersen TR, Wilhelmsen L, Faergeman O et al. Follow-up study of patients randomised in the Scandinavian Simvastatin Survival Study of cholesterol lowering. *Am J Cardiol* 2000; **86**: 257–62.

34. Shepherd J, Blauw GJ, Murphy MB et al. Pravastatin in elderly individuals at risk of vascular disease (PROSPER): a randomised controlled trial. *Lancet* 2002; **360**: 1623–30.

35. Pedersen TR, Kjekshus J, Pyörälä K et al. Effect of simvastatin on ischemic signs and symptoms in the Scandinavian Simvastatin Survival Study (4S). *Am J Cardiol* 1998; **81**: 333–5.

36. Plehn JF, Davis BR, Sacks FM et al. Reduction of stroke incidence after myocardial infarction with pravastatin: the Cholesterol and Recurrent Events (CARE) study. *Circulation* 1999; **99**: 216–23.

37. Shepherd J, Blauw GJ, Murphy MB et al. The design of a prospective study of pravastatin in the elderly at risk (PROSPER). *Am J Cardiol* 1999; **84**: 1192–7.

38. Folstein MF, Folstein SE, McHugh PR. Mini-Mental State: a practical method for grading the cognitive state of patients for the clinician. *J Psychiatr Res* 1975; **12**: 189–98.

39. Ford I, Blauw GJ, Murphy MB et al. A prospective study of pravastatin in the elderly at risk (PROSPER): screening experience and baseline characteristics. *Curr Controlled Trials Cardiovasc Med* 2002; **3**: 8–14.

40. Houx PJ, Shepherd J, Blauw GJ et al. Testing cognitive function in elderly populations: the PROSPER Study. *J Neurol Neurosurg Psychiatry* 2002; **73**: 385–9.

41. Macfarlane PW, Latif S. Automated serial ECG comparison based on the Minnesota Code. *J Electrocardiol* 1996; **29** (Suppl): 29–34.

42. Byington RP, Dans BR, Plehn JF et al. for the PPP investigators. Reduction of stroke events with pravastatin. *Circulation* 2001; **103**: 387–92.

43. Shipley MJ, Pocock, SJ, Marmot HG. Does plasma cholesterol concentration predict mortality from coronary heart disease in elderly people? 18-year follow-up of the Whitehall Study. *BMJ* 1991; **303**: 89–92.

44. Prospective Studies Collaboration. Cholesterol, diastolic blood pressure and stroke: 13,000 strokes in 450,000 people in 45 prospective cohorts. *Lancet* 1995; **346**: 1647–53.

45. Weverling-Rijnsburger AW, Blauw GJ, Lagaay MA et al. Total cholesterol and risk of mortality in the oldest old. *Lancet* 1997; **350**: 1119–23.

46. Bjerre LM, LeLorier J. Do statins cause cancer? A Meta-analysis of large randomised clinical trials. *Am J Med* 2001; **110**: 716–23.

13

Combination therapy with statins

Gilbert R Thompson

INTRODUCTION

Monotherapy with one of the statins does not always lower low-density lipoprotein (LDL) cholesterol and triglycerides or raise high-density lipoprotein (HDL) cholesterol to the required extent and it is sometimes necessary to combine their administration with other lipid-regulating drugs. For example, in severe familial hypercholesterolaemia (FH) even maximal doses of statins do not always lower LDL cholesterol sufficiently and an anion-exchange resin is often added. Also, in mixed dyslipidaemia, statin monotherapy may fail to reduce triglycerides and raise HDL cholesterol to the desired levels and it may be necessary to add either nicotinic acid (niacin) or a fibrate to achieve these objectives.

Mixed dyslipidaemia is especially common in type 2 diabetes and is a more important determinant of prognosis than is hyperglycaemia. Based on sub-group analyses of the Scandinavian Simvastatin Survival Study (4S)[1] and the Cholesterol and Recurrent Events (CARE) trial,[2] respectively, simvastatin and pravastatin have both been shown to be effective in reducing the risk of coronary heart disease (CHD) in diabetics. However, so too has gemfibrozil,[3] which suggests that lowering LDL cholesterol with a statin or reducing triglycerides and increasing HDL cholesterol with a fibrate are equally useful in this context. This raises the question as to whether a combination of the two approaches would provide even greater benefit in terms of secondary prevention than either alone. The safety of combined statin/fibrate therapy has been questioned because of the perception that

this may increase the risk of myositis. However, in the original report[4] all the cases developing this complication had received a statin combined with gemfibrozil. Other fibrates do not appear to carry the same risk and the chances of developing myositis with any of the statins combined with bezafibrate or fenofibrate seem to be acceptably low.

An additional reason for combination therapy is to improve the response of patients who are refractory to statins. Inter-individual variability in response to these drugs is well recognized and occurs to a similar extent in patients with FH as in those with non-familial hypercholesterolaemia; this suggests that variations in receptor-mediated LDL catabolism are not responsible. Instead it seems that genetic variability in cholesterol absorption is an important determinant of statin responsiveness. This is illustrated by the sub-group analysis conducted on the Finnish cohort of 4S, who were divided into quartiles according to their serum cholestanol-to-cholesterol ratio.[5] Cholestanol was used as an index of cholesterol absorption, those in the lowest quartile of the cholestanol-to-cholesterol ratio being regarded as hypo-absorbers, and those in the highest quartile as hyper-absorbers. As expected, there was an inverse correlation between cholesterol absorption and synthesis, the latter reflected by the lathosterol-to-cholesterol ratio. Values of serum cholesterol were similar in each quartile at baseline, but in subjects treated with simvastatin the subsequent reduction in serum cholesterol in the high absorbers and low synthesizers was less marked than in those who absorbed less cholesterol and synthesized more

Table 13.1 Comparative effects of lipid-regulating drugs

Daily dose [ref.]	Mean change (%)		
	LDL-C	HDL-C	TG
Atorvastatin 40 mg [10]	−51	+5	−32
Nicotinic acid 4 g [11]	−9	+43	−34
Gemfibrozil 1.2 g [12]	−18	+12	−40
Ezetimibe 10 mg [13]	−18.5	+3.5	−4.9

LDL-C, low-density lipoprotein cholesterol; HDL-C, high-density lipoprotein cholesterol; TG, triglycerides.

and there was a less marked decrease in their lathosterol-to-cholesterol ratio. Thus, those whose basal cholesterol synthesis rate was low showed a lesser decrease in synthesis when treated with simvastatin than those whose synthesis rate was initially high.

Using mevalonic acid rather than lathosterol as an index of cholesterol synthesis in refractory FH patients, Naoumova et al.[6] had also found that a poor response to statins was associated with a low basal rate of cholesterol synthesis. One possibility is that the latter was secondary to increased cholesterol absorption due to inheritance of the apoE4 allele.[7] An alternative explanation might be the inheritance of *ABC G5* and *G8* gene polymorphisms, which predispose to increased cholesterol absorption.[8] Combining statins with drugs such as ezetimibe, which block cholesterol absorption and up-regulate its synthesis, has obvious therapeutic potential in these circumstances.[9]

COMPARATIVE EFFICACY OF STATINS, NICOTINIC ACID, FIBRATES AND EZETIMIBE

Table 13.1 compares the lipid-regulating effects of monotherapy with nicotinic acid, gemfibrozil and ezetimibe versus atorvastatin. The latter is currently the most effective statin on the market in terms of LDL-lowering efficacy, and none of the other three drugs shown in Table 13.1 can match it in this respect. However, nicotinic acid and gemfibrozil each have a greater HDL cho-

lesterol raising effect and both lower triglycerides to a similar or more marked extent than atorvastatin 40 mg daily. Hence either nicotinic acid or a fibrate would be appropriate adjuvant therapy with a statin in mixed dyslipidaemia. In contrast, ezetimibe may be a more suitable choice in circumstances where there is a need to enhance the LDL-lowering effect of a statin or else just maintain it, but at a reduced dosage.

Nicotinic acid

The lipid-regulating effects of large doses of nicotinic acid (usually known as niacin in the USA) were first described in 1962. Long-term follow-up of patients who participated in the Coronary Drug Project showed a reduction in total mortality in those taking nicotinic acid during the trial and the drug would be more widely used were it not for its side-effects. The most prominent of these is cutaneous flushing, which is mediated by prostaglandins. Other adverse effects are skin rashes, gastrointestinal upsets, hyperuricaemia, hyperglycaemia and hepatic dysfunction. Sustained-release preparations reduce flushing but accentuate the risk of hepatitis.[14]

However, a recently developed extended-release form of nicotinic acid (Niaspan) seems to be free from this drawback.[15] At the maximum recommended dose of 2 g daily, decreases in LDL cholesterol, triglycerides and Lp(a) averaged 17%, 35% and 24% respectively, whereas HDL cholesterol increased by 26%. Although 30% of those randomized to Niaspan failed to complete the study because of side-effects, the frequency of abnormal liver function tests was similar to that on placebo.

EFFICACY, TOLERABILITY AND SAFETY OF STATIN/NICOTINIC ACID COMBINATION THERAPY

The combined administration of a statin and nicotinic acid was first described over ten years ago, lovastatin being the statin used in that instance.[14] In a retrospective survey, 22 patients receiving this combination for up to 18 months

Table 13.2   Lipid-regulating effects of statin/nicotinic acid combination therapy compared with statin monotherapy

Ref.	Statin (mg/day)	NA (g/day)	Patients	n	Weeks	Δ Statin + NA vs Statin		
						LDL-C	HDL-C	TG
18	L 80	3	HC	8	ns	−19%	+21%	−8%
19	P 40	1–2	HC	154	8	−9%	+3%	−21%
20	L 20	1.2	HC	25	12	−12%	+2%	−16%
21	P 20	3	HTG	39	6	−11%	+29%	−27%
22	A, S, P, F 5–80	1	HC or HTG	66	4–12	−8%	+23%	−24%

NA, nicotinic acid; L, lovastatin; P, pravastatin; F, fluvastatin; A, atorvastatin; S, simvastatin; HC, hypercholesterolaemic; HTG, hypertriglyceridaemic; ns, not stated.

showed no untoward side-effects and a statistical comparison in 11 of these patients showed that combination therapy decreased serum cholesterol to a significantly greater extent than nicotinic acid alone. A year-long, open-label study subsequently showed that concomitant administration of lovastatin, pravastatin or simvastatin with Niaspan decreased LDL cholesterol to a greater extent than Niaspan alone in hypercholesterolaemic patients (by 32% vs 18%) without unduly increasing the frequency of adverse events.[16] Flushing caused the withdrawal of 5% of patients taking Niaspan and 2% of those on a concomitant statin had to discontinue the latter because of an increased transaminase, but there were no cases of myositis. Similar results were observed in a placebo-controlled trial of fluvastatin and nicotinic acid versus nicotinic acid.[17]

Of greater interest are studies which have compared the effects of combination therapy with those of statin alone (Table 13.2). Three were placebo-controlled randomized trials,[19–21] one was an open-label study[18] and one was a retrospective analysis.[22] In all five studies the combination of nicotinic acid with a statin resulted in greater decreases in LDL cholesterol and triglycerides, and greater increases in HDL cholesterol than occurred with statin monotherapy. Decreases in LDL cholesterol and increases in HDL cholesterol tended to be more marked with high doses of nicotinic acid

whereas percentage decreases in triglyceride were greater in hypertriglyceridaemic than in hypercholesterolaemic patients.

In the two trials which used 1–1.2 g of nicotinic acid daily, the frequency of clinical and laboratory events did not differ between the statin monotherapy and combination therapy groups.[20,22] However, at higher doses of nicotinic acid, the frequency of clinical adverse events and of drop-outs was higher in those on combination therapy than in those on statin alone.[19,21] Likewise, increases in liver transaminases were more marked on combination therapy than on statin, although no significant increase in creatine phosphokinase levels was observed with either treatment regimen.[19]

The published data show that the addition of nicotinic acid 1–3 g daily lowers LDL cholesterol on average by 10% below the level achieved by statin monotherapy, but at the cost of decreased tolerability. Hence it is doubtful whether this combination could be recommended solely on the grounds of its LDL-lowering potential. However, in patients with raised triglycerides and/or low HDL cholesterol, a similar reduction in LDL cholesterol is accompanied by decreases in triglycerides and increases in HDL cholesterol in the region of 25%, which more than compensates for the side-effects of the nicotinic acid component of the combined regimen. An additional reason for using the latter is to treat raised levels of Lp(a), which are unresponsive to statin monotherapy but decrease markedly on nicotinic acid.[11]

The value of simultaneously lowering LDL cholesterol and raising HDL cholesterol has been clearly demonstrated in a trial of patients with coronary heart disease (CHD) associated with a low HDL cholesterol but normal LDL cholesterol.[23] Angiographic regression of coronary disease and a drastic reduction in clinical events were documented in those randomized to receive low-dose simvastatin combined with nicotinic acid 2.4 g daily. These benefits were attributable both to the 42% decrease in LDL cholesterol and to the 26% increase in HDL cholesterol which ensued. However, in patients given concomitant anti-oxidant vitamins, the increase in HDL cholesterol was attenuated[24] and the angiographic and clinical benefits were less marked than in those receiving simvastatin plus nicotinic acid without anti-oxidants. Although the mechanism of the adverse effect of the latter on HDL is unclear, these findings illustrate the importance of the HDL-raising effect of nicotinic acid. Despite the lack of a simvastatin monotherapy group in this trial, it is most unlikely that simvastatin used alone, in a dose which averaged only 13 mg daily, would have achieved changes in LDL and HDL cholesterol comparable to those seen on combination therapy. In the light of these findings, it is of interest that a formulation containing lovastatin 10 mg and extended-release nicotinic acid 0.5 g has recently been developed and shown to be well tolerated and effective.[25]

FIBRATES

The lipid-regulating properties of fibrates were first described almost 40 years ago. The five compounds marketed in the UK are clofibrate, bezafibrate, fenofibrate, gemfibrozil and ciprofibrate. All are effective in controlling hypertriglyceridaemia and in raising HDL cholesterol but they vary in their ability to reduce LDL cholesterol, fenofibrate and ciprofibrate being the most potent. Clofibrate, the prototype, is now obsolete because it increases biliary cholesterol secretion and doubles the risk of developing gallstones. A rare side-effect of clofibrate and of the other fibrates is an acute myositic syndrome accompanied by an increase in creatine phosphokinase (CK), patients with renal impairment being particularly vulnerable.

Gemfibrozil is a homologue of clofibrate but has a much shorter plasma half-life. During the Helsinki Heart Study, the average changes in serum lipids induced by gemfibrozil 1.2 g daily were a 10% decrease in LDL cholesterol, 43% decrease in triglyceride and 10% increase in HDL cholesterol.[26] Accompanying reductions in the incidence of primary CHD events by gemfibrozil were attributable both to the decrease in LDL cholesterol and the increase in HDL cholesterol and were most marked in individuals with triglyceride >2.3 mmol/l (200 mg/dl) and LDL:HDL cholesterol ratio >5.[27] Additional evidence of the benefits of gemfibrozil came from the Veterans Affairs High Density Lipoprotein Cholesterol Intervention Trial (VAHIT), which showed that the drug reduced the risk of secondary events in elderly men with a low HDL cholesterol.[3] More recently, the Bezafibrate Infarction Prevention (BIP) trial demonstrated the benefits of bezafibrate in secondary prevention of CHD in hypertriglyceridaemic subjects.[28]

EFFICACY AND TOLERABILITY OF STATIN/FIBRATE COMBINATION THERAPY

Comparison of statin/fibrate combination therapy with fibrate alone shows that the former achieves significantly greater reductions in LDL cholesterol[29,30] and triglyceride,[30] as would be expected. However, as with statins plus nicotinic acid, the comparison between combination therapy and statin monotherapy is of greater relevance.

Table 13.3 compares the lipid-regulating effects of statin/fibrate combination therapy with statin monotherapy which were observed in six trials. Four of these were randomized, placebo-controlled studies[30–33] and two were long-term open-label studies.[34,35] In the two trials involving hypercholesterolaemic patients, combination therapy resulted in mean decreases in LDL cholesterol and triglyceride and increases in HDL cholesterol which were 8%, 10% and 27% greater than those on statin monotherapy.[31,32] In

Table 13.3   Lipid-regulating effects of statin/fibrate combination therapy compared with statin monotherapy

Ref.	Statin (mg/day)	Fibrate (mg/day)	Patients	n	Weeks	Δ Statin + Fibrate vs Statin		
						LDL-C	HDL-C	TG
31	P 40	G 1200	HC	65	12	−3.5%	+11%	−27.5%
32	F 40	B 400	HC	19	6	−13%	+8%	−26%
33	F 40	G 1200	MHL	21	6	+8%	+8%	−51%
30	S 20	B 400	MHL	25	12	+4%	+7%	−26%
34	S 10, P 20	f 300, mf 200	MHL	80	104	+2%	+7%	−32%
35	S 20	B 400	MHL	100	52	+2%	+11%	−29%

P, pravastatin; F, fluvastatin; S, simvastatin; G, gemfibrozil; B, bezafibrate; f, fenofibrate; mf, micronized fenofibrate; HC, hypercholesterolaemia; MHL, mixed hyperlipidaemia.

contrast, in the four trials involving patients with mixed hyperlipidaemia,[30,33–35] combination therapy resulted in 2–8% increases in LDL cholesterol compared with statin monotherapy whereas changes in HDL cholesterol and triglycerides were similar in direction and magnitude to those seen in hypercholesterolaemic patients. One of the trials involved diabetic patients, in whom combination therapy resulted in significant decreases in fibrinogen and Lp(a), potentially beneficial changes which did not occur with statin monotherapy.[35]

In general, statin/fibrate drug combinations were well tolerated and the incidence of clinical and laboratory adverse events was similar to that observed with monotherapy with statins and fibrates. However, two of 75 patients on pravastatin/gemfibrozil combination therapy were withdrawn from one study on account of asymptomatic elevations of CK,[31] and in another study myopathy occurred in two of 48 subjects on simvastatin/bezafibrate combination therapy and in one of 100 subjects receiving simvastatin alone.[35] The extent to which combination therapy increases the risk of muscle damage is discussed in greater detail below.

SAFETY OF STATINS AND FIBRATES

Considering that they inhibit such a key enzyme as HMG-CoA reductase, statins are remarkably safe drugs. Theoretical concerns in the past related to cataract formation and liver damage but neither of these has materialized despite the administration of these drugs to millions of patients during the past 15 years. For example, in the recent Heart Protection Study (HPS), the incidence of asymptomatic increases in hepatic alanine aminotransferase (ALT) in over 10 000 patients given simvastatin 40 mg daily for five years was less than 1%.[36] The only potentially fatal side-effect of statins is myositis, which can lead to rhabdomyolysis and renal failure. Under certain circumstances the risk of myositis is enhanced by concomitant fibrate therapy.

The chances of myositis and rhabdomyolysis occurring during monotherapy with most statins is exceedingly low. Farmer recently analysed data from over 30 000 patients who had received pravastatin, simvastatin or lovastatin for periods of five years or more and found that the incidence of myositis was 0.1%, identical to that on placebo.[37] In the HPS the frequency of CK elevations over ten times the upper limit of normal was 0.09% in patients on simvastatin compared with 0.05% in those on placebo.[36] The likelihood of this complication occurring is dose-related and is increased by concomitant treatment with drugs which inhibit the cytochrome P450 3A4 pathway, via which most statins are metabolized. Prominent among these compounds is cyclosporin, which markedly increases statin blood levels and the risks of myositis and rhabdomyolysis.[38]

The fact that fibrates can increase the risk of myositis in patients on statins first came to light in 1990, when the US Food and Drug Administration (FDA) received 12 case reports of myositis associated with concomitant use of lovastatin and gemfibrozil.[4] All patients had CK levels over ten times the upper limit of normal and five developed acute renal failure. Subsequent estimates of the frequency of myositis in those on statin/fibrate combination therapy vary from 0.12%[39] to 1%.[40] In a third survey the incidence was 0.34%,[41] with gemfibrozil the culpable fibrate in every instance, as in the original FDA report.

The relevance of this observation became clear following 31 fatal cases of myositis associated with the use of cerivastatin in the USA, 12 of whom were also receiving gemfibrozil.[37] Most of the remainder were on a high dose of cerivastatin alone, which raises questions as to whether this statin is inherently more myotoxic than the others.[42] The drug has now been withdrawn by the manufacturers.

All fibrates can cause myositis[40] and there is nothing to suggest that gemfibrozil is especially prone to cause this complication on its own. However, concomitant administration of gemfibrozil with lovastatin or simvastatin leads to markedly elevated levels of these compounds via a non-cytochrome P450-dependent mechanism.[43,44] In contrast, bezafibrate has no effect on statin blood levels.[44] Therefore it seems clear that gemfibrozil should not be co-administered with any statin, apart possibly from fluvastatin,[45] whereas all the other fibrates appear to be relatively safe in this respect, except in patients with renal insufficiency.

CHOLESTEROL ABSORPTION AND EFFECTS OF INHIBITION

An association between the efficiency with which cholesterol is absorbed and the concentration of cholesterol in plasma, especially in LDL, has long been recognized. In part, this derives from observations in both experimen-

tal animals and man concerning the basis of the twin phenomena of hypo- and hyper-responsiveness to dietary cholesterol. Hypo-responders have been shown to absorb a lower percentage of cholesterol than do hyper-responders when the dietary intake is raised and exhibit a smaller increase in LDL cholesterol. As mentioned earlier, the likelihood is that these traits are genetically determined, possession of the apoE4 allele, for example, being associated with a hyper-absorptive and hyper-responsive tendency.[9] Another putative source of genetic variation is polymorphism of the ABC G8 transporter, which is involved in regulating intestinal cholesterol efflux.[8] Up-regulation of the latter mechanism could explain why the efficiency with which cholesterol is absorbed decreases when the intake is raised;[46] hyper-responders may lack this adaptive response.

Further evidence that cholesterol absorption efficiency and LDL cholesterol concentration are causally related comes from studies of pharmacological inhibitors of cholesterol absorption. For example, neomycin, a polycationic compound, interacts with bile acid and fatty acid anions to precipitate mixed micelles within the intestinal lumen whereas plant sterols and stanols reduce the micellar solubilization of cholesterol. Both mechanisms inhibit cholesterol absorption and a linear correlation has been shown between decreases in cholesterol absorption and LDL cholesterol in subjects given neomycin and sitostanol ester; this was accompanied by a doubling in the rate of cholesterol synthesis.[47]

Recently, a specific and saturable pathway has been identified which mediates the transport of cholesterol from mixed micelles into enterocytes.[48] A novel class of compounds, 2-azetidinone derivatives, has now been shown to interact with the protein in the intestinal brush border membrane which constitutes this putative cholesterol transporter, thereby providing a third mechanism for inhibiting cholesterol absorption.[49] The first of these cholesterol absorption inhibitors to undergo clinical trials, ezetimibe, has recently been launched.

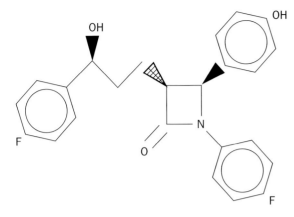

Fig. 13.1 Chemical structure of ezetimibe (SCH 58235).

EZETIMIBE

Ezetimibe (SCH 58235) is 1-(4-fluorophenyl)-(3R)-[3-(4-fluorophenyl)-(3S)-hydroxypropyl]-(4S)-(4-hydroxyphenyl)-2-azetidinone,[50] as shown in Fig. 13.1. Oral administration to rats showed that the compound is rapidly absorbed and extensively glucuronidated by the small intestine and then excreted as the glucuronide in bile.[51] The glucuronide localizes in the intestinal mucosa and inhibits cholesterol absorption more efficiently than the parent compound. Administration to apoE knockout mice showed that ezetimibe almost totally inhibited cholesterol absorption, markedly lowered plasma cholesterol and decreased the extent of aortic and carotid atherosclerosis.[52]

Randomized, placebo-controlled trials in hypercholesterolaemic subjects show dose-dependent reductions in LDL cholesterol over the range 0.25–10 mg daily.[53] The mean decrease in LDL cholesterol on ezetimibe 10 mg daily was 18.5%, which was accompanied by a 3.5% increase in HDL cholesterol and a non-significant 5% decrease in serum triglyceride. The drug has a half-life of 24 hours and is equally effective whether taken in the morning or evening and with or without food. Ezetimibe was well tolerated and the frequency of adverse events in more than 400 subjects over a period of 12 weeks was similar to that in the placebo group.

COMBINED THERAPY WITH EZETIMIBE AND STATINS

Studies in dogs show that ezetimibe caused only small decreases in plasma cholesterol, due to the compensatory increase in cholesterol synthesis engendered by the inhibition of dietary and biliary cholesterol absorption.[54] Statin monotherapy also had little effect, but the combined administration of ezetimibe and a statin to chow-fed animals resulted in decreases in plasma cholesterol of 30–60%.

Published data in humans are scanty but a preliminary report shows that concomitant administration of ezetimibe and simvastatin, each in a dose of 10 mg daily, decreased LDL cholesterol by 17% more than simvastatin alone.[55] These data were obtained in hypercholesterolaemic men on a low-fat diet and suggest an additive rather than a synergistic interaction between the two drugs, as was seen in dogs.

Further evidence of an additive effect has come from a study undertaken in 50 patients with homozgyous FH,[56] half of whom were undergoing LDL apheresis and continued to do so during the trial. The latter was designed to compare the effects of ezetimibe 10 mg plus atorvastatin or simvastatin 40 or 80 mg daily versus the effects of atorvastatin or simvastatin 80 mg daily, each regimen being tested by its ability to lower LDL cholesterol below baseline values achieved on atorvastatin or simvastatin 40 mg daily. Results in those on ezetimibe 10 mg plus statin 80 mg daily showed that the combined therapy lowered LDL cholesterol levels by an additional 20.5% compared with statin alone (Fig. 13.2). The drug combination was well tolerated and the only significant adverse event was an asymptomatic rise in aminotransferases in one patient, which was also observed in one patient on statin alone.

CONCLUSION

Statins provide a well-proven means of treating dyslipidaemia and preventing CHD, due mainly to their ability to lower LDL levels in a safe and effective manner. However, not everyone responds equally well to statins and a

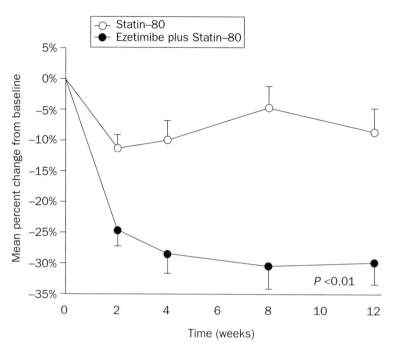

Fig. 13.2 Percentage change in LDL cholesterol from baseline (value on diet plus statin 40 mg daily) in FH homozygotes treated with atorvastatin or simvastatin 80 mg daily, with or without concomitant ezetimibe 10 mg daily. (Adapted with permission from ref. 56.)

significant minority fail to benefit from treatment.[57] Furthermore, statins have only moderate triglyceride-lowering and HDL-raising properties, and fibrates and nicotinic acid are both more effective when the pattern of dyslipidaemia to be treated is characterized by increases in triglyceride and decreases in HDL cholesterol without any increase in LDL. For these reasons the combined use of one or other of these compounds with statins provides a potential means of normalizing all the main lipoproteins which influence the progression of CHD.

Combined use of nicotinic acid and statins not only enables better control of mixed dyslipidaemia to be achieved than by statins alone but is uniquely able to lower Lp(a) levels. The main drawbacks of nicotinic acid are its side-effects, some of which are especially undesirable in patients with mixed dyslipidaemia and type 2 diabetes or obesity, notably aggravation of hyperglycaemia and hyperuricaemia. However, these and other side-effects such as flushing and hepatotoxicity seem to be less frequent with the extended-release form of nicotinic acid, Niaspan, than with other preparations, as was borne out recently by a trial in diabetics.[58]

Hence, for those who can tolerate it, the combination of Niaspan with a statin provides an attractive option, especially for those with low HDL levels and CHD.

Combined use of fibrates and statins offers an alternative means of treating mixed dyslipidaemia, except in those with renal impairment. Symptomatic side-effects are fewer than with nicotinic acid/statin combinations and the reduction in triglycerides even more marked. However, this is at the expense of a lesser rise in HDL cholesterol and a slight increase in LDL cholesterol. The main deterrent to combined use of statins and fibrates is the risk of myositis, although analysis of the data suggests that this can be minimized by avoiding the use of gemfibrozil. On the credit side, most fibrates tend to reduce fibrinogen levels, which are often raised in diabetics. However, unlike nicotinic acid and statins,[23] so far there have been no trials of fibrate/statin combination therapy in the prevention of CHD.

The most recent innovation in the therapeutic arena is ezetimibe. This compound's ability to block cholesterol absorption provides a novel means of complementing the inhibitory action of statins on cholesterol synthesis. This ability has already been demonstrated in patients with homozygous FH,[56] in whom it has always been notoriously difficult to lower LDL levels to anywhere near the normal range. It remains to be seen whether ezetimibe/statin combinations will be reserved for the minority whose raised LDL levels are refractory to statin monotherapy or whether they will be used as a means of keeping statin dosage to a minimum in a much broader range of patients, including those unable to tolerate high doses of statins. Either way, as has happened with anti-hypertensive agents, combination therapy with statins and other lipid-regulating drugs looks set to stay.

REFERENCES

1. Pyörälä K, Pedersen TR, Kjekshus J et al. and the Scandinavian Simvastatin Survival Study Group. Cholesterol lowering with simvastatin improves prognosis of diabetic patients with coronary heart disease. *Diabetes Care* 1997; **20**: 614–20.

2. Goldberg RB, Mellies MJ, Sacks FM et al. Cardiovascular events and their reduction with pravastatin in diabetic and glucose-intolerant myocardial infarction survivors with average cholesterol levels: subgroup analyses in the cholesterol and recurrent events (CARE) trial. The CARE Investigators. *Circulation* 1998; **98**: 2513–19.

3. Rubins HB, Robins SJ, Collins D et al. Gemfibrozil for the secondary prevention of coronary heart disease in men with low levels of high-density lipoprotein cholesterol. *New Engl J Med* 1999; **341**: 410–18.

4. Pierce LR, Wysowski DK, Gross TP. Myopathy and rhabdomyolysis associated with lovastatin–gemfibrozil combination therapy. *JAMA* 1990; **264**: 71–5.

5. Miettinen TA, Strandberg TE, Gylling H, for the Finnish Investigators of the Scandinavian Simvastatin Survival Study Group. Non-cholesterol sterols and cholesterol lowering by long-term simvastatin treatment in coronary patients. Relation to basal serum cholesterol. *Arterioscler Thromb Vasc Biol* 2000; **20**: 1340–6.

6. Naoumova RP, Marais AD, Mountney J et al. Plasma mevalonic acid, an index of cholesterol synthesis *in vivo*, and responsiveness to HMG-CoA reductase inhibitors in familial hypercholesterolaemia. *Atherosclerosis* 1996; **119**: 203–13.

7. O'Neill FH, Patel DD, Knight BL et al. Determinants of variable response to statin treatment in patients with refractory familial hypercholesterolemia. *Arterioscler Thromb Vasc Biol* 2001; **21**: 832–7.

8. Berge KE, von Bergmann K, Lutjohann D et al. Heritability of plasma noncholesterol sterols and relationship to DNA sequence polymorphism in ABCG5 and ABCG8. *J Lipid Res* 2002; **43**: 486–94.

9. Thompson GR, O'Neill F, Seed M. Why some patients respond poorly to statins and how this might be remedied. *Eur Heart J* 2002; **23**: 200–6.

10. Jones P, Kafonek S, Laurora I et al., for the CURVES Investigators. Comparative dose efficacy study of atorvastatin versus simvastatin, pravastatin, lovastatin, and fluvastatin in patients with hypercholesterolemia (the CURVES study). *Am J Cardiol* 1998; **81**: 582–7.

11. Carlson LA, Hamsten A, Asplund A. Pronounced lowering of serum levels of lipoprotein Lp(a) in hyperlipidaemic subjects treated with nicotinic acid. *J Int Med* 1989; **226**: 271–6.

12. Tikkanen MJ, Helve E, Jaattela A et al. Comparison between lovastatin and gemfibrozil in the treatment of primary hypercholesterolemia: the Finnish Multicenter Study. *Am J Cardiol* 1988; **62**: 35J–43J.

13. Bays HE, Moore PB, Drehobl MA et al. Effectiveness and tolerability of ezetimibe in patients with primary hypercholesterolemia: pooled analysis of two phase II studies. *Clin Ther* 2001; **23**: 1209–30.

14. Henkin Y, Oberman A, Hurst DC, Segrest JP. Niacin revisited: clinical observations on an important but underutilized drug. *Am J Med* 1991; **91**: 239–46.

15. Goldberg A, Alagona P Jr, Capuzzi DM et al. Multiple-dose efficacy and safety of an extended-release form of niacin in the management of hyperlipidemia. *Am J Cardiol* 2000; **85**: 1100–5.

16. Guyton JR, Goldberg AC, Kreisberg RA et al. Effectiveness of once-nightly dosing of extended-release niacin alone and in combination for hypercholesterolemia. *Am J Cardiol* 1998; **82**: 737–43.

17. Jacobson TA, Chin MM, Fromell GJ et al. Fluvastatin with and without niacin for hypecholesterolemia. *Am J Cardiol* 1994; **74**: 149–54.

18. Illingworth DR, Bacon S. Treatment of heterozygous familial hypercholesterolemia with lipid-lowering drugs. *Arteriosclerosis* 1989; **9** (Suppl 1): I121–I134.

19. Davignon J, Roederer G, Montigny M et al. Comparative efficacy and safety of pravastatin, nicotinic acid and the two combined in patients with hypercholesterolemia. *Am J Cardiol* 1994; **73**: 339–45.

20. Vacek JL, Dittmeier G, Chiarelli T et al. Comparison of lovastatin (20 mg) and nicotinic acid (1.2 g) with either drug alone for type II hyperlipoproteinemia. *Am J Cardiol* 1995; **76**: 182–4.

21. O'Keefe JH Jr, Harris WS, Nelson J, Windsor SL. Effects of pravastatin with niacin or magnesium on lipid levels and postprandial lipemia. *Am J Cardiol* 1995; **76**: 480–4.

22. Wolfe ML, Vartanian SF, Ross JL et al. Safety and effectiveness of Niaspan when added sequentially to a statin for treatment of dyslipidemia. *Am J Cardiol* 2001; **87**: 476–9.

23. Brown BG, Zhao XQ, Chait A et al. Simvastatin and niacin, antioxidant vitamins, or the combination for the prevention of coronary disease. *N Engl J Med* 2001; **345**: 1583–92.

24. Cheung MC, Zhao XQ, Chait A et al. Antioxidant supplements block the response of HDL to simvastatin–niacin therapy in patients with coronary artery disease and low HDL. *Arterioscler Thromb Vasc Biol* 2001; **21**: 1320–6.

25. Kashyap ML, McGovern ME, Berra K et al. Long-term safety and efficacy of a once-daily niacin/lovastatin formulation for patients with dyslipidemia. *Am J Cardiol* 2002; **89**: 672–8.

26. Manninen V, Elo MO, Frick MH et al. Lipid alterations and decline in the incidence of coronary heart disease in the Helsinki Heart Study. *JAMA* 1988; **260**: 641–51.

27. Manninen V, Tenkanen L, Koskinen P et al. Joint effects of serum triglyceride and LDL cholesterol and HDL cholesterol concentrations on coronary heart disease risk in the Helsinki Heart Study. *Circulation* 1992; **85**: 37–45.

28. Secondary prevention by raising HDL cholesterol and reducing triglycerides in patients with coronary artery disease: the Bezafibrate Infarction Prevention (BIP) study. *Circulation* 2000; **102**: 21–7.

29. Papadakis JA, Ganotakis ES, Jagroop IA et al. Statin + fibrate combination therapy fluvastatin with bezafibrate or ciprofibrate in high-risk patients with vascular disease. *Int J Cardiol* 1999; **69**: 237–44.

30. Kehely A, MacMahon M, Barbir M et al. Combined bezafibrate and simvastatin treatment for mixed hyperlipidaemia. *Q J Med* 1995; **88**: 421–7.

31. Wiklund O, Bergman M, Bondjers G et al. Pravastatin and gemfibrozil alone and in combination for the treatment of hypercholesterolemia. *Am J Med* 1993; **94**: 13–20.

32. Leitersdorf E, Muratti EN, Eliav O et al. Efficacy and safety of a combination fluvastatin–bezafibrate treatment for familial hypercholesterolemia: comparative analysis with a fluvastatin–cholestyramine combination. *Am J Med* 1994; **96**: 401–7.

33. Smit JWA, Jansen GH, de Bruin TWA, Erkelens DW. Treatment of combined hyperlipidemia with fluvastatin and gemfibrozil, alone or in combination, does not induce muscle damage. *Am J Cardiol* 1995; **76**: 126A–128A.

34. Ellen RL, McPherson R. Long-term efficacy and safety of fenofibrate and a statin in the treatment of combined hyperlipidemia. *Am J Cardiol* 1998; **81**: 60B–65B.

35. Gavish D, Leibovitz E, Shapira I, Rubinstein A. Bezafibrate and simvastatin combination therapy for diabetic dyslipidemia: efficacy and safety. *J Intern Med* 2000; **247**: 563–9.

36. Heart Protection Study Collaborative Group. MRC/BHF Heart Protection Study of cholesterol lowering with simvastatin in 20536 high-risk individuals: a randomised placebo-controlled trial. *Lancet* 2002; **360**: 7–22.

37. Farmer JA. Learning from the cerivastatin experience. *Lancet* 2001; **358**: 1383–4.

38. Gruer PJK, Vega JM, Mercuri MF et al. Concomitant use of cytochrome P450 3A4 inhibitors and simvastatin. *Am J Cardiol* 1999; **84**: 811–15.

39. Ferrill SA. Statin–fibrate combination therapy. *Ann Pharmacother* 2001; **35**: 908–17.

40. Shepherd J. Fibrates and statins in the treatment of hyperlipidaemia: an appraisal of their efficacy and safety. *Eur Heart J* 1995; **16**: 5–13

41. Thompson GR, Dean J, Wilson PWF. *Dyslipidaemia in Clinical Practice*. London: Martin Dunitz, 2002.

42. Evans M, Rees A. The myotoxicity of statins. *Curr Opin Lipidol* 2002; **13**: 415–20.

43. Backman JT, Kyrklund C, Kivisto KT et al. Plasma concentrations of active simvastatin acid are increased by gemfibrozil. *Clin Pharmacol Ther* 2000; **68**: 122–9.

44. Kyrklund C, Backman JT, Kivisto KT et al. Plasma concentrations of active lovastatin acid are markedly increased by gemfibrozil but not by bezafibrate. *Clin Pharmacol Ther* 2001; **69**: 340–5.

45. Spence JD, Munoz CE, Hendricks L et al. Pharmacokinetics of the combination of fluvastatin and gemfibrozil. *Am J Cardiol* 1995; **76**: 80A–83A.

46. Ostlund RE Jr, Bosner MS, Stenson WF. Cholesterol absorption efficiency declines at moderate dietary doses in normal human subjects. *J Lipid Res* 1999; **40**: 1453–8.

47. Gylling H, Miettinen TA. The effect of cholesterol absorption inhibition on low-density lipoprotein cholesterol level. *Atherosclerosis* 1995; **117**: 305–8.

48. Hernandez M, Montenegro J, Steiner M et al. Intestinal absorption of cholesterol is mediated by a saturable inhibitable transporter. *Biochim Biophys Acta* 2000; **19**: 232–42.

49. Kramer W, Glombik H, Petry S et al. Identification of binding proteins for cholesterol absorption inhibitors as components of the intestinal cholesterol transporter. *FEBS Lett* 2000; **487**: 293–7.

50. Rosenblum SB, Huynh T, Afonso A et al. Discovery of 1-(4-fluorophenyl)-(3*R*)-[3-(4-fluorophenyl)-(3*S*)-hydroxypropyl]-(4*S*)-(4-hydroxyphenyl)-2-azetidinone (SCH 58235): a designed, potent, orally active inhibitor of cholesterol absorption. *J Med Chem* 1998; **41**: 973–80.

51. Van Heek M, Farley C, Compton DS et al. Comparison of the activity and disposition of the novel cholesterol absorption inhibitor, SCH58235, and its glucuronide, SCH60663. *Br J Pharmacol* 2000; **129**: 1748–54.

52. Davis HR Jr, Compton DS, Hoos L, Tetzloff G. Ezetimibe, a potent cholesterol absorption inhibitor, inhibits the development of atherosclerosis in apoE knockout mice. *Arterioscler Thromb Vasc Biol* 2001; **21**: 2032–8.

53. Bays HE, Moore PB, Drehobl MA et al. Effectiveness and tolerability of ezetimibe in patients with primary hypercholesterolemia: pooled analysis of two phase II studies. *Clin Ther* 2001; **23**: 1209–30.

54. Davis HR Jr, Pula KK, Alton KB et al. The synergistic hypocholesterolemic activity of the potent cholesterol absorption inhibitor, ezetimibe, in combination with 3-hydroxy-3-methylglutaryl coenzyme A reductase inhibitor in dogs. *Metabolism* 2001; **50**: 1234–41.

55. Kosoglou T, Meyer I, Musiol B et al. Pharmacodynamic interaction between the new selective cholesterol absorption inhibitor ezetimibe and simvastatin. *Atherosclerosis* 2000; **151**: 135.

56. Gagne C, Gaudet D, Bruckert E for the Ezetimibe Study Group. Efficacy and safety of ezetimibe coadministered with atorvastatin or simvastatin in patients with homozygous familial hypercholesterolemia. *Circulation* 2002; **105**: 2469–75.

57. Miettinen TA, Gylling H, Strandberg T et al. Baseline serum cholestanol as predictor of recurrent coronary events in subgroup of Scandinavian Simvastatin Survival Study. *BMJ* 1998; **316**: 1127–30.

58. Grundy SM, Vega GL, McGovern ME et al. Efficacy, safety, and tolerability of once-daily niacin for the treatment of dyslipidaemia associated with type 2 diabetes: results of the assessment of diabetes control and evaluation of niaspan trial. *Arch Int Med* 2002; **162**: 1568–76.

14

Guidelines for clinical use of the statins

Christopher J Packard

INTRODUCTION

With the publication of landmark statin-based cholesterol-lowering trials described earlier in this book, a new certainty has entered the language of those who formulate guidelines for best practice in coronary prevention. Trials from the pre-statin era, the Lipid Research Clinics Primary Prevention Trial and the Helsinki Heart Study (HHS),[1,2] provided evidence of the benefits of lipid correction for the enthusiasts but left the vast majority of clinicians unconvinced as to the net gain to be obtained from widespread use of cholesterol-lowering agents. These studies demonstrated reductions in coronary morbidity with bile acid sequestrant (cholestyramine) or fibrate (gemfibrozil) treatments but had no clear effect on coronary or total mortality. Indeed there were calls for a moratorium on the use of lipid-lowering drugs outside those at very high risk of coronary heart disease (CHD);[3] increased risk of cancer, suicide or violent death was touted as the downside of cholesterol lowering, and opinion leaders became polarized and the general physician confused.

Guidelines for the use of lipid-lowering diets and drugs were devised and promulgated in this difficult environment by expert committees adopting a consensual but often optimistic view of the existing trial data.[4,5] However, the recent demonstration in major clinical trials of reductions in coronary events, cardiovascular mortality and overall death rates on statin treatment removed the doubts about the benefits of cholesterol lowering. This in turn has led to a revision of the early guidelines which for the most part has been a clarification and confirmation of

their recommendations rather than a complete rewrite, much to the relief of the original authors.

As recommendations concerning the utility of statin therapy have become increasingly upbeat there has been a parallel waning of the enthusiasm for dietary measures to lower plasma cholesterol. In the population approach to coronary prevention it is suggested that since the majority of subjects at risk of CHD have 'normal' cholesterol levels, the only way to tackle the problem is by encouraging a change in the general dietary intake of cholesterol and saturated fat.[6] However, carefully designed studies of the effectiveness of dietary intervention on cholesterol lowering in free-living subjects have yielded limited benefits.[7] Average cholesterol reductions in subjects given dietary advice and followed up for one year were small.[7] Thus, for the physician attempting to achieve a diet-induced cholesterol reduction, the effort can be as 'rewarding' as persuading people to stop smoking or lose weight. That said, population lifestyles do change but it takes time and the dissemination of a much more integrated message than can be achieved by physicians working alone or even on a regional basis. Nevertheless, lifestyle modification is still the cornerstone of coronary prevention – the adoption of a prudent Mediterranean-style diet, smoking cessation and weight loss with increased uptake of exercise are sensible first steps in those at risk of CHD and useful adjunctive therapy in those with established disease. An aspect of growing concern is the 'epidemic' of obesity in the population, especially in the young. This is likely to lead to increased incidence of diabetes and CHD in Western countries in the future. Only fairly dramatic lifestyle changes will head off this public health disaster.

The following discussion focuses on three questions and attempts to derive answers from the findings of recent landmark studies. The issues are: who benefits most from statin therapy; to whom should such drug treatment be directed; and what are the goals of treatment? Answering these questions provides the conceptual framework for current guidelines of coronary prevention. In the last section new, existing and, in some cases, recently revised published guidelines are reviewed with the object of identifying common recommendations and any important differences.

WHO BENEFITS MOST FROM STATIN THERAPY?

It is often the case that the imposition of specific inclusion and exclusion criteria in clinical trials so moulds the cohort recruited that the findings, if positive, may not apply to the typical patient attending the physician for the condition under investigation. Fortunately, the nature of the groups used in the major statin trials is now so wide that conclusions can be drawn regarding the efficacy of treatment for most segments of the population. The effects of baseline lipid phenotype, age, gender and other risk factors have been addressed either in the original reports or in subsequent publications. Perhaps the single issue on which conclusions cannot be drawn is the influence of ethnicity. Not enough subjects from ethnic minorities in the countries where the trials were conducted were included to examine this question properly and at present we have to extrapolate from findings in Caucasians. Hopefully, this shortcoming will be resolved soon. Parenthetically, it should be noted that until recently virtually no outcome data were available for the effects of cholesterol-lowering medication in women or older patients.

Influence of baseline lipid phenotype

Hyperlipidaemia is commonly divided into three types: raised cholesterol; raised trigly-

ceride; and combined (or mixed) hyperlipidaemia where both are elevated. The combined phenotype appears to carry a particularly high risk of CHD.[8] Low high-density lipoprotein (HDL) is also considered a powerful independent predictor of risk. It is usually found associated with a raised plasma triglyceride but can also occur as an isolated abnormality. In the HHS, analysis revealed that the group of subjects who at baseline had a raised triglyceride/low HDL cholesterol pattern achieved the greatest relative risk reduction of about 70%.[9] Those who presented with simple elevation in low-density lipoprotein (LDL) experienced less benefit from gemfibrozil treatment. The West of Scotland Coronary Prevention Study (WOSCOPS) and the Scandanavian Simvastatin Survival Study (4S) were conducted in subjects who exhibited moderate hypercholesterolaemia (mean LDL cholesterol on entry was about 5.0 mmol/l in both studies).[10,11] Division of subjects into quartiles or quintiles of baseline LDL revealed that the drugs employed produced a relative uniform relative risk reduction across the entire range of values.[12,13] As in the Helsinki study, we observed that subjects in the top quintile of plasma triglyceride (>2.0 mmol/l) had virtually double the CHD risk of those in the lowest quintile,[12] but variation in plasma triglyceride or HDL was not associated with any change in beneficial effects of pravastatin therapy. Likewise, splitting subjects into the same lipid phenotypes as used in HHS (high or low plasma triglyceride, high or low LDL/HDL ratio) revealed no difference in the relative risk reduction induced by the drug (WOSCOPS Study Group, unpublished observations). Recruits to the Air Force/Texas Coronary Atherosclerosis Prevention Study (AFCAPS)[14] and the Cholesterol and Recurrent Events trial (CARE)[15] had typically average plasma cholesterol levels and a low HDL cholesterol. Here again, the risk reduction in the entire trial cohort was in line with that seen in the studies in hypercholesterolaemics. Thus, the broad picture emerges whether one examines sub-groups or entire trial populations that the risk reduction accompanying statin therapy is independent of lipid phenotype. The practical outcome of this

Table 14.1   Effects of gender on CHD prevention with statins

Study	Gender	No. of subjects	Placebo event rate* (%)	Risk reduction** (%)
4S	Women	827	21.7	35 (9–53)
	Men	3617	29.4	34 (24–42)
CARE	Women	576	28	46 (22–62)
	Men	3583	26	20 (8–30)
LIPID	Women	1516	14	11 (−18–33)
	Men	7498	16	26 (17–35)
AFCAPS	Women	997	1.3	46 (ns)
	Men	5608	3.0	36 (significant)
HPS	Women	5082	17.7	19% (significant)
	Men	15454	27.6	22% (significant)
PROSPER***	Women	3000	12.9	4% (ns)
	Men	2804	19.8	23% (8–35)

* Placebo event rates are comparable within trials but not between trials since different events are included.
** Confidence limits, where known are shown in parentheses.
*** PROSPER event rates are over 3.2 years; other trials are five-year rates.
ns, not significant.

finding is that guidelines need not take into consideration detailed lipid measurements before embarking on treatment.

The uniformity of benefit from statin therapy was illustrated with particular clarity in the BHF/MRC Heart Protection Study (HPS).[16] This is the largest lipid-lowering trial to date, with over 20 000 participants. Recruits were those with vascular disease or those at high risk who attended hospital clinics; the latter were mostly diabetics and hypertensives. Subjects had a broad range of LDL cholesterol levels on entry and it was observed that the relative risk reduction was the same for all tertiles of plasma LDL concentration at baseline. In particular, clear benefit was documented for patients with an LDL cholesterol below 3.0 mmol/l, i.e. below the current target in European and UK guidelines. The information from this well-powered trial largely overturns the previous suggestion from analysis of the CARE trial that patients with a low LDL cholesterol (<125 mg/dl; 3.2 mmol/l) do not experience a reduction in CHD risk on statin therapy.[15]

Similar data are not present from primary prevention studies. AFCAPS[14] studied subjects with low-to-average cholesterol levels who

were CHD-free, but the number of events was too small to address satisfactorily the risk reduction attendant on treating very low LDL cholesterol levels. Looking at epidemiological surveys, it can be seen that the association of absolute risk with LDL in populations is curvilinear, i.e. the relationship is flat below a plasma cholesterol level of about 5.0 mmol/l (equivalent to an LDL cholesterol of about 3.0 mmol/l).[17] Thus, even if a relative risk reduction of 20–30% can be achieved by statin therapy, the absolute decrement in risk in primary prevention may be too small to be worthwhile.

Influence of age and gender

Women were included in six of the seven major statin outcome trials and the results, compared with men, are presented in Table 14.1. In the primary prevention study AFCAPS, the event rate in females was less than half that of males, in keeping with the known gender difference in CHD incidence in the general population. Risk reduction estimates were similar in this trial for both genders and the test for interaction was not significant.[14] It is noteworthy that in

Table 14.2   Effects of age on CHD prevention with statins

Study	Age range (years)	No. of subjects	Placebo event rate* (%)	Risk reduction** (%)
4S	>65	1021	33.4	34 (16–48)
	<65	3423	26.4	34 (24–43)
CARE	>60	2129	27	27 (12–38)
	<60	2030	26	20 (4–33)
LIPID	65–69	2168	19	28 (11–41)
	54–64	3414	14	20 (3–34)
HPS	<65	9839	22.1	24 (significant)
	65–70	4891	27.2	23 (significant)
	≥70	5806	28.7	18 (significant)
PROSPER***	70–82	5804	12.2	19 (6–31)

* Placebo event rates are comparable within trials but not between trials, since different events are included.
** Confidence limits, where known, are shown in parentheses.
*** PROSPER event rates are over 3.2 years; other trials are five-year rates.

secondary prevention studies event rates on placebo are similar between the genders, suggesting that once a woman has had a myocardial infarction (MI) or similar event she should be treated with the same vigour as a man; the putative protective effect of endogenous oestrogen on the cardiovascular system appears to be present no longer. Fortunately, as for primary prevention, the benefits of statin treatment do not differ in men and women who have established CHD; in the trials listed in Table 14.1 there was no heterogeneity of treatment effect with respect to gender. The clearest evidence comes from HPS, which included a large group of women (>5000) in which the benefit of statin therapy was equivalent to that seen in men.[16] Thus once a woman is identified as at high CHD risk she should enter the same treatment algorithm as a man, at least for secondary prevention. Hormone replacement therapy (HRT) was once considered an option in women but the results of the HERS trial[18] and the recently published Women's Health Initiative[19] indicate that the effects of HRT on CHD risk are, if anything, adverse. Thus, statin therapy is at the moment the regimen of choice for coronary disease prevention in both sexes.

Age is an important factor in any treatment strategy. First, it is the most powerful determinant of absolute CHD risk and hence of the likelihood that a patient will cross the threshold for aggressive (i.e. drug) treatment laid out in European and US guidelines. Second, the strength of the association between cholesterol and CHD risk diminishes in older people and so the benefit of statin-induced LDL lowering may be less. Table 14.2 summarizes the findings in the prevention trials that included sufficient numbers of older subjects to allow conclusions to be drawn as to the efficacy of treatment. In each study older participants experience a risk reduction of a magnitude similar to that seen in middle age. The recently published PROSPER (Prospective Study of Pravastatin in the Elderly at Risk) trial was designed to address this specific issue.[20] It recruited men and women who had a history of, or were at risk for, vascular disease. Treatment for a period of just over three years produced a reduction of 19% in the risk of MI ($p = 0.006$) and 24% in the risk of CHD death ($p = 0.043$). No effect was seen in the risk of stroke, but this may be due to the short follow-up. The HPS investigators reported results recently[21] which showed that 70- to 75-year-old subjects treated with simvastatin had a 21% reduction in the risk of a vascular event ($p < 0.0001$) and an 18% decrease in incidence of stroke ($p = 0.0003$). This direct evidence therefore supports the view that no upper age limit should be applied in prevention strategies. Given the weakened relationship between LDL cholesterol and risk in the elderly (in PROSPER, LDL cholesterol was not a predictor of CHD events) it is remarkable that statin treatment produced these substantial risk reductions.

Other risk factors

In each of the statin trials it was reported that smokers were at substantially greater risk than non-smokers or former smokers and that a risk reduction with statin treatment was independent of smoking status. For example, in WOSCOPS 10.4% of current smokers versus 6.0% of non-smokers experienced a coronary event, but a 31% risk reduction pertained in both groups. However, it was noteworthy that smokers on statin still had a higher event rate than non-smokers on placebo.[10] Hypertension is the other major, highly prevalent risk factor for CHD; i.e. alongside cholesterol and smoking. In CARE hypertensives had a similar risk reduction to non-hypertensives[15] and the same was broadly true in the Long-term Intervention with Pravastatin in Ischemic Disease (LIPID) trial, AFCAPS, HPS and PROSPER (WOSCOPS and 4S do not report data for this categorization).[14,16,20,22]

Diabetes carries a high risk of CHD, although its low prevalence (at least in Western countries) means that it does not register as a major population factor. CARE, 4S and HPS were trials that included enough diabetics to evaluate the potential benefits of statin therapy.[16,23,24] Since the characteristic dyslipidaemia in non-insulin-dependent diabetes is a raised plasma triglyceride/low HDL pattern, it was not obvious a priori that statins would generate a clinically useful risk reduction. Furthermore, an adverse influence of hyperinsulinaemia on atherosclerosis might over-ride any effect of statin-induced cholesterol lowering. However, all report that the drugs are effective in diabetics with established CHD, with a risk reduction at least as great as that seen in non-diabetics. Indeed, the incidence of recurrent coronary events in a diabetic who has survived a MI is so

great that aggressive intervention is mandatory. HPS also provides information on the effectiveness of statin therapy in primary prevention of CHD in diabetics. A group of 3982 diabetics with no prior history of CHD were recruited into the trial. Those assigned to statin therapy had a significant risk reduction of about 26% for the first major vascular event.[16]

HPS recruited a substantial number of patients in whom vascular disease at baseline affected the cerebral and peripheral vessels rather than coronary arteries. These too benefited from therapy, with relative risk reductions in future vascular events that were in line with those seen in patients with pre-existing coronary disease.[16] It was noteworthy in this trial that the risk of a further vascular event in patients with established cerebrovascular or peripheral vascular disease was as high as the risk in a patient with coronary disease (Table 14.3).

There is increasing recognition that chronic inflammation plays a central role in atherogenesis. Inflammatory cells such as lymphocytes and macrophages are found in abundance in atherosclerotic lesions, and indeed are the key feature of unstable lesions that are prone to rupture and precipitate an acute coronary event. Plasma markers of a pro-inflammatory state such as C-reactive protein (CRP) and interleukin-6 are elevated in subjects at high risk of CHD.[25,26] CRP in particular has been proposed as a risk factor to be added to the classic constellation of age, sex, blood pressure, smoking and plasma cholesterol.[25] Further support for this concept comes from an analysis of the AFCAPS trial in which it was observed that subjects with low LDL but raised CRP experienced benefit from statin therapy whereas those with low LDL and low CRP did not.[27] However, not all investigators agree that CRP is truly independent of other factors such as HDL (CRP and HDL show a strong negative association) and question how much its measurement adds to the assessment of global risk.[26,28]

Conclusions from an evaluation of who benefits most from statin therapy are, on the basis of the preceding discussion, easy to draw.

Table 14.3 Absolute risk reduction and numbers needed to treat (NNT) with statin therapy

Subject history	Absolute risk per five years of fatal/non-fatal MI (%)	NNT*
Primary prevention		
Male, female, low HDL, average cholesterol (AFCAPS)	2.8	102
Male, moderate LDL ↑, no other risk factor, age <55 years (WOSCOPS)	3.5	82
Male, moderate LDL ↑, no other risk factor, age >55 years (WOSCOPS)	5.3	54
All WOSCOPS men	9.3	31
Male, moderate LDL ↑, multiple risk factors (WOSCOPS)	12.8	22
Male, ECG abnormalities, age <55 years (WOSCOPS)	11.9	24
Diabetic no prior CHD (HPS)	18.6	15
Secondary prevention		
Female, post-MI, average cholesterol (CARE)	11.4	25
All CARE subjects	13.2	22
Female, post-MI/angina, ↑ LDL (LIPID)	21.7	13
All 4S subjects	22.6	13
Prior CHD (HPS)	22.5	13
Prior cerebrovascular disease (HPS)	23.6	12
Prior peripheral vascular disease (HPS)	30.5	9
Male or female, age >65 years (4S)	33.4	9
Diabetic with CHD (HPS)	37.8	8
Diabetic with CHD, ↑ cholesterol (4S)	41.1	7

* Assuming a 35% risk reduction across all subjects.

Remarkably, it appears that the treatment effect is independent of lipid phenotype, age, gender and the presence of other risk factors. A relative reduction of 20–40% in CHD risk was experienced across the wide range of subjects recruited to the major statin trials. It may be argued therefore that statin treatment should be available to all. However, economics and the desire not to medicalize large sections of the population dictate, at least for the moment, that the use of these drugs should be targeted.

TO WHOM SHOULD STATIN THERAPY BE TARGETED?

If all enjoy the same relative risk reduction on statin therapy then the most logical means of targeting treatment is to direct it to those at highest risk, i.e. individuals with the greatest absolute risk of a coronary event over a given period of time. The range of risk can be wide even in a relatively homogeneous group of subjects chosen for an intervention trial.[29] Table 14.3 provides indicative ranking of subject types who might be considered as candidates for statin treatment. Absolute risk of a future fatal/non-fatal MI rises over ten-fold when comparing the typical recruit to AFCAPS with the diabetics in the 4S trial. Interestingly, there is considerable overlap in risk between groups randomized in WOSCOPS, i.e. high-risk primary prevention, and those in CARE or LIPID who fall into the secondary prevention category. Indeed, middle-aged, moderately hypercholesterolaemic men with signs or symptoms of coronary artery disease have a five-year risk of an event that approaches that seen in 4S. Thus, if absolute CHD risk is chosen as the arbiter of who is to be treated, then the distinction between primary and secondary prevention blurs. This is no bad thing since the identification of individuals at high risk who have not yet suffered a potentially fatal first event is a key objective of any prevention programme. Recognition of the importance of risk assessment has led to the development of computer and paper-based instruments to calculate absolute CHD risk. These are based on epidemiological surveys and include the major common risk factors (age, sex, blood pressure, smoking, cholesterol and HDL levels) together with new additions: Lp(a), fibrinogen, etc.[30,31] Setting the risk threshold for prescription of a statin is as much a social and economic decision as a medical one.

Knowledge of the absolute risk reduction expected from an intervention (i.e. absolute risk multiplied by relative risk reduction) permits calculation of a simple index – number needed to treat to prevent one event (NNT, the reciprocal of the absolute risk reduction) – that allows different therapeutic regiments to be compared without resorting to a formal cost–benefit or cost-effectiveness analysis. NNT for various categories of subject are presented in Table 14.3. They give an indication of the clinical benefit that follows from statin therapy in primary and secondary prevention. Treating over 100 patients for five years, as in AFCAPS, to prevent a single MI would be considered by many physicians too little return for a great deal of effort and expense. On the other hand, treatment of ten or 20 subjects to prevent a major coronary event is good medical practice and a worthwhile use of resources. This level of return from intervention compares very favourably with other medical regimens used to prevent vascular disease.[29,32]

GOALS OF STATIN TREATMENT

In determining the optimal treatment strategy for correction of raised LDL levels in those at risk of CHD, it is important to bear in mind that the goal is CHD reduction, not LDL change for its own sake. The relationship between plasma cholesterol level and CHD risk in the general population is curvilinear, i.e. relatively flat below 5.0 mmol/l (193 mg/dl), with a shallow gradient as cholesterol rises to 6.5 mmol/l (251 mg/dl) and then a steep association thereafter.[17] The changing nature of the association gave rise to the treatment thresholds promulgated in early guidelines.[4] However, epidemiology can provide only a crude estimate of the benefit to be gained from a given cholesterol reduction. More definitive information comes from clinical trials.

Three publications appeared in 1998 which described the findings of the WOSCOPS, CARE and 4S trials with regard to the association between change in LDL on statin therapy and the subsequent risk of a major coronary event.[12,33,34] In the report of the WOSCOPS investigators[12] it was seen that subjects on pravastatin exhibited a wide range of LDL lowering, from a few percent to nearly 60% reduction. Treated subjects were divided into quintiles according to extent of the LDL fall in either percentage or absolute amounts. It appeared that optimal reduction in CHD risk of about 40% occurred in the mid-quintile, where LDL was decreased 25% or about 1.0 mmol/l (39 mg/dl). Further LDL reduction (up to about 40% in quintile 5) gave no measurable additional decrement in risk. On the basis of these findings it was concluded that a curvilinear relationship existed between fall in LDL and risk reduction.

Secondary prevention trials such as 4S and CARE also reported a curvilinear association between LDL fall on statin treatment and CHD risk reduction.[33,34] In 4S, however, the attenuation of benefit appeared less marked than in other trials, This is possibly due to the much higher starting LDL levels in these subjects. It is difficult on the basis of CARE, LIPID and 4S to extract definitive information about the potential benefit of treating post-MI patients with low LDL levels because of limited subject numbers in this LDL range. HPS on the other hand had a substantial number of subjects with low-baseline LDL cholesterol. Its publication has led to a more aggressive stance with regard to the use of statins in patients with vascular disease who have low LDL levels. Clear benefit was observed in those whose starting LDL cholesterol was below 3.0 mmol/l (116 mg/dl). Indeed the relative risk reduction of 19% was uniform across the LDL range in the trial. In the lowest tertile of baseline LDL, the mean achieved LDL cholesterol on statin was 1.8 mmol/l (70 mg/dl). This is considerably less than the current UK and European target of below 3.0 mmol/l (116 mg/dl)[35] and more in line with the US guideline that LDL be reduced to below 100 mg/dl (2.6 mmol/l). This 100 mg/dl target was set in ATPII[5] and reinforced in a recent revision (ATPIII).[36] It was based (pre publication of HPS) on a meta-analysis of small clinical trials. One of note was the post-CABG study[37] which provided evidence for fewer new lesions on grafts and fewer events if LDL was maintained below 100 mg/dl.

The new findings in HPS strongly suggest that subjects with arteriosclerotic vascular disease (regardless of site) should be treated with a statin even if LDL levels are low. However, no trial to date provides clear evidence that even greater reductions in LDL produce larger benefits. As noted above, some suggest that there is a law of diminishing returns with respect to relative risk reduction as LDL is reduced further, while others argue that the findings in 4S and HPS support clearly a 'lower is better' philosophy. The answer to this controversy will come from outcome trials such as Treat to New Targets (TNT) study in which subjects are titrated to differing LDL levels.

CURRENT GUIDELINES AND THEIR IMPLEMENTATION

Composing guidelines, particularly for the management of hyperlipidaemia and coronary prevention, has become something of a medical speciality in its own right. Documents are produced at a continental (Europe), national (UK), regional (Scottish) and local level, e.g. the Greater Glasgow Health Board has its own set. For the non-expert physician, attempting to follow best practice can be daunting since in many instances minor and sometimes major differences exist in the recommendations of expert bodies. The size of the guideline documents varies from a single page to over 50 pages and the subject matter can focus entirely on lipids or present a more integrated approach with rec-

ommendations for the management of other risk factors, including blood pressure. In an attempt to eliminate the variable, possibly arbitrary, nature of the material included in guideline documents some expert groups such as the Scottish Intercollegiate Guidelines Network (SIGN) have generated guidelines on how to write guidelines – an approach that carries a lot of merit!

Differences in approach have existed between US and European guidelines. The former focused on banding risk according to LDL cholesterol and had a low target of below 100 mg/dl (2.6 mmol/l) for those at highest risk (i.e. secondary prevention) while the latter emphasized the importance of global risk assessment and used a moderate LDL goal. With publication of the third revision of the US guidelines (ATPIII),[36] the conceptual differences are narrowed. Risk assessment including calculation of global risk is seen as the first key step in patient management on both sides of the Atlantic. Further, following publication of HPS it is likely that the next revision of the European guidelines will recommend a more aggressive LDL target of about 2.5 mmol/l (97 mg/dl).

The NCEP ATPIII guidelines[36] maintain the key features of ATPII, i.e. banding of LDL cholesterol levels and assignment to a risk category dependent on a risk factor count. These factors are cigarette smoking, hypertension (BP >140/90), low HDL cholesterol (<40 mg/dl; 1.05 mmol/l), family history of premature CHD in a first-degree relative and age (men ≥45 years; women ≥55 years).

Noteworthy features in the recent revision are as follows. First the definition of low HDL is altered from <35 to <40 mg/dl. This has the effect of increasing substantially the number of subject who broach this risk criterion. Second, physicians are encouraged to assess the global risk of a coronary event using the charts developed from the Framingham epidemiological study. A risk of over 20% over ten years is counted as 'CHD equivalent' and identifies a patient who should be treated as though they had established disease (secondary prevention), i.e. the LDL goal is then <100 mg/dl rather than the more moderate <130 mg/dl (3.4 mmol/l) target used if global risk is 10–20% over ten years. Third, diabetes is considered a 'CHD equivalent' risk. There are now substantial data to support the view that a patient with diabetes who has not yet had a MI is at approximately the same risk of a future coronary event as a non-diabetic patient with established CHD (see Table 14.3).[36] Fourth, the particular constellation of risk factors comprising the 'metabolic syndrome' (abdominal obesity, moderately elevated triglyceride, low HDL, raised blood pressure and elevated glucose) is recognized as identifying individuals at risk of CHD in the absence of elevated LDL. This syndrome is associated with insulin resistance and has also been termed Syndrome X. To qualify for this category individuals have to display three of the five characteristics noted above. The use of this pragmatic method of finding subjects with metabolic syndrome is an important step forward in targeting diabetes and CHD prevention strategies in the general population.

European guidelines propose a holistic approach to risk assessment. The first step is to estimate the ten-year risk of a coronary event from tables based on the Framingham risk equation.[30] Variables to be evaluated are the total cholesterol/HDL cholesterol ratio, age, sex, blood pressure, smoking and diabetic status. A threshold risk level of 20% (or 30% in the UK) identifies those who require aggressive intervention, usually drug (statin) treatment. Cognisance should be taken of the over-riding impact of age on risk in these tables, and if a younger person with significant risk factors does not currently broach the 20% threshold then his or her risk should be estimated at the age of 60 years. If the threshold is now crossed, a more aggressive intervention policy should be adopted.

In practice, an assessment of risk is only needed for asymptomatic patients. Those with signs or symptoms of established CHD, i.e. MI survivors, patients complaining of angina or those who have undergone or await coronary artery bypass grafting (CABG) or percutaneous transluminal coronary angioplasty (PTCA), are held to be at sufficiently increased risk without taking other factors into account. Certainly, the event rates seen in the placebo arms of statin

trials (see Table 14.3) bear this out and these studies provide solid evidence for the benefit of therapy almost regardless of the state of the myocardium. Further, although most secondary prevention trials began statin therapy some months after the qualifying event, demonstration of very early benefit from drug therapy has led to the conclusion that treatment should be initiated as soon as possible in patients with CHD. Recent evidence for this approach comes from the MIRACL study, which initiated statin therapy within days of an acute coronary event.[38] Correction of lifestyle factors and the adoption of a prudent diet can be introduced concurrently. There are benefits other than LDL reduction to be obtained from diet manipulation in secondary prevention, e.g. addition of fish oil[39] and possibly vitamin E[39,40] has been shown to be beneficial.

A conundrum arises when global risk is used as the trigger for statin treatment. An asymptomatic middle-aged man who smokes may present with moderate hypertension and average LDL levels. Does the clinician use drugs to correct the raised blood pressure for which the evidence of benefit is less strong or is a statin prescribed on the basis of the findings of the above trials? An integrated approach to the correction of all modifiable risk factors is clearly needed to guide physicians in these difficult decisions. The recently published joint guidelines from the British Cardiac, Hyperlipidaemia, Hypertension and Diabetic societies are a start in tackling the problem of the patient at risk, not just risk factors.[41] It is likely that the next generation of treatment recommendations will also include input from neurologists since the prevention of stroke is now accepted as a property of statin therapy, at least in the post-MI situation.

Templates for guidelines in primary and secondary prevention are offered in Figs 14.1 and 14.2. In primary prevention the mood, in the UK at least, is not to indulge in population screening for cholesterol. This would identify individuals with moderate cholesterol elevations who may have no other risk factors and thus do not merit drug therapy. They may become the 'worried well' and suffer a negative impact on quality of life from the screening

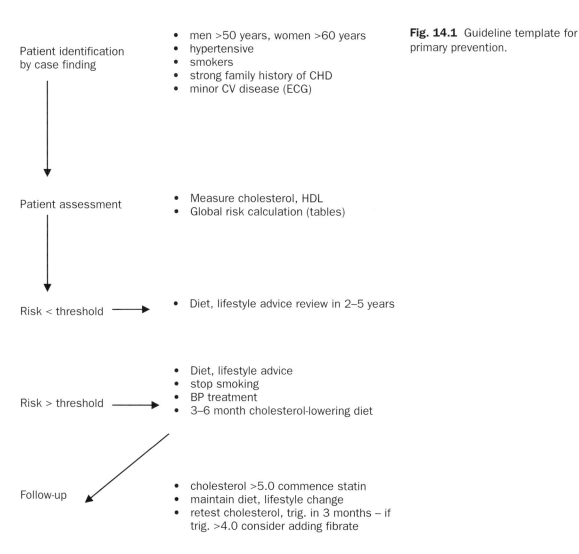

Patient identification
by case finding

- men >50 years, women >60 years
- hypertensive
- smokers
- strong family history of CHD
- minor CV disease (ECG)

Fig. 14.1 Guideline template for primary prevention.

Patient assessment

- Measure cholesterol, HDL
- Global risk calculation (tables)

Risk < threshold

- Diet, lifestyle advice review in 2–5 years

Risk > threshold

- Diet, lifestyle advice
- stop smoking
- BP treatment
- 3–6 month cholesterol-lowering diet

Follow-up

- cholesterol >5.0 commence statin
- maintain diet, lifestyle change
- retest cholesterol, trig. in 3 months – if trig. >4.0 consider adding fibrate

exercise for little overall medical benefit. The consensus is to influence such people through population-based health education. Case finding in older adults by GPs and practice nurses may represent the most cost-effective method of identifying those at risk for CHD. Assessment of their global risk can then be carried out at Well Man or Well Woman clinics with measurements of random cholesterol and HDL. The tables in the new guideline documents[36,41] permit the assignment of an approximate absolute risk of a coronary event which is the criterion used to decide if drug treatment is required once lifestyle changes have proven inadequate. From the above discussion it is clear that aggressive treatment of the high-risk primary prevention subject is as important as treatment of those who have had a MI.

In secondary prevention (see Fig. 14.2) patients identify themselves. The wealth of evidence for benefit from statin therapy indicates that this should be instituted as soon as possible. This often means in the case of a MI survivor discharging the patient on a statin (as well as other key medications such as aspirin and beta-blocker where indicated). Diet and lifestyle changes can follow in the framework of a cardiac rehabilitation programme. Patients on waiting lists for revascularization or immediately post intervention should be treated with equal vigour. When patients present with combined hyperlipidaemia, statins alone may not

Patient identification
– self-selecting

- post-MI
- pre/post-CABG
- pre/post-angioplasty
- angina
- post-stroke
- PVD
- diabetic

Patient assessment

- General risk factor evaluation
- random cholesterol

Early treatment

- aspirin, beta-blocker, statin
- if MI, discharge on statin
- if PTCA/CABG, begin statin before procedure

Follow-up

- lifestyle, diet advice
- enrol in cardiac rehabilitation
- retest cholesterol, trig. in 3 months – if trig. >4.0 consider adding fibrate

Fig. 14.2 Guideline template for secondary prevention.

generate a satisfactory correction of the lipid profile. In these instances the addition of a fibrate can be helpful in correcting the lipid pattern.

CONCLUSION

Coronary artery disease is an area of medicine where abundant clinical trial data exist to support aggressive intervention with medical, specifically statin, therapy to prevent a first or recurrent event. The uniformity of benefit seen in major outcome studies regardless of the status of the patient provides a simple conceptual framework for the drawing up of guidelines for coronary prevention in general and the use of statins in particular. All with established CHD merit early statin treatment. Asymptomatic subjects require global risk assessment to determine

their need for drug therapy. This is a medical but also socio-economic decision given the current cost of statins. Future developments will be the widespread availability of computer-based multifactorial risk assessment programmes, the identification of novel risk factors, the development of new ways of detecting occult CHD and the expiry of patents on first generation statins.

ACKNOWLEDGEMENT

The author thanks Ms Shelley Wilkie for her excellent secretarial assistance in the preparation of this manuscript.

REFERENCES

1. The Lipid Research Clinics Coronary Primary Prevention Trial Results. I. Reduction in incidence

of coronary heart disease. *JAMA* 1984; **251**: 351–64.

2. Frick MH, Elo O, Haapa K et al. Helsinki Heart Study : primary-prevention trial with gemfibrozil in middle-aged men with dyslipidemia : safety of treatment, changes in risk factors and incidence of coronary heart disease. *N Engl J Med* 1987; **317**: 1237–45.

3. Davey Smith G, Pekkanen J. Should there be a moratorium on the use of cholesterol-lowering drugs? *BMJ* 1992; **304**: 431–4.

4. Pyörälä K, de Backer G, Graham I et al., on behalf of the Task Force. Prevention of coronary heart disease in clinical practice. Recommendations of the Task Force of the European Society of Cardiology, European Atherosclerosis Society and European Society of Hypertension. *Eur Heart J* 1994; **15**: 1300–1.

5. Summary of the second report of the national cholesterol education program (NCEP) expert panel on detection, evaluation, and treatment of high blood cholesterol in adults (adult treatment panel II). *JAMA* 1993; **269**: 3015–23.

6. International Task Force for Prevention of Coronary Heart Disease. Prevention of Coronary Heart Disease: scientific background and new clinical guidelines. *Nutrition Metabolism Cardiovasc Dis* 1992; **2**: 113–56.

7. Imperial Cancer Research Fund OXCHECK Study Group. Effectiveness of health checks conducted by nurses in primary care: final results of the OXCHECK study. *BMJ* 1995; **310**: 1099–104.

8. Manninen V, Tenkanen L, Koskinen P et al. Joint effects of serum triglyceride and LDL cholesterol and HDL cholesterol concentrations on coronary heart disease risk in the Helsinki Heart Study. *Circulation* 1992; **85**: 37–45.

9. Huttunen JK, Manninen V, Manttari M et al. The Helsinki Heart Study. Central findings and clinical implications. *Ann Med* 1991; **23**: 155–9.

10. Shepherd J, Cobbe SM, Isles CG et al. Prevention of coronary heart disease with pravastatin in men with hypercholesterolemia. *N Engl J Med* 1995; **333**: 1301–7.

11. The Scandinavian Simvastatin Survival Study Group. Randomized trial of cholesterol lowering in 4444 patients with coronary heart disease: the Scandinavian Simvastatin Survival Study (4S). *Lancet* 1994; **344**: 1383–9.

12. West of Scotland Coronary Prevention Study Group. Influence of pravastatin and plasma lipids on clinical events in the West of Scotland

Coronary Prevention Study (WOSCOPS). *Circulation* 1998; **97**: 1440–5.

13. Pedersen TR, Kjeksus J, Berg K et al. Baseline serum cholesterol and treatment effect in the Scandinavian Simvastatin Survival Study (4S). *Lancet* 1995; **345**: 1274–5.

14. Downs JR, Clearfield E, Weis S et al. Primary prevention of acute coronary events with lovastatin in men and women with average cholesterol levels. *JAMA* 1998; **279**: 1615–22.

15. Sacks FM, Pfeffer MA, Lemuel AM et al., for the Cholesterol and Recurrent Event Trial Investigators. The effect of pravastatin on coronary events after myocardial infarction in patients with average cholesterol levels. *N Engl J Med* 1996; **335**: 1001–9.

16. Heart Protection Study Collaborative Group. MRC/BHF Heart Protection Study of cholesterol lowering with simvastatin in 20536 high-risk individuals: a randomised placebo-controlled trial. *Lancet* 2002; **360**: 7–22.

17. Grundy SM. Statin trials and goals of cholesterol-lowering therapy. *Circulation* 1998; **97**: 1436–9.

18. Hulley SB, Grady D, Bush T et al., for the HERS Research Group. Randomized trial of estrogen plus progestin for secondary prevention of coronary heart disease in post-menopausal women. *JAMA* 1998; **280**: 605–13.

19. Writing Group for the Women's Health Initiative Investigators. Risks and benefits of estrogen plus prostegin in healthy post-menopausal women: principal results from the Women's Health Initiative randomised controlled trial. *JAMA* 2002; **288**: 321–33.

20. Shepherd J, Blauw GJ, Murphy MB et al. on behalf of the PROSPER Study Group. Pravastatin in elderly individuals at risk of vascular disease (PROSPER): a randomised controlled trial. *Lancet* 2002; **360**: 1623–30.

21. Collins R, Armitage J. High-risk elderly patients PROSPER from cholesterol-lowering therapy. *Lancet* 2002; **360**: 1618–19.

22. Long-term Intervention with Pravastatin in Ischemic Disease (LIPID) Study Group. Prevention of cardiovascular events and death with pravastatin in patients with coronary heart disease and a broad range of initial cholesterol levels. *N Engl J Med* 1998; **339**: 1349–57.

23. Goldberg RB, Mellies MJ, Sacks FM et al. Cardiovascular events and their reduction with pravastatin in diabetic and glucose intolerant myocardial infarction survivors with average cholesterol levels. *Circulation* 1998; **98**: 2513–19.

24. Pyörälä K, Pedersen TJ, Kjerkshus J et al. and the Scandinavian Simvastatin Survival Study (4S) Group. Cholesterol lowering with simvastatin improves prognosis of diabetic patients with coronary heart disease. *Diabetes Care* 1997; **20**: 614–20.

25. Ridker PM, Hennekens CH, Buring JE, Rifai N. C-reactive protein and other markers of inflammation in the prediction of cardiovascular disease in women. *N Engl J Med* 2000; **342**: 836–43.

26. Danesh J, Whincup P, Waljer M et al. Low-grade inflammation and coronary disease: prospective study and updated meta-analyses. *BMJ* 2000; **321**: 199–204.

27. Ridker PM, Rifai N, Clearfield M et al. Measurement of C-reactive protein for the targeting of statin therapy in the primary prevention of acute coronary events. *N Engl J Med* 2001; **344**: 1959–65.

28. Shah PK. Circulating markers of inflammation for vascular risk prediction: are they ready for prime time? *Circulation* 2000; **105**: 1758–9.

29. West of Scotland Coronary Prevention Study Group. Identification of high-risk groups and comparisons with other cardiovascular intervention trials. *Lancet* 1996; **348**: 1339–42.

30. Wilson PW, D'Agostino RB, Levy D et al. Prediction of coronary heart disease using risk categories. *Circulation* 1998; **97**: 1837–47.

31. Assmann G, Culler P, Schulte H. The Muster heart study (PROCAM). Results of follow-up at 8 years. *Eur Heart J* 1998; **19** (Suppl A): A2–A11.

32. Jonsson B, Johansson M, Kjekshus J et al. Cost-effectiveness of cholesterol lowering. Results from the Scandinavian Simvastatin Survival Study (4S). *Eur Heart J* 1996; **17**: 1001–7.

33. Sacks FM, Moyé LA, Davis BR et al. Relationship between plasma LDL concentrations during treatment with pravastatin and recurrent coronary events in the Cholesterol and Recurrent Events trial. *Circulation* 1998; **97**: 1446–52.

34. Pedersen TR, Olsson AG, Faergerman O et al. Lipoprotein changes and reduction in the inci-dence of major coronary heart disease events in the Scandinavian Simvastatin Survival Study (4S). *Circulation* 1998; **97**: 1453–60.

35. Wood D, de Backer G, Faergerman O et al. Prevention of coronary heart disease in clinical practice: summary of recommendations of the Second Joint Task Force of European and Other Societies on Coronary Prevention. *Atherosclerosis* 1998; **140**: 199–220.

36. Expert Panel on Detection, Evaluation and Treatment of High Blood Cholesterol in Adults. Executive summary of the Third Report of the National Cholesterol Education Program (NCEP) Expert Panel on Detection, Evaluation and Treatment of High Blood Cholesterol in Adults (Adult Treatment Panel III). *JAMA* 2001; **285**: 2486–97.

37. Knatterud GL, Rosenberg Y, Campeau L et al. and Post-CABG Investigators. The long-term effects on clinical outcomes of aggressive lowering of low-density lipoprotein cholesterol levels and low-dose anti-coagulation in the Post Coronary Artery Bypass Graft Trial. *Circulation* 2000; **102**: 157–65.

38. Schwartz GG, Olsson AG, Ezekowitz MD et al. Effects of atorvastatin on early recurrent ischemic events in acute coronary syndromes. The MIRACL Study: a randomised controlled trial. *JAMA* 2001; **285**: 1711–18.

39. GISSI Prevenzione Investigators. Dietary supplementation with n–3 polyunsaturated fatty acids and vitamin E after myocardial infarction: results of the GISSI-Prevenzione trial. *Lancet* 1999; **354**: 447–55.

40. Stephens NG, Parsons A, Schofield PM et al. Randomised controlled trial of vitamin E in patients with coronary heart disease: Cambridge Heart Antioxidant Study (CHAOS). *Lancet* 1996; **347**: 781–6.

41. Wood D, Durrington O, McInnes G et al. for the British Cardiac Society, British Hyperlipidaemia Association, British Hypertension Society. Joint British recommendations on prevention of coronary heart disease in clinical practice. *Heart* 1998; **80** (Suppl 2): S1–S29.

15

The cost-effectiveness of statin use

J Jaime Caro and Krista F Huybrechts

INTRODUCTION

For the first edition of this book, it was felt necessary to justify the very need for cost-effectiveness information and even the basic methods had to be described. Since then, economic analysis of healthcare interventions has become mainstream and there have been considerable advances in the evaluations of statin use and other interventions to reduce the risk of cardiovascular disease, both in methodological terms and in the number of interventions, populations and countries that have been analysed.[1–52] Indeed, there are now several reviews of the published cost-effectiveness analyses,[21–28] and these have generally concluded that statin use can be cost-effective in many situations. Now decision makers face the challenge of dealing with the profusion of information in order to assess the implications for local budgets[29–47] and even the choice of statin.[4,7,9,15,26,28,44] Despite the numerous publications on the subject, however, the standards to be used in such judgements remain ill defined.

Through the many evaluations that have been carried out, it has become clear that the issue is no longer whether but rather in whom the statins are cost-effective, and this depends predominantly on the level of cardiovascular risk manifest without their use. In this new chapter, we address this cost-effectiveness as a function of risk in light of the new guidelines for managing hyperlipidaemia. We begin with a delineation of an economic evaluation and its key components.

ELEMENTS OF 'COST-EFFECTIVENESS' ANALYSIS

General considerations

Economic analyses of medical interventions, particularly of pharmacological ones such as the statins, are today mostly about their efficiency; in other words, they address the amount of health 'produced' for a given cost.[53] This approach is typically known as 'cost-effectiveness analysis' (though this general use of the term conflicts with its proper technical application to an analysis where health gains are valued in natural units rather than monetary units or utilities). The virtue of these kinds of evaluations is that they allow, at least in principle, the ranking of interventions according to their efficiency and, thus, they provide the decision-maker with a metric for judging their worth. Apart from the lack of consensus on the minimum efficiency required (leading to the pronouncement of arbitrary thresholds such as $50 000 per life-year gained), these types of analyses do not take into account the availability of the resources required to implement the intervention.

Thus, a second major type of analysis has begun to appear. In these evaluations, the acceptability of the intervention's efficiency is taken for granted and the assessment focuses on the impact its implementation will have on the available budgets and other resources.[54] Properly done, this kind of economic analysis delves in depth into the delivery of healthcare and the changes that might result. This makes its results extremely local, however, even more so than those of cost-effectiveness studies, and thus reduces their scientific usefulness.

Components

The efficiency of any medical intervention is typically analysed in terms of its incremental health consequences relative to the net health-care costs. By convention, this is expressed as a ratio of the net costs to the value of the health gains: the cost-effectiveness ratio. Despite this ratio's popularity in pharmacoeconomic circles, it is flawed because it does not provide for decision making the way a proper cost–benefit calculation, which expresses both the numerator and denominator in monetary units, would.[55] Given the discomfort induced in many, the predilection has been, however, to stop short of the direct equation of health with money.

Effectiveness
Health outcomes
The end-points used for statistical reasons in trials (i.e. one end-point or a pre-defined cluster of a few key ones perceived to be sufficiently objective) are usually too narrow to be meaningful to patients, and thus presumably to the decision makers – numerous, if not all, cardiovascular end-points are consequential. Indeed, the object of lipid-lowering therapy is to retard or even reverse the progression of atherosclerotic disease. An economic analysis, therefore, should not be confined solely to the health consequences defined as primary end-points in the trials. This expansion of the end-point must be tempered by the need to stay within the bounds set by available data and reasonable projections they may give rise to. Even a single end-point has multiple implications: pain and suffering; life expectancy; financial; social; etc. Thus, to fully address the decision, an economic analysis should consider all of these. This proves very difficult, however, as there is no obvious way to put all these aspects together and neither utilities nor 'quality of life' measures are sufficiently developed to be a practical alternative at this point.

Instead, many economic analyses focus on the change in life expectancy. This simplifies the end-point but brings on new problems. None of the trials are sufficiently long to provide for reasonable quantification of the life-years gained. Although some have nonetheless advocated use of the trial data alone,[56] this is clearly not a tenable position.[57] It would involve accepting the clinically absurd proposition that cardiovascular disease that is not fatal within the few years of a trial will have no detrimental impact on life expectancy (and is thus not worth preventing!).

A much more credible premise is that the implications of these non-fatal events must also be taken into account. To do so requires data external to the trials which permit quantification of the full survival curve following an event and the comparable curve in the absence of an event.

Risk reduction
To quantify the health consequences – known commonly as the 'effectiveness' – of a preventive intervention like a statin, the reduction in risk is required. For theoretical reasons, supported by some empirical results, it is thought that the relative risk reduction applies broadly to populations beyond those studied in the trials. The same, however, cannot be said for the absolute risk reduction, the measure required in economic analysis. The procedures employed to ensure validity in a trial – particularly patient selection, consent and mandated management – tend to yield a healthier, better cared for population than that extant in routine practice. This means that the absolute risk reductions derived from trial data tend to be underestimates.

The absolute risk reduction can be calculated easily from the relative risk reduction obtained from a properly conducted clinical trial by multiplying the latter by the reference risk. The reference risk, then, can be derived using other data from epidemiologic studies with fewer constraints and more applicability to other settings and populations. Although the applicability of the relative risk reduction across populations lies at the root of much of current clinical research, one could legitimately question whether it is justified to assume the same risk reduction for all individuals when the risk can vary over such a broad range. More importantly, it is typically assumed that the same relative risk reduction applies regardless of which risk factors – treatment-modifiable or not – constitute that risk. For example, a 77-year-old male smoker with total cholesterol 190 mg/dl, HDL cholesterol 47 mg/dl and (untreated) systolic blood pressure 123 mmHg has a 20% ten-year risk. It is unlikely, however, that the relative risk reduction due to statin treatment observed in this person will be the same as that in a 46-year-old male non-smoker with total cholesterol 285 mg/dl, HDL cholesterol 38 mg/dl and (treated) systolic blood pressure 136 mmHg who also experiences a 20% risk. This differential effect of treatment depending on what constitutes the risk is not currently accounted for in cost-effectiveness analyses.

Costs

Although many aspects of statin use might be considered under the rubric costs, most analyses confine this element to the direct use of healthcare resources. This includes medical activities, hospitalizations, medicines and laboratory testing, and might extend to paramedical areas such as stays in nursing homes. It does not encompass resources typically covered by patients and their families (e.g. transportation) nor the indirect costs of lost productivity and other such implications of illness. In general, the criterion is that the expenses be borne by the decision maker to whom the analysis is directed, i.e. the 'perspective'. To estimate the direct costs, two separate types of data are required. One is the pattern of use of healthcare resources following an event, the other is the expense of a unit of each type of resource used. By aggregating the product of the two, an overall cost is estimated.

The cost of statin use to prevent cardiovascular disease is offset somewhat by the savings produced by avoiding this disease in a proportion of the patients. Cardiovascular events typically consume substantial healthcare resources. Nearly always they lead to hospitalization and frequently this involves a stay in special care

units and the use of invasive procedures or surgery. Moreover, patients discharged alive will tend to require additional services, at least initially, and some events may imply care for long-term disability. Determination of the resource use pattern following each event involves knowing the type of healthcare services used by the patient, the frequency and duration of use for each service, and the proportion of patients with the condition who use the service. These patterns of resource use may be highly dependent on the country or even physician at issue. Thus, it is important to cite the country or region to which the patterns apply.

The methods used to estimate offsetting costs vary considerably among economic evaluations. A large source of the differences is the availability of information about the cost of managing cardiovascular events. Data on resource patterns are still very scanty and, even when available, they can be difficult to obtain. Although recently it has become somewhat easier to estimate the cost of the acute hospitalization as many organizations collect this information for administrative purposes, subsequent care remains difficult to quantify.

For the treatment itself, variations in dose and compliance must not be ignored. Compliance data are necessary so as to not overestimate the cost of treatment – only the proportion actually taking the medication should incur its cost. Measuring compliance can prove difficult, however, and trials typically report only drop-outs, which can result from many protocol-related reasons other than non-compliance. Nevertheless, using these proxy measures to estimate compliance is better than ignoring it altogether.

Assigning a unit cost is somewhat easier as lists of prices tend to exist in many places. These are rarely the actual cost of a service as they tend to reflect other items, but are frequently used, sometimes with correction factors applied, e.g. a cost-to-charge ratio in the USA. When the source data are older than the reporting year of the analysis, most researchers choose to inflate the values. Not only must the inflation rate and procedure used be noted but this practice can lead to distortions in the estimates as the unit costs of individual items often fail to follow average inflation rates.

As obtaining each of these components can be quite difficult, investigators sometimes resort to using standard aggregate measures, most commonly based on Diagnosis Related Groups (DRGs). Although easier to find, these types of estimates have a serious deficiency for economic analysis – few (<10%) DRGs are disease- or procedure-specific. Thus, they reflect conditions that have nothing to do with the disease at hand.

All estimates must be reported in terms of a currency and are thus subject to fluctuations in that currency. It is important, therefore, to cite both the year to which the source data correspond and the year used for the currency.

ECONOMIC IMPLICATIONS IN RELATION TO RISK

Cardiovascular disease has been and will likely continue to be one of the most costly diseases. It has been estimated that in 2002 alone, $329 billion will have been spent on treatment costs and lost productivity in the USA.[58] The mean first-year costs for acute in-patient and post-acute care for cardiovascular events have previously been estimated to vary between $7399 and $54 848 (1998 US$), depending on the type of event.[59] Given the large number of people affected and the seriousness of the consequences, primary prevention offers the greatest opportunity for decreasing the burden of cardiovascular disease.

The National Cholesterol Education Program (NCEP) in the USA released in May 2001 its most recent guidelines for the management of hyperlipidaemia, known as NCEP ATPIII.[60] Its major new feature, compared with previous reports published in 1988 and 1993, is a focus on primary prevention in persons with multiple risk factors, many of which have a relatively high risk for coronary heart disease (CHD) and are expected to benefit from rather intense low-density lipoprotein (LDL)-lowering therapy. A primary aim of the guidelines is indeed to match intensity of LDL-lowering therapy with

absolute risk. Out of concern for the budgetary implications of widespread drug use, the risk cut-points are based on cost-effectiveness as well as risk–benefit considerations.

A similar approach has been taken in European guidelines.[61–66] In this section, we assess the practical implications of the NCEP approach. Specifically, the cost-effectiveness of drug treatment is estimated across a broad range of CHD risk levels. This provides a numerical context in which to interpret the qualitative statements about cost-effectiveness included in the guidelines and allows further validation of the recommended cut-points from an efficiency point of view. In addition, to help inform the budgetary implications, the potential size and characteristics of the populations in the USA that would be affected according to the guidelines are examined.

Continuum Of Risk Evaluation

The cost-effectiveness of statin therapy was assessed using the Continuum Of Risk Evaluation (CORE), an economic model of prevention of cardiovascular disease that allows balancing the major clinical benefits of treatment against the cost of its provision across a broad range of cardiovascular disease risk. CORE, described in detail elsewhere,[67] is a simulation of the course of individual patients. The simulations are carried out in two sub-models: one evaluates the transition from health to cardiovascular disease (i.e. primary prevention); the other evaluates the implications of additional events (i.e. secondary prevention). Each month of the individual's life is simulated based on the risks they are expected to face, given their characteristics. As the surviving patient moves through the model, the number and type of events, as well as their time of occurrence, are tallied. This process is replicated for a given number of patients. To assess the implications of a particular treatment, pharmacological or other, the same patients are modelled again but the risks are adjusted to accord with the new treatment strategy. The cumulative difference in events reflects the effectiveness of the intervention.

The efficacy of statin use was estimated by re-analysing data from the West of Scotland Coronary Prevention Study (WOSCOPS),[68] the Cholesterol and Recurrent Events trial (CARE)[69] and the Long-term Intervention with Pravastatin in Ischemic Disease study (LIPID).[70] This led to estimates of 22% reduction of cardiovascular disease risk in patients without pre-existing disease and 20% in secondary prevention. To accord with NCEP guidelines, a time horizon of ten years was considered in the analyses. It was therefore assumed that the treatment effect observed in the trials, which had an average follow-up of five years, would extend to ten years.

To determine the implications of cardiovascular events for life expectancy – and thus permit estimation of the life-years gained – the remaining duration of life beyond the model's time horizon must be estimated for patients still alive at the end of the simulation. This was realized by exposing the patient to death hazards appropriate for the age, gender and cardiovascular status at that time. The hazard functions were derived using data from the USA life table,[71] the Scottish record linkage system,[72] and Saskatchewan Health,[73] and allow for the tendency of the death hazard to decrease with time from the acute cardiovascular event as well as for the natural increasing trend with age. Discounting is applied at 3% per year. Duration was not adjusted by quality of life, owing to a lack of appropriate data.

The costs of treatment and of cardiovascular disease were assessed from the perspective of a payer providing full healthcare coverage. Only direct medical costs are included. In-patient cost estimates for initial events and specific patterns of subsequent events were developed using data from five all-payer state discharge databases (California, Florida, Massachusetts, Maryland and Washington),[74–78] supplemented with information from the literature for in-patient physician services. The costs of subsequent care comprise post-discharge sub-acute in-patient care, community care and hospital readmissions related to the cardiovascular events, and are based on a variety of sources, including Medicare Ambulatory Payment Groups, government reports, clinical practice guidelines and other literature.

For consistency with the efficacy data, the drug cost was based on the Average Wholesale Price for pravastatin, reduced by 18.3% to reflect the actual pharmacy acquisition costs.[79] The cost of a lipid profile and a visit to the general practitioner every six months for monitoring purposes was also included. As there was no evidence in the trials of important side-effects caused by treatment,* no costs for their management were included. All estimates are reported in 1998 US$ and were discounted at 3% per year.

Cost-effectiveness by risk

The cost-effectiveness of drug treatment – expressed as cost per discounted life-year gained – for primary and secondary prevention was estimated for the various age categories considered in NCEP ATPIII. The primary prevention analyses make use of the full, integrated model; that is, subjects who start on primary prevention continue treatment if an initial non-fatal cardiovascular event occurs. Results are provided separately for males and females.

For primary prevention, a range of reference risks is considered to allow evaluation of the impact of treatment in the various risk strata likely to occur in a primary prevention population. For secondary prevention, on the other hand, the occurrence of a previous event is considered a marker of disease, and discrimination of treatment between patient groups based on poorly understood subsequent risk markers seems harder to justify. The population's average reference risk was therefore estimated by calculating the hazard of recurrent cardiovascular events over the five years of the CARE trial in the placebo group on an 'intention-to-treat' basis. These five-year reference risks amount to 53.5% for males, and 60.6% for females (approximately ten-year risks of 78.1% and 84.5%, respectively).

---

* It should be noted that the body of evidence supporting the association between statin use and the very rare condition rhabdomyolysis is growing.

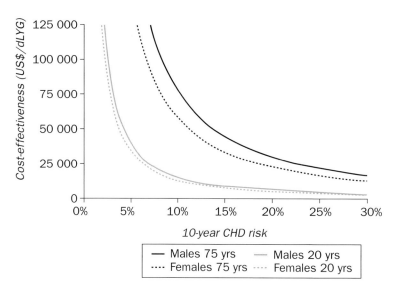

Fig. 15.1 Cost-effectiveness by ten-year coronary disease risk.

Figure 15.1 illustrates the cost-effectiveness of primary prevention with a statin for various risk levels over a ten-year time horizon. The curves for the youngest and oldest age groups considered in the ATPIII guidelines are displayed. The cost-effectiveness ratios for other age groups fall within the band bordered by these two extreme curves. For risks above 20%, the cost-effectiveness generally remains well below $20 000 per dLYG (discounted life year gained – the threshold frequently used to classify programmes as having strong evidence of cost-effectiveness) with a maximum around $30 000 per LYG for the oldest age groups. At a 10% risk – an important risk level in view of the NCEP ATPIII recommendations – the cost-effectiveness varies between $13 400 and $79 200 per LYG, depending on the age and, to a lesser extent, the gender of the individual. From an efficiency point of view, treatment would be hard to justify for risks much below 5% as the cost-effectiveness ratios rise steeply beyond this level for all ages considered.

Although there is no clear threshold value that determines when a therapy is or is not cost-effective, it is informative to view the results in light of the values that are commonly used for strong ($20 000 per LYG) and moderate ($50 000 per LYG) evidence of cost-effectiveness. The ten-year risks at which these thresholds are crossed are displayed for the various age groups in Fig. 15.2. If the strictest criterion were used, the lowest risk at which treatment seems warranted (from an efficiency viewpoint) varies between about 7% for the youngest and 25% for the oldest candidates. The 10% cut-point is crossed at the age of about 30 for males and 35 for females. For a threshold of $50 000 per LYG, treatment of patients with a ten-year risk above 10% would certainly seem justified in almost all cases.

The cost-effectiveness of secondary prevention with a statin was estimated to vary between $1263/dLYG and $5276 for males, and between $360/dLYG and $1530/dLYG for females, depending on the age at which treatment is initiated, again using a ten-year time horizon. Drug therapy can therefore be fully supported on cost-effectiveness grounds.

Budget implications

Decision making on the affordability of a specific therapy, in this case statins, depends not only on considerations about cost-effectiveness but also on the total costs to the community given the size of the potential populations. Data from the 1988–1994 National Health and Nutrition Examination Survey (NHANES III)[80] were employed to characterize the populations that would fall within each of the risk and treatment categories specified in NCEP ATPIII. All indi-

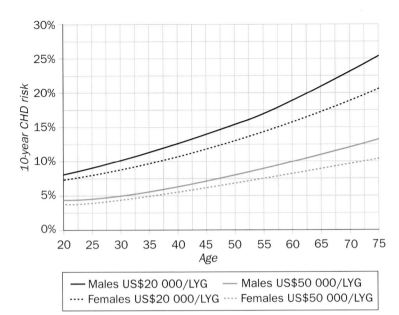

Fig. 15.2 Risks at which cost-effectiveness thresholds are crossed.

viduals between 20 and 79 years of age were used as the starting population for the analyses. First, patients in the highest-risk category, with clinically manifest cardiovascular disease, defined as a prior stroke, myocardial infarction or congestive heart failure, were identified. Next, patients with a diagnosis of peripheral arterial disease, abdominal aortic aneurysm, symptomatic carotid artery disease or diabetes were selected, as NCEP considers them equivalent to patients with established cardiovascular disease in terms of risk level. The risk status in the remaining persons was determined by a two-step procedure as described in the guidelines. First, the number of risk factors was counted. These include cigarette smoking, hypertension (blood pressure ⩾140/90 mmHg or on anti-hypertensive medication), low high-density lipoprotein (HDL) cholesterol (<40 mg/dl), family history of premature CHD (CHD in male first-degree relative <55 years; CHD in female first-degree relative <65 years) and age (men ⩾45 years; women ⩾55 years). High HDL cholesterol (i.e. ⩾60 mg/dl) counts as a 'negative' risk factor as its presence removes one risk factor from the total count. Information on all these risk factors was available in NHANES with the exception of family history of premature death. The closest variable in the NHANES dataset

asked whether the individual had 'Any relative with a heart attack before the age of 50?' which was therefore used as a proxy for the more specific definition considered in ATPIII. Second, the ten-year CHD risk was estimated for these patients based on the risk scoring system provided in the guidelines. The risk factors included in the calculation of ten-year risk are age, total cholesterol, HDL cholesterol, systolic blood pressure, treatment for hypertension and cigarette smoking. All of these variables were available in the NHANES dataset. Based on this information, individuals could be classified in one of the three risk categories that determine the LDL cholesterol goal. Finally, the individuals' LDL cholesterol levels were obtained to determine the recommended treatment: lifestyle changes or drug therapy.

Twenty-seven percent of the adult US population (about 188 million) falls into the highest-risk category, i.e. established CHD, CHD risk equivalent or a ten-year risk greater than 20%. Of those, about 8.7 million patients (5.3 million males and 3.5 million females) have overt cardiovascular disease. Another 27% have multiple risk factors; the remainder constitutes the lowest-risk category (0–1 risk factor). Some level of treatment – therapeutic lifestyle changes or drug therapy – is recommended for 46% of the population: 39% of

Table 15.1   Breakdown of the US population according to various risks and treatment recommendations

Risk category	Therapeutic lifestyle changes	Drug therapy
CHD or CHD risk equivalents (10-year risk >20%)	15 843 574	26 915 386
2+ risk factors (10-year risk 10–20%)	5 498 622	8 614 737
2+ risk factors (10-year risk >10%)	10 181 077	6 212 034
0–1 risk factor	6 432 911	3 313 430
All	**37 956 184**	**45 055 586**

females and 50% of males. Table 15.1 presents the breakdown of the population according to the various risk and treatment categories. As NCEP ATPIII provides only one LDL cholesterol cut-point for differentiating treatment in individuals with 2+ risk factors and a ten-year risk between 10% and 20%,[60] it was assumed that lifestyle changes would be recommended for everyone with an LDL cholesterol below 130 mg/dl, which will likely overestimate the number of people in this sub-group.

Only about 2% of the population without CHD or CHD risk equivalent – that is, those individuals for whom the CHD risk can be estimated using the risk scoring provided in NCEP ATPIII – have a ten-year risk above 20%. About three-quarters of the population has a risk less than 5%. The overall risk distribution for males and females is provided in Fig. 15.3a.

Not surprisingly, the distribution in females is clearly shifted towards the lower risk levels compared with males. The same holds within specific risk categories. For example, 47% of females with two or more risk factors have a risk ≤1% versus 16% of males (see Fig. 15.3c–e).

For the majority of people in the lowest-risk category, treatment does not seem necessary. Drug therapy is recommended for only about 4% of males and females, interestingly spread fairly evenly across all risk levels (see Fig. 15.3b and e). About one-third of individuals with multiple risk factors would be advised to start drug therapy, but this is largely driven by those with a 10–20% risk: 58% of males and 75% of females, compared with 17% of those with a risk <10% (see Fig. 15.3b and d).

Whereas the differences in cost-effectiveness of drug therapy between males and females at a given age and risk are relatively minor (and mainly due to gender differences in life expectancy), the distribution of individuals across the various age and risk categories differs substantially, as illustrated in Fig. 15.4. As many as 49% of females – for whom drug therapy would be indicated according to ATPIII – have a ten-year risk below 5% and thus unfavourable cost-effectiveness. The corresponding number for males is 15%. Likewise, only about 4% of females are at very high risk (>20%), compared to 16% of males. These findings suggest that treatment of hypercholesterolaemia in females following the NCEP ATPIII will, on average, be somewhat less cost-effective than in their male counterparts.

CONCLUSION

Developments in healthcare have placed pressure on proponents of new therapies to defend the reasonableness of the associated expense. The use of statins to prevent cardiovascular disease is no exception. Unfortunately, these economic concerns occasion a whole new set of data requirements – needs for which the field has been ill prepared. For the most part, the massive prevention clinical trials did not collect these types of information. Nevertheless, economic analyses of the trials have been undertaken and many have been published. Although several methodological concerns may be raised, these analyses, in general, remove economic efficiency as the basis for rejecting use of the statins to prevent cardiovascular disease – invariably, the

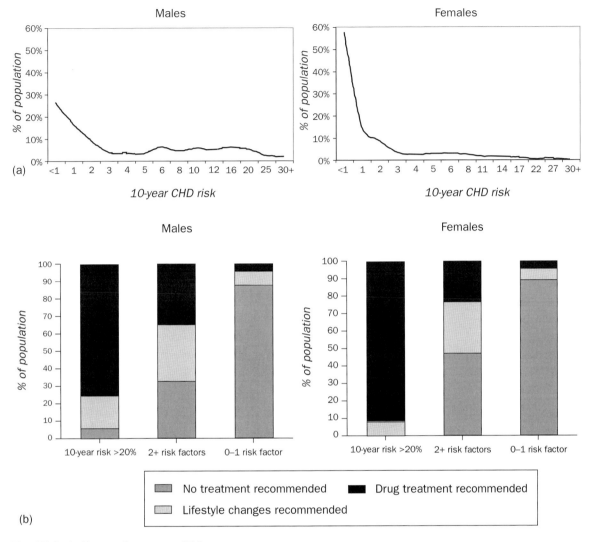

Fig. 15.3a,b For caption, see p. 223.

cost-effectiveness is well within the bounds typically felt to demarcate 'acceptable' therapies.

This admissible, even desirable, economic efficiency poses a dilemma for those who set health policy. Hypercholesterolaemia is a common condition and the trials have shown that nearly all those affected can benefit. Indeed, some of the trials suggest even lower thresholds at which treatment should be considered. Implementing these results thus leads to very large numbers of people receiving statins and – though this may represent an economically efficient intervention – the total expense may well exceed the capacity of many healthcare systems. Accordingly, more precise targeting of treatment has become an important consideration. This targeting assumes, however, that equity is not an issue. Even if a therapy is shown to be more cost-effective in a particular group of people, the question remains whether it is fair to withhold beneficial therapy from other insured people simply because, on average, it is less economically efficient. This is an area that has not received much attention but may become the focus as decision makers attempt to make full use of economic information.

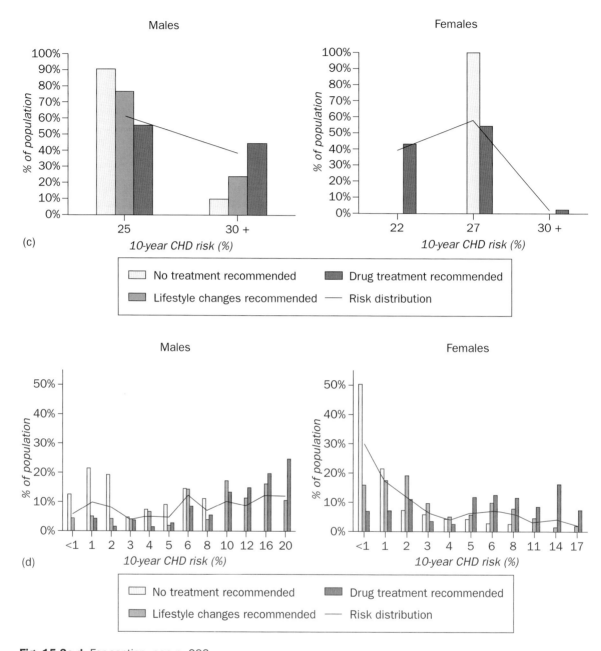

Fig. 15.3c,d For caption, see p. 223.

REFERENCES

1. Glasziou PP, Eckermann SD, Mulray SE et al. Cholesterol-lowering therapy with pravastatin in patients with average cholesterol levels and established ischaemic heart disease: is it cost-effective? *Med J Aust* 2002; 21: **177**: 428–34.

2. Athyros VG, Papageorgiou AA, Mercouris BR et al. Treatment with atorvastatin to the National Cholesterol Educational Program goal versus usual care in secondary coronary heart disease prevention. The GREek Atorvastatin and Coronary heart disease Evaluation (GREACE) study. *Curr Med Res Opin* 2002; **18**: 20–8.

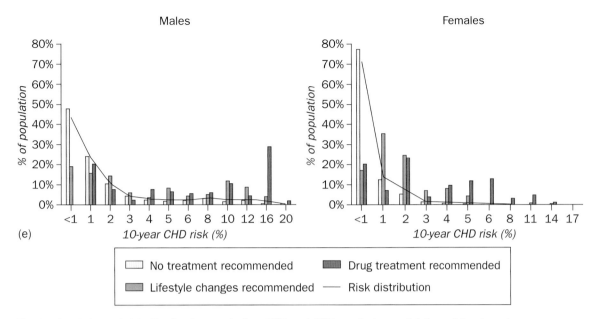

Fig. 15.3 (a) Overall risk distribution, excluding CHD and CHD equivalents. (b) Overall treatment recommendations by risk category (c) Risk distribution and breakdown of treatment recommendations by risk level for subjects with ten-year CHD risk greater than 20%. (d) Risk distribution and breakdown of treatment recommendations by risk level for subjects with 2 or more risk factors. (e) Risk distribution and breakdown of treatment recommendations by risk level for subjects with less than two risk factors.

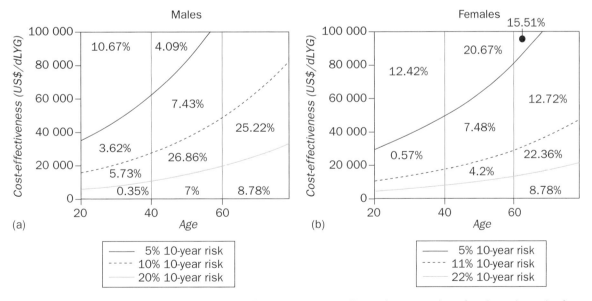

Fig. 15.4 Cost-effectiveness by age and risk. The percentages indicate the proportion of patients in each of the areas delineated by the vertical gridlines and the risk curves.

3. Wendland G, Klever-Deichert G, Lauterbach K. Cost-effectiveness of lipid-lowering therapy. *Herz* 2001; **26**: 552–60.

4. McPherson R, Hanna K, Agro A, Braeken A for the Canadian Cerivastatin Study Group. Cerivastatin versus branded pravastatin in the treatment of primary hypercholesterolemia in primary care practice in Canada: a one-year, open-label, randomized, comparative study of efficacy, safety, and cost-effectiveness. *Clin Ther* 2001; **23**: 1492–507.

5. Taylor AJ, Grace K, Swiecki J et al. Lipid-lowering efficacy, safety, and costs of a large-scale therapeutic statin formulary conversion program. *Pharmacotherapy* 2001; **21**: 1130–9.

6. Maclaine GD, Patel H. A cost-effectiveness model of alternative statins to achieve target LDL-cholesterol levels. *Int J Clin Pract* 2001; **55**: 243–9.

7. Attanasio E, Russo P, Allen SE. Cost-minimization analysis of simvastatin versus atorvastatin for maintenance therapy in patients with coronary or peripheral vascular disease. *Clin Ther* 2001; **23**: 276–83; discussion 274–5.

8. Russell MW, Huse DM, Miller JD et al. Cost-effectiveness of HMG-CoA reductase inhibition in Canada. *Can J Clin Pharmacol* 2001; **8**: 9–16.

9. Tarraga Lopez PJ, Celada Rodriguez A, Cerdan Oliver M et al. Cost-effectiveness of atorvastatin against simvastatin as hypolipemic treatment in hypercholesterolemic patients in primary care. *Aten Primaria* 2001; **27**: 18–24.

10. Garcia-Altes A, Jovell AJ. Which statin is more efficient? Concepts and applications in economic evaluation. *Aten Primaria* 2000; **26**: 333–8.

11. Perreault S, Levinton C, Le Lorier J. Efficacy and cost of HMG-CoA reductase inhibitors in the treatment of patients with primary hyperlipidemia. *Can J Clin Pharmacol* 2000; **7**: 144–54.

12. Szucs TD, Berger K, Marz W, Schafer JR. Cost-effectiveness of pravastatin in secondary coronary prevention in patients with myocardial infarct or unstable angina in Germany. An analysis on the basis of the LIPID trial. *Herz* 2000; **25**: 487–94.

13. Grover SA, Coupal L, Zowall H, Dorais M. Cost-effectiveness of treating hyperlipidemia in the presence of diabetes: who should be treated? *Circulation* 2000; **102**: 722–7.

14. Hilleman DE, Heineman SM, Foral PA. Pharmacoeconomic assessment of HMG-CoA reductase inhibitor therapy: an analysis based on the CURVES study. *Pharmacotherapy* 2000; **20**: 819–22.

15. Cobos A, Jovell AJ, Garcia-Altes A et al. Which statin is most efficient for the treatment of hypercholesterolemia? A cost-effectiveness analysis. *Clin Ther* 1999; **21**: 1924–36.

16. Szucs TD, Bertel O, Darioli R et al. Pharmacoeconomic evaluation of pravastatin in coronary secondary prevention in patients with myocardial infarct or unstable angina pectoris. An analysis based on the LIPID Study. *Schweiz Rundsch Med Prax* 2000; **89**: 745–52.

17. Prosser LA, Stinnett AA, Goldman PA et al. Cost-effectiveness of cholesterol-lowering therapies according to selected patient characteristics. *Ann Intern Med* 2000; **132**: 769–79.

18. Jonsson B, Cook JR, Pedersen TR. The cost-effectiveness of lipid lowering in patients with diabetes: results from the 4S trial. *Diabetologia* 1999; **42**: 1293–301.

19. Hilleman DE, Phillips JO, Mohiuddin SM et al. A population-based treat-to-target pharmacoeconomic analysis of HMG-CoA reductase inhibitors in hypercholesterolemia. *Clin Ther* 1999; **21**: 536–62.

20. Grover SA, Coupal L, Paquet S, Zowall H. Cost-effectiveness of 3-hydroxy-3-methylglutaryl-coenzyme A reductase inhibitors in the secondary prevention of cardiovascular disease: forecasting the incremental benefits of preventing coronary and cerebrovascular events. *Arch Intern Med* 1999; **159**: 593–600.

21. Durrington P. The human and economic costs of undertreatment with statins. *Int J Clin Pract* 2002; **56**: 357–68.

22. Jonsson B. Economics of drug treatment: for which patients is it cost-effective to lower cholesterol? *Lancet* 2001; **358**: 1251–6.

23. Shepherd J. Economics of lipid lowering in primary prevention: lessons from the West of Scotland Coronary Prevention Study. *Am J Cardiol* 2001; **87**: 19B–22B.

24. Rockson SG. Benefits of lipid-lowering agents in stroke and coronary heart disease: pharmacoeconomics. *Curr Atheroscler Rep* 2000; **2**: 144–50.

25. Marks D, Wonderling D, Thorogood M et al. Screening for hypercholesterolaemia versus case finding for familial hypercholesterolaemia: a systematic review and cost-effectiveness analysis. *Health Technol Assess* 2000; **4**: 1–123.

26. Elliott WJ, Weir DR. Comparative cost-effectiveness of HMG-CoA reductase inhibitors in secondary prevention of acute myocardial infarction. *Am J Health Syst Pharm* 1999; **56**: 1726–32.

27. Hay JW, Yu WM, Ashraf T. Pharmacoeconomics of lipid-lowering agents for primary and secondary prevention of coronary artery disease. *Pharmacoeconomics* 1999; **15**: 47–74.

28. Schwartz JS. Economics and cost-effectiveness in evaluating the value of cardiovascular therapies. Comparative economic data regarding lipid-lowering drugs. *Am Heart J* 1999; **137**: S97–S104.

29. Wettermark B, Hjemdahl P. Can we afford good cholesterol-lowering therapy? Budgeting of statin costs versus medical needs in the county of Stockholm. *Lakartidningen* 2001; **98**: 5472–3, 5476–8, 5481–3.

30. Mullins CD. The economics of lipid management. *Manag Care* 2001; **10** (11 Suppl): 17–8; discussion 19–24.

31. Lim SS, Vos T, Peeters A et al. Cost-effectiveness of prescribing statins according to pharmaceutical benefits scheme criteria. *Med J Aust* 2001; **175**: 459–64.

32. Beaird J. Using cost-effectiveness to target cholesterol reduction. *Ann Intern Med* 2001; **135**: 299–300.

33. Johannesson M. At what coronary risk level is it cost-effective to initiate cholesterol lowering drug treatment in primary prevention? *Eur Heart J* 2001; **22**: 919–25.

34. Pickin DM, McCabe CJ, Ramsay LE et al. Cost-effectiveness of HMG-CoA reductase inhibitor (statin) treatment related to the risk of coronary heart disease and cost of drug treatment. *Heart* 1999; **82**: 325–32.

35. Van Hout BA, Simoons ML. Cost-effectiveness of HMG coenzyme reductase inhibitors: whom to treat? *Eur Heart J* 2001; **22**: 751–61.

36. Cates C. A vote of no confidence in the precision of the estimated cost-effectiveness of lipid lowering. *Br J Gen Pract* 2000; **50**: 917.

37. Wilcock M. A vote of no confidence in the precision of the estimated cost-effectiveness of lipid lowering. *Br J Gen Pract* 2000; **50**: 917–18.

38. Hippisley-Cox J, Pringle M. The cost-effectiveness of lipid lowering in patients with ischaemic heart disease: an intervention and evaluation in primary care. *Br J Gen Pract* 2000; **50**: 699–705.

39. Barry M, Heerey A, Sheehan O et al. Pharmacoeconomics of lipid lowering therapy in Ireland. *Ir Med J* 1999; **92**: 430–2.

40. Reckless JP. Cost-effectiveness of statins. *Curr Opin Lipidol* 2000; **11**: 351–6.

41. Klever-Deichert G, Hinzpeter B, Wendland G, Lauterbach K. Cost–benefit analysis of an evidence-based secondary prevention of coronary heart diseases by statins. An analysis for Germany from a social security perspective. *Med Klin* 2000; **95**: 305–13.

42. Pearson TA. Population benefits of cholesterol reduction: epidemiology, economics, and ethics. *Am J Cardiol* 2000; **85**: 20E–3E.

43. Garber AM. Using cost-effectiveness analysis to target cholesterol reduction. *Ann Intern Med* 2000; **132**: 833–5.

44. Patel RJ, Gray DR, Pierce R, Jafari M. Impact of therapeutic interchange from pravastatin to lovastatin in a Veterans Affairs Medical Center. *Am J Manag Care* 1999; **5**: 465–74.

45. Bonneux L, Barendregt JJ. Primary prevention remains expensive, notwithstanding the consensus on lowering serum cholesterol levels. *Ned Tijdschr Geneeskd* 1999; **143**: 772–5.

46. Kessler JM. Economics and cost-effectiveness in evaluating the value of cardiovascular therapies. Lipid-lowering drugs, cost-effectiveness data, and the formulary system: a health systems perspective. *Am Heart J* 1999; **137**: S111–S114.

47. Jackson JD. Economics and cost-effectiveness in evaluating the value of cardiovascular therapies. Economics and cost-effectiveness in evaluating the value of cardiovascular therapy: lipid-lowering therapies – an industry perspective. *Am Heart J* 1999; **137**: S105–S10.

48. Delahanty LM, Sonnenberg LM, Hayden D, Nathan DM. Clinical and cost outcomes of medical nutrition therapy for hypercholesterolemia: a controlled trial. *J Am Diet Assoc* 2001; **101**: 1012–23.

49. Brunner E, Cohen D, Toon L. Cost-effectiveness of cardiovascular disease prevention strategies: a perspective on EU food-based dietary guidelines. *Public Health Nutr* 2001; **4**: 711–15

50. Finkelstein EA, Troped PJ, Will JC, Palombo R. Cost-effectiveness of a cardiovascular disease risk reduction program aimed at financially vulnerable women: the Massachusetts WISEWOMAN project. *J Womens Health Gend Based Med* 2002; **11**: 519–26.

51. Nyman JA, Martinson MS, Nelson D et al., for the VA-HIT Study Group. Cost-effectiveness of gemfibrozil for coronary heart disease patients with low levels of high-density lipoprotein cholesterol: the Department of Veterans Affairs High-Density Lipoprotein Cholesterol Intervention Trial. *Arch Intern Med* 2002; **162**: 177–82.

52. Ellis SL, Carter BL, Malone DC et al. Clinical and economic impact of ambulatory care clinical pharmacists in management of dyslipidemia in older adults: the IMPROVE study. Impact of Managed Pharmaceutical Care on Resource Utilization and Outcomes in Veterans Affairs Medical Centers. *Pharmacotherapy* 2000; **20**: 1508–16.

53. Marwick C. Pharmacoeconomics: is a drug worth its cost? *JAMA* 1994; **272**: 1395.

54. Trueman P, Drummond M, Hutton J. Developing guidance for budget impact analysis. *Pharmacoeconomics* 2001; **19**: 609–21.

55. Garber AM, Phelps CE. Economic foundations of cost-effectiveness analysis. *J Health Econ* 1995; **1**: 1–46.

56. Pharoah PDP, Hollingworth W. Cost-effectiveness of lowering cholesterol concentration with statins in patients with and without pre-existing coronary heart disease: life table method applied to health authority population. *BMJ* 1996; **312**: 1443–8.

57. Drummond M, Davies L. Economic analysis alongside clinical trials: Revisiting the methodological issue. *Intl J Tech Assess Health Care* 1991; **7**: 561–73.

58. American Heart Association. *2002 Heart and Stroke Statistical Update*. Dallas, Texas: American Heart Association, 2001.

59. Caro Research. *Weighing the Costs and Benefits of Preventing Cardiovascular Disease with Pravastatin*. Economic dossier submitted to the FDA under the FDA Modernization Act (Section 114), 1999.

60. Expert Panel on Detection, Evaluation, and Treatment of High Blood Cholesterol in Adults. Executive Summary of the Third Report of the National Cholesterol Education Program (NCEP) Expert Panel on Detection, Evaluation, and Treatment of High Blood Cholesterol in Adults (Adult Treatment Panel III). *JAMA* 2001; **285**: 2486–97.

61. Fretheim A, Bjorndal A, Oxman AD et al. Guidelines for pharmacological primary prevention of cardiovascular diseases – who should be treated? *Tidsskr Nor Laegeforen* 2002; **122**: 2277–81.

62. Scottish Intercollegiate Guidelines Network (SIGN). *Lipids and the Primary Prevention of Coronary Heart Disease. A National Clinical Guideline*. Edinburgh (Scotland): SIGN 1999: 60.

63. Simoons ML. Cholesterol-lowering therapy; a recommendation from the Health Council. *Ned Tijdschr Geneeskd* 2000; **144**: 2442–4.

64. Wood D, Durrington F, Poulter N et al. on behalf of the British Cardiac Society, British Hyperlipidaemia Association, British Hypertension Society and endorsed by the British Diabetic Association. Joint British recommendations on prevention of coronary heart disease in clinical practice. *Heart* 1998; **80** (Suppl 2): S1–S29.

65. Wood D, de Backer G, Faergeman O et al. Prevention of coronary heart disease in clinical practice. Recommendations of the Second Joint Task Force of European and Other Societies on Coronary Prevention. *Eur Heart J* 1998; **19**: 1434–503.

66. Faergeman O. The revised joint guidelines. *Atheroscler Suppl* 2000; **1**: 3–7.

67. Caro JJ, Huybrechts KF, Klittich WS et al. for the CORE Study Group. Allocating funds to prevention of cardiovascular disease in light of the NCEP ATPIII guidelines. *Am J Man Care* 2003; **9**: 477–89.

68. Shepherd J, Cobbe SM, Ford I et al. Prevention of coronary heart disease with pravastatin in men with hypercholesterolemia. *N Engl J Med* 1995; **333**: 1301–7.

69. Sacks FM, Pfeffer MA, Moye LA et al. The effect of pravastatin on coronary events after myocardial infarction in patients with average cholesterol levels. *N Engl J Med* 1996; **335**: 1001–9.

70. The LIPID Study Group. Prevention of cardiovascular events and death with pravastatin in patients with coronary heart disease and a wide range of initial cholesterol levels. *N Engl J Med* 1998; **339**: 1349–57.

71. US Department of Health and Human Services. Centers for Disease Control and Prevention. *National Vital Statistics Reports* 1998; **47**; 1–20.

72. Kendrick S, Clarice J. The Scottish Record Linkage System. *Health Bull (Edin)* 1993; **51**: 72–9.

73. Malcomb E, Downey W, Strand LM et al. Saskatchewan Health's linkable databases in pharmacoepidemiology. *Post Marketing Surveillance* 1993; **6**: 175–264.

74. 1996 Discharge Data, Version A. California Office of Statewide Health Planning and Development Databases.

75. 1996 Hospital Patient Discharge Data (Statewide). State of Florida. Agency for Health Care Administration, State Center for Health Statistics.

76. 1996 Maryland Standard Public Use File. CHARS Public Data File. St Paul Computer Center, Inc., 1996.

77. Fiscal Year 1996 Merged Case Mix and Charge Data. Massachusetts Division of Health Care Finance and Policy.

78. Washington State Department of Health. Comprehensive Hospital Abstract Reporting System, 1996.

79. Cardinale V. 1998 *Drug Topics Red Book.* Montvale, NJ: Medical Economics Company, Inc., 1998.

80. US Department of Health and Human Services (DHHS). National Center for Health Statistics. *Third National Health and Nutrition Examination Survey, 1988–1994,* NHANES III (CD-ROM Series 11). Public Use Data File Documentation Number 76200. Hyattsville, MD: Centers for Disease Control and Prevention, 1996.

16

Unanswered questions about the use of statins

Mehmet Cilingiroglu and Christie M Ballantyne

INTRODUCTION

The predictive relation between plasma cholesterol and coronary heart disease (CHD) has been well established by numerous observational and clinical trials. The concept of risk factors, introduced by the Framingham Heart Study more than 50 years ago, serves as the 'gold standard' in risk assessment for CHD. The major risk factors account for over 80% of excess risk for premature CHD according to follow-up data from the Multiple Risk Factor Intervention Trial (MRFIT).[1] The findings from Framingham have contributed greatly to the recommendations for CHD prevention published by the National Cholesterol Education Program (NCEP).[2] In May 2001, the National Heart, Lung and Blood Institute (Bethesda, MD) released updated cholesterol guidelines for the adult US population, and simultaneously, the executive summary of the Adult Treatment Panel III (ATP III) was published in the *Journal of the American Medical Association*. This report updated clinical guidelines for cholesterol testing and management and is the most recent component of the NCEP. Two previous panels have issued guidelines for adult treatment, and other panels of the NCEP have previously issued reports detailing other aspects of cholesterol measurement and management (including population recommendations, laboratory guidelines and standards for the treatment of children and adolescents). Also, since the first Joint European Societies – European Society of Cardiology, European

Atherosclerosis Society and European Society of Hypertension – Task Force recommendations on CHD prevention in clinical practice were published in 1994 new scientific evidence has emerged in both primary and secondary coronary prevention, particularly in relation to lipid-lowering therapy. Therefore, a second Task Force was convened by the three major societies, including professional representatives from behavioural medicine, primary care and the European Heart Network, to revise the recommendations, which were published in 1998.[3]

'Expert' groups in the USA and Europe have issued hundreds of guidelines in the last century. For decades, these publications found themselves gathering dust on shelves or quickly discarded. Only over the last one to two decades have clinical guidelines increasingly become part of the daily life of practising clinicians. The importance of such guidelines can be tracked to at least two concurrent developments: increasing attention to the practice of what is called evidence-based medicine and the increasing complexity of contemporary medical management. With regard to the latter, lipid management is no exception.

Our understanding of the complexity of lipid metabolism has been paralleled by the development of a wide array of laboratory tests and pharmacological interventions. Additionally, publications of large and important epidemiological observational studies evaluating the impact of cholesterol and lipoproteins on the development of CHD events has been partly eclipsed by 'mega-trials' of pharmacological interventions in individuals both with and without evident CHD. There have also been numerous smaller supplementary studies focused on specific sub-groups and on atherosclerosis progression. In their totality, these studies clearly document a favourable impact for lipid-modifying therapies.

For coronary prevention to become an integral part of everyday clinical practice, national societies of cardiology, atherosclerosis and hypertension, in collaboration with other professional organizations within each country, must take responsibility for developing their own guidelines, appropriate for their political, social and medical circumstances. The common challenge for cardiologists, physicians and other health professionals is to realize the potential for coronary prevention for all our patients and to contribute to wider public health efforts to reduce the enormous burden of cardiovascular disease. Despite established guidelines and major clinical trials and research data, there are several unanswered questions about the management of lipids in individuals with and without evident CHD.

WHO SHOULD BE TREATED?

For several years following the release of US and European initial guidelines, the co-ordinating committees felt that the importance of implementing the guidelines outweighed the need to develop new guidelines. Eventually, however, it became clear that the quantity of new information available from recent trials made it imperative that new guidelines be issued.

An over-riding approach in ATP III and Recommendations of the Second Joint Task Force of European and other Societies on Coronary Prevention is immediately evident when the full report is compared with the previous reports, namely, a series of evidence statements, followed by specific evidence-based recommendations. The evidence type includes four categories:

- major randomized controlled clinical trials
- smaller controlled trials and meta-analyses
- observational and metabolic studies
- clinical experience.

As the basic principle of prevention consists of matching the intensity of risk-reducing interventions to the level of the risk, the new guidelines have focused on those at higher risk. This necessarily blurs the distinction between primary and secondary prevention. A number of specific components aid particularly in both the identification and management of persons at high absolute risk without clinically evident coronary or other vascular disease. There are three key groups of patients without evident vascular disease who are nevertheless at high risk. The first is patients with diabetes. The multiple metabolic and lipid abnormalities present in such patients places them at particularly high risk for vascular disease events. Furthermore, among patients with diabetes who do have CHD events, their mortality and morbidity is much higher than age-matched non-diabetic patients. The second group includes patients whose ten-year CHD risk is over 20% by using Framingham scoring. Those two groups are considered to be CHD risk equivalents. That is, their ten-year risk is similar to the ten-year risk of an individual with stable angina, thus equivalent to a CHD patient.

The third high-risk group that attracts specific attention in the new guidelines contains those patients with multiple metabolic risk factors; this is known as metabolic syndrome. While the absolute ten-year risk of such patients varies widely and has not been as intensively studied as the other sub-groups noted previously, such patients are at markedly increased risk. Furthermore, they are optimal patients for intensified therapeutic lifestyle changes.

A complete lipid profile is now preferred for all patients 20 years and older for primary prevention. Furthermore, new guidelines have modified lipid and lipoprotein classifications so that a low-density lipoprotein cholesterol (LDL-C) of <100 mg/dl in ATP III is defined as optimal for the entire population, low high-density lipoprotein cholesterol (HDL-C) as a categorical risk factor has been raised from <35 mg/dl to 40 mg/dl and there are lower triglyceride cut-points, with more attention to moderate elevations. While the LDL-C remains the primary target for these patients, once the

LDL-C target has been achieved, then a non-HDL-C target is also specified for patients with triglycerides ≥200 mg/dl.

The Second Joint Task Force of E uropean and other Societies on Coronary Prevention identified a goal of LDL-C <115 mg/dl and total cholesterol <190 mg/dl for patients with CHD or other atherosclerotic disease, and for healthy high-risk individuals.

The new guidelines take an important step forward by placing considerable focus on the concept of risk and risk assessment, with attention to both long-term or lifetime risk, as well as short-term or ten-year-risk. It is important to consider lifetime or long-term risk in people who initially seem to be at relatively low short-term risk but have a single dominant risk factor. While such patients will not fall into the higher-risk sub-groups mentioned earlier, they will be at higher long-term risk. This highlights the importance of treating healthy individuals with abnormalities of even one risk factor. It is, however, recognized that it is clearly appropriate to focus more intensive risk-lowering strategies (especially drug therapies) on individuals at higher short-term (ten years) levels of risk. To estimate ten-year risk, the Framingham investigators have developed a sophisticated mathematical model that integrates the presence and levels of multiple clinical risk factors into a precision model.

While many aspects of the new guidelines generated considerable discussion and some controversy during the panel's deliberations, several key issues can be highlighted.

Some have raised the concern about targeting the metabolic syndrome for increased vigilance. Put simply, why isn't the metabolic syndrome elevated to the high-risk status, just as diabetes or a 20% ten-year risk is? Unfortunately, there is uncertainty about the precise risk associated with the metabolic syndrome and its components. While attention clearly does need to be directed to this important constellation of risk factors, in the evidence-based ATP III and Recommendations of the Second Joint Task Force of European and other Societies on Coronary Prevention reports, the panel could not confidently point to a level of risk associated with the metabolic syndrome

with any precision. Hopefully, in subsequent reports and as future research emerges, the contribution to risk of this syndrome and its key components can be known more precisely so that the goals associated with the presence of the metabolic syndrome can become more specific.

Some have raised concern about not including the family history in the Global Risk Score as a risk factor. When the Framingham investigators used family history (as assessed in the Framingham Heart Study), it did not add materially to the prediction of ten-year risk. This is probably for two reasons: firstly, family history operates through other risk factors, either environmental ones or inherited risk factors, such as high blood pressure and abnormal lipids; secondly, family history in Framingham was determined by asking a simple question that was not validated.

The results of the Heart Protection Study (HPS)[4] raised controversy about current guidelines. The largest cholesterol-lowering trial yet performed, this included over 20 000 patients with coronary disease, other vascular disease, diabetes and/or hypertension, randomized to 40 mg of simvastatin or matching placebo over a five-year treatment period. The primary endpoint (total mortality), as well as all pre-specified secondary end-points (the incidence of non-fatal myocardial infarction (MI), stroke and revascularization, and the incidence of a first major vascular event) in all pre-specified sub-groups, produced similar risk reductions of approximately 25%. In HPS there was also a definite 24% reduction in the first occurrence of any of the major vascular events (first stroke, non-fatal and fatal MI). The proportional reduction in the event rate was similar (and significant) in each category or sub-category of participants studied. Included in the pre-specified sub-group were patients with a baseline LDL-C of <115 mg/dl and <100 mg/dl, groups currently not recommended for further lipid-lowering therapy by current European and US guidelines, respectively. In HPS, about 3500 participants presented with a pre-treatment LDL-C measurement that was already below the 'target' level recommended by the current US and European guidelines. In these groups, there was a risk reduction similar to that

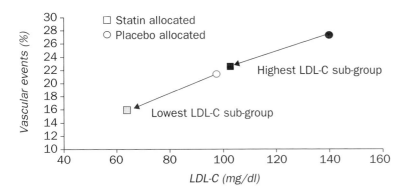

Fig. 16.1 Event reductions in Heart Protection Study patients with lower and higher low-density lipoprotein cholesterol (LDL-C) levels at baseline. (Adapted from http://www.hpsinfo.org.)

seen in all other sub-groups (Fig. 16.1), raising the suggestion that even CHD patients with baseline LDL-C of <100 mg/dl should be treated with statins. These findings indicate that current guidelines may inadvertently lead to substantial under-treatment of high-risk patients who present with LDL-C concentrations below, or close to, particular targets (such as <100 mg/dl in ATP III guidelines or <115 mg/dl in the Second European Joint Task Force recommendations).

Previous randomized trials of cholesterol-lowering therapy tended to include people with pre-existing heart disease and exclude older individuals, so they mainly involved middle-aged men (since women tend to develop heart disease at an older age than men). In HPS, proportional reduction in the rate of major cardiovascular events with allocation to simvastatin also seemed to be about one-quarter irrespective of sex and age of the participants. Indeed, even among the 1263 individuals aged 75–80 years at entry, and so aged about 80–85 years by the end of the study, the reduction in the event rate was substantial and definite. Much larger numbers of participants suffered a stroke in the HPS than in any previous cholesterol-lowering trial, resolving any remaining uncertainties about the effects of statin therapy on the incidence of stroke.

The HPS raises the following question: since <100 mg/dl or <115 mg/dl is defined as optimal LDL-C for all adults, why shouldn't everyone be treated to a target of 100 mg/dl whenever drug therapy is indicated? A key principle of current guidelines is matching the intensity of the treatment to the level of the risk. While epidemiological information tells us that

LDL-C <100 mg/dl or <115 mg/dl is ideal for our population as a whole, some persons with LDL-C levels over 100 mg/dl remain at low risk and, therefore, it is appropriate not to consider drug therapy in persons at otherwise low risk (people with 0–1 risk factor who have a ten-year risk below 10%). In the HPS, the size of the five-year benefit depends mainly on each individual's overall risk of major vascular events, rather than on their blood lipid concentrations alone. There were highly significant risk reductions among the participants whose pre-treatment measurements of LDL-C were below 100 mg/dl. Defining an optimal level for the whole population is very different than specifying specific LDL-C goals and cut-points for the therapy in individuals with varying degrees of risk. Hence, the absolute size of the risk reduction produced by lowering LDL-C may be determined more by an individual's overall risk of cardiovascular disease than simply by their initial blood lipid concentrations. The HPS has shown that statin therapy prevents not just coronary events and coronary revascularizations but also ischaemic strokes and peripheral revascularizations. Hence, decisions about whether to initiate therapy should perhaps now be guided by the estimated risk of suffering any such major vascular event, and not just a coronary event as used in the ATP III risk assessment tool. If the benefit of lipid-modifying therapy is primarily related to the future risk for any cardiovascular event, then improved methods to assess global risk are essential to identify individuals who will benefit from statin therapy. Refining treatment guidelines will continue to be one of the most important challenges for atherosclerosis researchers in the 21st century.

WHAT ARE THE OPTIMAL RISK ASSESSMENT METHODS TO IDENTIFY HIGH-RISK INDIVIDUALS?

The concept of risk assessment and reduction, introduced by the Framingham Heart Study and redefined in other models, forms the cornerstone of preventive cardiology. Risk factor assessment determines the therapeutic strategy because the intensity of the preventive intervention is tailored to the patient's risk of CHD. Calculations of short-term (or absolute) versus long-term (lifetime) risk do influence therapeutic decision making in the context of primary prevention. Aggressive risk reduction, formerly used exclusively in secondary prevention, may be pivotal to optimal patient management in high-risk primary prevention.

Non-invasive imaging techniques and novel serum markers have the potential to directly or indirectly measure and monitor atherosclerosis in asymptomatic individuals and to empirically identify appropriate candidates for aggressive primary prevention. These modalities may be best used after global risk assessment with traditional risk factors, to identify persons at moderate risk (e.g. ten-year risk of 10–20%) for whom additional testing may resolve whether or not they are at high risk and deserving aggressive intervention. However, most of these modalities are not recommended yet for population screening. Simple office-based screening modalities such as 12-lead ECG, urinary albumin, ankle–brachial blood pressure index and others are under-utilized for optimal risk assessment and identifying high-risk individuals.

NON-INVASIVE IMAGING: CARDIODIAGNOSTIC MODALITIES

Resting and exercise ECG testing

In asymptomatic persons, exercise ECG testing generates a high rate of false-positive responses and is thus not considered suitable as a widespread population-screening tool. However, an ischaemic ECG response at low workloads in asymptomatic patients has been associated with a higher risk of cardiac events.[5] Although ST depression over 1 mm within six minutes on the Bruce protocol has been linked to an increased risk of CHD events in men, the absolute risk in the absence of risk factors is low. Routine use of exercise ECG to screen unselected asymptomatic patients before in-office risk assessment is not recommended. At present, the role of exercise ECG is limited to the cardiovascular work-up of asymptomatic men over 40 years old with one or more risk factors in whom a vigorous exercise programme is being considered, in the absence of contraindications to the stress testing. Additional data are required before exercise testing can be recommended in women or the elderly (over 75 years old). Middle-aged men with hypercholesterolaemia and abnormal ECG had a markedly increased risk for cardiovascular events and benefited from statin therapy in the West of Scotland Coronary Prevention Study (WOSCOPS).[6]

Electron beam computed tomography (EBCT)

EBCT is a highly sensitive modality for quantifying calcium, as a marker of atherosclerosis within the coronary vasculature, particularly within the context of multivessel disease.[7] EBCT generates scans more rapidly than helical CT through the use of an electron beam and stationary tungsten target. A major limitation of EBCT, poor reproducibility between scans, appears to have been overcome by the introduction of a new volumetric scoring system useful in detecting small lesions.[8] However, the correlation between arterial calcification and the risk of plaque rupture has not been established, and EBCT is not yet recommended for widespread population screening. Compared with invasive modalities such as intravascular ultrasound, EBCT is less sensitive in the detection of single-vessel disease.[7] The vulnerable plaque and severe coronary artery stenosis may be present even in the absence of calcium. The risk associated with a normal or low calcified coronary artery calcium (CAC) score in the presence of multiple risk factors is unclear. In general, however, a high calcium score indicates the probability of vulnerable plaques but fails to identify the site of specific vulnerable lesions. Although EBCT has been associated with sensitivities as high as 95% for detection of any 50% narrowing, its specificity (ranging from 45% to 50%) is well below that desired in a screening test. A large study showed that an EBCT calcium score did not contribute additional information to the traditional Framingham risk assessment in predicting future coronary events in high-risk individuals.[8,9]

In some studies EBCT was able to detect the regression of atherosclerotic lesions in response to lipid-lowering therapy.[10] Therefore, serial EBCT may evolve into an important modality if additional studies demonstrate that differences in calcium scores over time, particularly in response to lipid-lowering therapy, correlate with the differences in the rate of coronary events.

A recent consensus statement concluded that insufficient data exist to recommend EBCT for general population screening or routine clinical use.[7] The clinical role of EBCT is yet to be established in terms of screening for disease or risk assessment. Unfortunately, despite these recommendations, the use of EBCT to evaluate asymptomatic individuals for risk of developing obstructive CHD has been highly commercialized over the past ten years. In fact, a high calcium score on EBCT frequently leads to invasive and expensive tests and subsequent revascularization, thereby creating a coronary event in an asymptomatic individual.

Magnetic resonance coronary angiography (MRCA)

Primarily a research tool, MRCA is still under investigation.[11] MRCA has shown promise in relative risk of detecting large stenosis and may overcome the obstacle of motion artifact to provide 3D visualization of the coronary arteries.[12] Sensitivity and specificity are highly variable, with sensitivities of 50% and 100% and specificities of 85% and 90% reported in the detection of left anterior descending stenosis.[12] However, MRCA has the potential to image plaque composition and size, thereby specifically pinpointing areas vulnerable to plaque rupture. Unfortunately, MRCA cannot accurately detect smaller stenoses, an important determinant of risk in primary prevention.

Positron emission tomography (PET)

PET can be used to assess coronary flow and flow reserve; however, its use is limited by its inability to detect coronary stenosis below 50%.[5] In studies of patients with hypercholesterolaemia, PET has documented decreased myocardial blood flow in conjunction with increased serum and LDL cholesterol and improved flow reserve after lipid-lowering therapy.[13] In the future, PET may have a role in the detection of early endothelial dysfunction and in the non-invasive monitoring of aggressive lipid-lowering therapy and risk factor modification in asymptomatic high-risk patients.

Ankle–brachial blood pressure index testing (ABI)

A simple and inexpensive diagnostic test, ABI testing requires only a blood pressure cuff and a Doppler ultrasonic sensor to reliably identify lower-extremity peripheral artery disease (PAD) in asymptomatic persons over 50 years of age.[14] The systolic pressure in both arms taken with the blood pressure cuff and Doppler probe, is averaged and divided into the systolic blood pressure in the posterior tibial or dorsalis pedis artery in the leg. The higher reading is used to determine the ABI. ABI should be calculated separately for each leg. An ABI below 0.90 in either leg indicates PAD; the lower the ABI value, the more severe the obstruction.[14]

ABI-detectable PAD has been shown to correlate with a higher prevalence of CHD, which confirms that atherosclerosis is a systemic disease in which PAD signifies disease throughout the vasculature.[15] When performed by well-trained technicians, the accuracy of ABI testing for stenosis over 50% in leg arteries is very high (sensitivity 90%, specificity 98%).

An abnormal ABI adds to the information provided by traditional risk assessment and elevates asymptomatic patients to a higher-risk category, justifying therapeutic intervention in primary prevention equivalent to that of secondary prevention. ABI testing is particularly useful in patients with multiple risk factors for CHD, such as smokers or those with diabetes mellitus.

B-mode ultrasound

B-mode ultrasound is a safe, non-invasive and relatively inexpensive technique for the visualization of intima–media thickness (IMT) in the lumen of selected arteries, including the carotid, aortic and femoral arteries.[14,16] At least five studies have demonstrated that carotid IMT measurements correlate with the presence of coronary atherosclerosis and represent an independent risk factor for CHD events and stroke. Impressive data from two large studies[17,18] in over 15 000 persons without CHD at baseline showed that the higher the IMT, the greater the risk of CHD and stroke. It has been well established that carotid IMT is an independent predictor of transient cerebral ischaemia, stroke and coronary events. Serial B-mode ultrasound measurements of the carotid artery also have the potential to monitor changes in IMT in response to therapy. However, standardized protocols for serial IMT measurements require considerable technician training and quality control before B-mode ultrasound can be widely used in the clinical follow-up of patients undergoing lipid-lowering therapy.[14]

SERUM MARKERS

As a result of advanced research and clinical trials in atherosclerosis several new serum markers have been discovered to be associated with CHD risk but have not been recommended in European or American guidelines for routine screening. Two novel serum markers, C-reactive protein (CRP) and homocysteine, have been studied to determine their usefulness in risk assessment.

C-reactive protein

CRP is an established marker of low-grade inflammation, reflecting elevated levels of proinflammatory cytokines such as interleukins, fibrinogen and soluble vascular adhesion molecules. The association of CRP with CHD has been documented in multiple large studies,[19] including the Physicians' Health Study and the Women's Health Study.[20,21] In the Physicians' Health Study, physicians in the highest quartile of hs-CRP at baseline had a two-fold higher risk of stroke, a three-fold higher risk of MI and a four-fold higher risk of severe PAD. Furthermore, the risk associated with hs-CRP was independent of other CHD risk factors. Similar results were observed in the Women's Health Study; half of all MIs occurred in previously healthy women in whom plasma lipid levels were normal. The levels of hs-CRP were significant predictors of cardiovascular risk even in the sub-group of women with LDL-C levels below 130 mg/dl, the target for primary prevention by current guidelines.[21]

In addition, the secondary prevention Cholesterol and Recurrent Events (CARE) trial demonstrated that CRP elevation was associated with a higher risk for recurrence of cardiovascular events; the relative risk was 75% higher in patients in the highest hs-CRP quintile compared with those in the lowest hs-CRP quintile.[22] The risk reduction was greatest in statin-treated patients with evidence of inflammation as indicated by elevated CRP. Whether these results obtained in secondary prevention can be extrapolated to primary prevention was studied in AFCAPS/TexCAPS, in which an elevated hs-CRP added to the risk estimation and identified a sub-group with relatively low lipid levels who still benefited from statin therapy (Table 16.1).[23] Recent studies raised a question regarding the optimal standardization of the high-sensitivity methods. Because the CRP value of an individual patient is interpreted within the context of cut-off points established by the prospective clinical studies, standardization of CRP assays is crucial. CRP screening may potentially be used to target statin therapy for the primary prevention of cardiac events among individuals without overt hyperlipidaemia. The Justification for the Use of statins in Primary prevention: an Intervention Trial Evaluating Rosuvastatin (JUPITER) study will directly test whether

Table 16.1 C-reactive protein in addition to low-density lipoprotein cholesterol level or total cholesterol/high-density lipoprotein cholesterol ratio as methods of targeting statin therapy in primary prevention: data from the Air Force/Texas Coronary Atherosclerosis Prevention Study

Sub-group	Lovastatin patients		Placebo patients		Relative risk (95% CI)	Number needed to treat
	n	Event rate	n	Event rate		
Low LDL-C, low CRP	726	0.025	722	0.022	1.08 (0.56–2.08)	–
Low LDL-C, high CRP	718	0.029	710	0.051	0.58 (0.34–0.98)	48
High LDL-C, low CRP	709	0.020	711	0.050	0.38 (0.21–0.70)	33
High LDL-C, high CRP	741	0.038	705	0.055	0.68 (0.42–1.10)	58
Low TC/HDL-C, low CRP	762	0.024	763	0.025	0.88 (0.47–1.67)	983
Low TC/HDL-C, high CRP	650	0.025	696	0.050	0.47 (0.27–0.85)	43
High TC/HDL-C, low CRP	673	0.021	670	0.050	0.42 (0.23–0.77)	35
High TC/HDL-C, high CRP	809	0.041	719	0.057	0.72 (0.46–1.13)	62

Low, below the median (149.1 mg/dl for LDL-C; 0.16 mg/dl for CRP; 5.96 for total cholesterol/HDL-C); high, above the median; CRP, C-reactive protein; HDL-C, high-density lipoprotein cholesterol; LDL-C, low-density lipoprotein cholesterol.
Adapted with permission from ref. 23.

patients with low LDL-C levels but high CRP levels also achieve a substantial benefit from statin therapy.

Homocysteine

Homocysteine is a mixed amino acid intermediary on the catabolic pathway between methionine and cysteine, and is the sum of the reduced form of the amino acid homocysteine and the homocysteinyl moiety of the oxidized disulphide homocystine–homocysteine. Several B vitamins are cofactors in the methionine catabolic pathway; in particular, deficiencies in folic acid, vitamin B_{12} and pyridoxine have been associated with mildly elevated homocysteine levels in healthy populations.[24] Individuals with highly elevated homocysteine are prone to severe, premature vascular disease in childhood.[25]

Case-control studies of patients presenting with CHD, cerebrovascular disease and peripheral vascular disease have demonstrated that homocysteine levels are significantly higher in cases than in controls, even after statistical adjustment for other cardiovascular risk factors.

More recently, observational studies have found that mildly elevated homocysteine is associated with increased incidence of both CHD and stroke. However, additional follow-up of the Physicians' Health Study cohort found no significant association between homocysteine and incidence of MI.[26] Alfthan et al. found no association between homocysteine and either MI or stroke in a Finnish prospective, population-based study,[27] and a nested case-control study involving men participating in the MRFIT showed no association between homocysteine and non-fatal MI or CHD.[28] Also, the ARIC study reported a lack of association between homocysteine and incident CHD over an average of 3.3 years of follow-up.[29] As a result, routine general population screening for homocysteine levels is not recommended at this time.[30] However, homocysteine testing should be considered in CHD patients who have no CHD risk factors and in asymptomatic patients with a strong family history of premature CHD. On-going clinical trials are addressing the key clinical issue of whether treatment of elevated homocysteine with high-dose folic acid and vitamins B_6 and B_{12} will reduce CHD events.

WHAT SHOULD THE LIPID TARGETS BE FOR STATIN THERAPY?

In addition to their use in CHD risk assessment, lipid measurements are used to guide the selection and intensity of lipid-modifying therapy. Although the evidence from clinical trials supports the current US and European guidelines for initiation of drug therapy based on both LDL-C and global risk for CHD, the HPS has recently shown benefit of therapy in high-risk patients with LDL-C levels well below the current threshold for initiation of therapy.

As CHD is multifactorial in origin it is important, in estimating CHD risk for an individual, to consider all the risk factors simultaneously. Traditionally, risk factor guidelines have focused on single factor assessment, particularly in the management of hyperlipidaemia. This has resulted in undue emphasis being placed on elevations of single risk factors rather than on overall level of risk based on a combination of risk factors.

Epidemiological studies have consistently demonstrated a dose–response relation between total cholesterol level and CHD risk. Despite a strong and consistent association within populations, elevated total cholesterol alone is not a very useful test to identify high-risk patients. In the Framingham Heart Study, total cholesterol distribution curves for men developing CHD and those remaining free of disease show considerable overlap between the levels of 150 mg/dl and 300 mg/dl, suggesting that additional factors influence the development of CHD.

LDL-C is generally believed to be the principal atherogenic lipoprotein in the development of atherosclerosis. Epidemiological studies and clinical trials have clearly established that elevations of LDL-C are associated with increased CHD risk and that aggressive LDL-C reduction with statins and other therapies in the primary and secondary prevention of CHD has been associated with significant mortality and morbidity benefits. The Framingham Heart Study suggested that LDL-C was a better predictor of CHD than total cholesterol level in both men and women; the strength of association may be greater in men than women. The relative risk associated with

LDL-C declines with age; hence the LDL-C value has less power to define risk in older persons.

While LDL-C remains the primary target for CHD prevention in the current US and European guidelines, determining the need for diet and drug therapy as well as being the goal of the therapy, many individuals who develop CHD do not have substantially elevated LDL-C but have derangements of other lipid fractions, most commonly low levels of HDL-C. In the ATP III guidelines, HDL-C is important in risk stratification in primary prevention, influencing the need for and intensity of treatment of LDL-C, and both HDL-C and triglyceride are defined as risk factors for the metabolic syndrome, a secondary target of therapy.

The ATP III guidelines define optimal LDL-C as <100 mg/dl but whether there is any clinical benefit from dietary or drug therapy to lower LDL-C below current guideline target levels has been answered by the data from HPS.[4] In HPS, about 3500 participants presented with a pretreatment LDL-C measurement that was already below the 'target' level recommended by the current US and European guidelines. In this group, there was a risk reduction similar to that seen in all other sub-groups, raising the suggestion that even CHD patients with baseline LDL-C of below 100 mg/dl should be treated with statins. These findings indicate that the current target levels of LDL-C <100 mg/dl and LDL-C <115 mg/dl in the US and European guidelines are clearly inadequate for many high-risk patients and that optimal LDL-C levels are probably well below these targets. On-going statin trials will provide evidence as to whether the optimal LDL-C is below 70 mg/dl versus the current US target of below 100 mg/dl.

The inverse relation between HDL-C level and CHD risk has been consistently confirmed in epidemiological observational studies. This relation may be due, at least in part, to the association of low HDL-C with other components of the metabolic syndrome, such as insulin resistance. An analysis of four prospective US studies demonstrated a consistent protective effect of HDL-C, such that each 1 mg/dl increment was associated with a 2–3% decrease in CHD.[31]

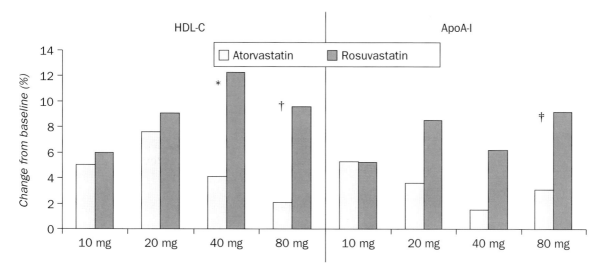

Fig. 16.2 Differing effects of statins on HDL-C and apolipoprotein (apo) A-I: atorvastatin versus rosuvastatin. *$p < 0.001$, †$p < 0.01$, ‡$p < 0.05$ for atorvastatin versus rosuvastatin. (Adapted with permission from ref. 35.)

Controversy has also arisen about the lack of an HDL-C target. While the current guidelines clearly recognized that HDL-C is a key risk predictor and elucidated in careful detail the therapeutic approach to patients with low HDL-C, the panel felt it was not appropriate to define a target of therapy for HDL-C. There are several reasons for this. It is well known that HDL-C metabolism is extraordinarily complex and that high levels are not always protective and low levels in genetic syndromes are not always associated with increased risk for CHD. Since there is no clinical trial based primarily on raising HDL-C, no target level was included in the guidelines. However, the Veterans Affairs HDL Cholesterol Intervention Trial (VA-HIT) clearly showed benefit in a low HDL-C population with CHD who had a modest 6% increase in HDL-C with gemfibrozil.[32] Statins vary in their ability to raise HDL-C and apolipoprotein (apo) A-I, as has been shown in previous studies (Fig. 16.2).[33–35]

While there is much evidence to suggest that triglyceride-rich lipoproteins are atherogenic, triglyceride level was found to be more predictive of CHD risk in women than men in the Framingham[36] and ARIC studies.[37] Elevated triglycerides are often accompanied by other metabolic disturbances that may predispose to CHD, including reduced HDL-C, increased

small, dense LDL-C particles and insulin resistance. These inter-relationships make it difficult to assess the independent risk conferred by triglyceride levels. The combined elevations of triglyceride and LDL-C may confer a greater risk for CHD than isolated increases in either.

Non-HDL-C, which includes cholesterol in LDL-C and triglyceride-rich lipoproteins, is identified as secondary target of therapy in persons with triglycerides ≥200 mg/dl by current guidelines. In the Lipid Research Clinics (LRC) Follow-up Study, the non-HDL-C level was a better predictor of mortality than the LDL-C level, particularly in women.[38]

Lipid parameters can be combined into ratios that reflect the proportion of atherogenic to anti-atherogenic lipid and lipoproteins. Proposed lipid ratios for CHD risk assessment include total cholesterol (TC)/HDL-C, LDL-C/HDL-C, triglyceride/HDL-C and apoB/apoA-I. For example, in AFCAPS/TexCAPS, following adjustment for non-lipid risk factors, the apoB/apoA-I ratio was the best discriminator of baseline risk and a value of ≥1.0 was associated with an increased risk for a first major coronary event of 38% (Fig. 16.3).[39] In the Apolipoprotein-related Mortality Risk (AMORIS) study, apoB/apoA-I ratio and levels of apoB and apoA-I were strong predictors of fatal MI in

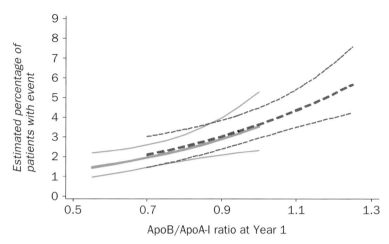

Fig. 16.3 Logistic regression model (adjusted for age, sex, marital status, hypertension, smoking and family history) of relation between on-treatment apoB/apoA-I ratio, with 95% confidence interval, in the Air Force/Texas Coronary Atherosclerosis Prevention Study. ——, lovastatin; - - - -, placebo. (Adapted with permission from ref. 39.)

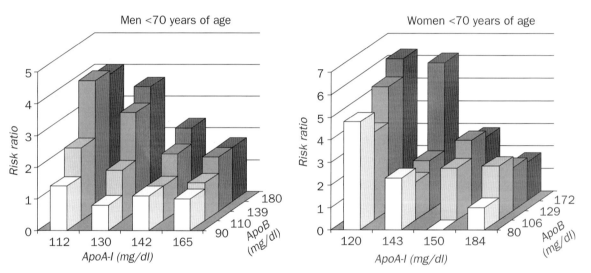

Fig. 16.4 Combined influence of apoB and apoA-I on risk ratios in men and women in the Apolipoprotein-related Mortality Risk study. (Adapted with permission from ref. 40.)

multivariate analyses adjusted for age, TC and triglycerides (Fig. 16.4).[40]

Perhaps the most widely used ratios are LDL-C/HDL-C and TC/HDL-C. Retrospective analysis of the Helsinki Heart Study revealed that LDL-C/HDL-C values greater than 5 were associated with increased coronary risk,[41] while an analysis of five-year data from the Program on the Surgical Control of Hyperlipidemias (POSCH) study found that the highest hazard ratios were for LDL-C/HDL-C, with each one-unit increment associated with a 1.2-fold increase in CHD risk.[42] On the basis of observational data, the TC/HDL-C ratio appears to be a

better predictor of subsequent CHD than LDL-C level. As well as being the best predictor of CHD risk in epidemiological studies, the TC/HDL-C ratio or apoB-100/apoA-I ratio may have value as a therapeutic target.

Although the ratios of TC/HDL-C and apoB-100/apoA-I have been useful in large epidemiological studies to identify high-risk individuals, these ratios are not addressed in the current US and European guidelines. Although multiple epidemiological and clinical trials are addressing optimal methods for identifying high-risk patients and the optimal target level for LDL-C, there are currently no large interventional studies designed to test whether improving lipid ratios would provide optimal reductions in risk for CHD events. On-going and future clinical trials with dietary and pharmacological lipoprotein modification are needed to determine whether apolipoproteins and lipid ratios that reflect comprehensive modifications of lipid profile are better therapeutic targets than LDL-C alone.

REFERENCES

1. Stamler J, Wentworth D, Neaton JD. Is the relationship between serum cholesterol and risk of premature death from coronary heart disease continuous and graded? Findings in 356,222 primary screenees of the Multiple Risk Factor Intervention Trial (MRFIT). *JAMA* 1986; **256**: 2823–8.
2. Expert Panel on Detection, Evaluation, and Treatment of High Blood Cholesterol in Adults. Summary of the third report of the National Cholesterol Education Program (NCEP) Expert Panel on Detection, Evaluation, and Treatment of High Blood Cholesterol in Adults (Adult Treatment Panel III). *JAMA* 2001; **285**: 2486–97.
3. Prevention of Coronary Heart Disease in Clinical Practice. Recommendations of the Second Joint Task Force of European and other Societies on Coronary Prevention. *Atherosclerosis* 1998; **140**: 199–270.
4. Heart Protection Study Collaborative Group. MRC/BHF Heart Protection Study of Cholesterol lowering with simvastatin in 20 536 high-risk individuals: a randomized placebo-controlled trial. *Lancet* 2002; **360**: 7–22.
5. Smith SC, Amsterdam E, Balady GJ et al. Prevention Conference V. Beyond secondary prevention. Identifying the high-risk patient for primary prevention. Tests for silent and inducible ischemia. Writing Group II. *Circulation* 2000; **101**: e12–e15.
6. West of Scotland Coronary Prevention Study Group. Baseline risk factors and their association with outcome in the West of Scotland Coronary Prevention Study. *Am J Cardiol* 1997; **79**: 756–62.
7. O'Rourke RA, Brundage BH, Froelicher VG. American College of Cardiology/American Heart Association expert consensus document on electron-beam computed tomography for the diagnosis and prognosis of coronary artery disease. *Circulation* 2000; **102**: 126–40.
8. Detrano RC, Wong ND, Doherty TM et al. Coronary calcium does not accurately predict near-term future coronary events in high-risk adults. *Circulation* 1999; **99**: 2633–8.
9. Taylor AJ, Feuerstein I, Wong H et al. Do conventional risk factors predict subclinical coronary artery disease? Results from the Prospective Army Coronary Calcium Project. *Am Heart J* 2001; **141**: 463–8.
10. Callister TQ, Raggi P, Cooil B et al. Effect of HMG-Co reductase inhibitors on coronary artery disease as assessed by electron-beam computed tomography. *N Engl J Med* 1998; **339**: 1972–8.
11. Benitez RM, Vogel RA. Assessment of subclinical atherosclerosis and cardiovascular risk. *Clin Cardiol* 2001; **24**: 642–50.
12. Van Geuns RJ, de Bruin HG, Rensing BJ et al. Magnetic resonance imaging of the coronary arteries: clinical results from three-dimensional evaluation of a respiratory gated technique. *Heart* 1999; **82**: 515–19.
13. Baller D, Notohamiprodjo G, Gleichmann U et al. Improvement in coronary flow reserve determined by positron emission tomography after 6 months of cholesterol-lowering therapy in patients with early stages of coronary atherosclerosis. *Circulation* 1999; **99**: 2871–5.
14. Greenland P, Abrahams J, Aurigemma GP et al. Prevention Conference V. Beyond secondary prevention. Identifying the high-risk patient for primary prevention. Noninvasive tests of atherosclerotic burden. Writing Group III. *Circulation* 2000; **101**: e16–e22.
15. Criqui MH, Deneberg JO, Langer RD et al. The epidemiology of peripheral arterial disease: importance of identifying the population at risk. *Vasc Med* 1997; **2**: 221–6.
16. Ioannis EK, Costas PT et al. Close relation between carotid and ascending aortic atherosclerosis in cardiac patients. *Circulation* 2000; **102**: 263–8.
17. Chambless LE, Heiss G, Folsom AR et al. Association of coronary heart disease incidence with carotid arterial wall thickness and major risk factors: the Atherosclerosis Risk in Communities (ARIC) Study, 1987–1993. *Am J Epidemiol* 1997; **146**: 483–94.
18. O'Leary DH, Polak JF, Dronmal RA et al. Carotid-artery intima and media thickness as a risk factor for myocardial infarction and stroke in older adults: Cardiovascular Health Study. *N Engl J Med* 1999; **340**: 14–22.
19. Rifai N, Ridker PM. Inflammatory markers and coronary heart disease. *Curr Opin Lipidol* 2002; **13**: 383–9.

20. Ridker PM, Cushman M, Stampfer MJ et al. Inflammation, aspirin, and risk of apparently healthy men. *N Engl J Med* 1997; **336**: 973–9.

21. Ridker PM, Buring JE, Shih J et al. Prospective study of C-reactive protein and the risk of future cardiovascular events among apparently healthy women. *Circulation* 1998; **98**: 731–3.

22. Ridker PM, Rifai N, Pfeffer MA et al. for the Cholesterol and Recurrent Events (CARE) Investigators. Inflammation, pravastatin, and the risk of coronary events after myocardial infarction in patients with average cholesterol levels. *Circulation* 1998; **98**: 839–44.

23. Ridker PM, Rifai N, Clearfield M et al. Measurement of C-reactive protein for targeting of statin therapy in the primary prevention of acute coronary events. *N Engl J Med* 2001; **344**: 1959–66.

24. Kang SS, Wong PWK, Norusis M. Homocysteinemia due to folate deficiency. *Metabolism* 1987; **36**: 458–62.

25. Boers GHJ, Smals AGH, Trijbels FJ et al. Heterozygocity for homocystinuria in premature peripheral and cerebrovascular occlusive arterial disease. *N Engl J Med* 1985; **313**: 709–15.

26. Chasan-Taber L, Selhub J, Rosenberg IH et al. A prospective study of folate and vitamin B6 and risk of myocardial infarction in US physicians. *J Am Coll Nutr* 1996; **15**: 136–43.

27. Alfthan G, Pekkanen J, Jauhiainen M et al. Relation of serum homocysteine and lipoprotein(a) concentrations to atherosclerotic disease in a prospective Finnish population based study. *Atherosclerosis* 1994; **106**: 9–19.

28. Evans RW, Shaten BJ, Hempel JD et al. Homocyst(e)ine and risk of cardiovascular disease in the Multiple Risk Factor Intervention Trial. *Arterioscler Thromb Vasc Biol* 1997; **17**: 1947–53.

29. Folsom AR, Nieto FJ, McGovern PG et al. Prospective study of coronary heart disease incidence in relation to fasting total homocysteine, related genetic polymorphisms, and B vitamins: the Atherosclerosis Risk in Communities (ARIC) study. *Circulation* 1998; **98**: 204–10.

30. Malinow MR, Bostom AG, Krauss RM. Homocysteine, diet, and cardiovascular diseases: a statement for healthcare professionals from the Nutrition Committee, American Heart Association. *Circulation* 1999; **99**: 178–82.

31. Gordon DJ, Probstfield JL, Garrison RJ et al. High-density lipoprotein cholesterol and cardiovascular disease: four prospective American studies. *Circulation* 1989; **79**: 8–15.

32. Rubins HB, Robins SJ, Collins D et al. for the Veterans Affairs High-Density Lipoprotein Cholesterol Intervention Trial Study Group. Gemfibrozil for the secondary prevention of coronary heart disease in men with low levels of high-density lipoprotein cholesterol. *N Engl J Med* 1999; **341**: 410–18.

33. Illingworth DR, Crouse JR III, Hunninghake DB et al. A comparison of simvastatin and atorvastatin up to maximal recommended doses in a large multicenter randomized clinical trial. *Curr Med Res Opin* 2001; **17**: 43–50.

34. Ballantyne CM, Hustad CM, Yuan Z et al. Efficacy and safety of simvastatin versus atorvastatin: results of the comparative HDL-C efficacy and safety study (CHESS) [Abstract P2197]. *Eur Heart J* 2002; **4** (Abstract Suppl): 420.

35. Schneck DW, Knopp RH, Ballantyne CM et al. Comparative effects of rosuvastatin and atorvastatin across their dose ranges in patients with hypercholesterolemia and without active arterial disease. *Am J Cardiol* 2003; **91**: 33–41.

36. Castelli WP. Epidemiology of triglycerides: a view from Framingham. *Am J Cardiol* 1992; **70**: 3H–9H.

37. Sharrett AR, Ballantyne CM, Coady SA et al. Coronary heart disease prediction from lipoprotein cholesterol levels, triglycerides, lipoprotein (a), apolipoproteins A-I and B, and HDL density subfractions: the Atherosclerosis Risk in Communities (ARIC) study. *Circulation* 2001; **104**: 1108–13.

38. Cui Y, Blumenthal RS, Flaws JA et al. Non-high-density lipoprotein cholesterol level as a predictor of cardiovascular disease mortality. *Arch Intern Med* 2001; **161**: 1413–19.

39. Gotto AM Jr, Whitney E, Stein EA et al. Relation between baseline and on-treatment lipid parameters and first acute major coronary events in the Air Force/Texas Coronary Atherosclerosis Prevention Study (AFCAPS/TexCAPS). *Circulation* 2000; **101**: 477–84.

40. Walldius G, Jungner I, Holme I et al. High apolipoprotein B, low apolipoprotein A-I, and improvement in the prediction of fatal myocardial infarction (AMORIS study): a prospective study. *Lancet* 2001; **358**: 2026–33.

41. Manninen V, Tenkanen L, Koskinen P et al. Joint effects of serum triglyceride and LDL cholesterol and HDL cholesterol concentrations on coronary heart disease risk in the Helsinki Heart Study: implications for treatment. *Circulation* 1992; **85**: 37–45.

42. Buchwald H, Boen JR, Nguyen PA et al. Plasma lipids and cardiovascular risk: a POSCH report. Program on the Surgical Control of the Hyperlipidemias. *Atherosclerosis* 2001; **154**: 221–7.

17

Statin therapy for the 21st century

James Shepherd

INTRODUCTION

The introduction of statin therapy into clinical practice has revolutionized the management of lipid disorders and, at a stroke, silenced the critics of cholesterol management as a means to vascular disease prevention. Yamamoto et al.[1] and Mabuchi et al.[2] were the first to take their courage in both hands and apply Endo's discovery (see Chapter 3) of the progenitor statin, compactin, to hypercholesterolaemic men. Their initiative paved the way for a raft of clinical trials (see Chapters 7 and 8) which tied statin therapy to virtually guaranteed lipid-lowering efficacy with a negligible side-effect profile. Contrary to the jaundiced expectations of some, there was no increased risk of cancer or of the likelihood of dying of accidental, suicidal or violent death. On the contrary, statins were the first lipid-lowering agents which, within the framework of a clinical trial, actually extended life by mechanisms which probably go beyond cholesterol reduction alone and which favourably affect blood flow through all major arterial conduits, including the coronary, cerebral and peripheral vessels. In fact the benefits of statins are so impressive that some enthusiasts have been emboldened to write that they 'are to atherosclerosis what penicillin was to infectious disease.'[3] Taking that analogy one step further might lead us to wonder whether statins represent the pinnacle of our needs as far as cholesterol lowering is concerned. If antibiotics have taught us anything it must surely be that nature is not as easily tamed as we might imagine. But, does atherosclerosis share the pleiotropic features that characterize infections? Advances in experimental pathology suggest that it may do[4] and some have implied from these findings that cholesterol lowering with statin therapy might not be the whole answer to atherosclerosis and vascular disease prevention, arguing that if it were, coronary events would have been eliminated in the published trials rather than 'merely' reduced by 30–50%. The flaw in this logic is of course that no clinical trial can truly reflect the multifaceted biology of real life and to eliminate a disease which crucially depends on the insidious tissue accumulation of cholesterol over a lifetime would probably require action over a longer timespan than is dictated by the exigencies of trial design. However, there is another more cogent reason why we should gain comfort from continuing lipid-lowering drug development. The primary pharmacological action of statins (see Chapter 4) is to promote the physiological clearance of low-density lipoprotein (LDL) from the circulation via its specific high-affinity receptor located particularly on hepatocyte membranes. However, the practising cardiologist will quickly point out that the majority of dyslipidaemic patients admitted to the coronary care unit usually exhibit raised plasma cholesterol and triglyceride levels rather than hypercholesterolaemia alone. This combined hyperlipidaemia results from over-production of triglyceride-rich very low-density lipoprotein (VLDL) particles coupled with defective catabolism of LDL. While the statins were specifically designed to deal with the latter problem, their ability to lower plasma triglyceride levels is much more limited. Head-to-head comparisons of the statins show that, at best, they can be expected to lower triglyceride by no more than about 20%, their efficacy perhaps being greater at higher triglyceride values. In an attempt to address this issue, the pharmaceutical industry has embarked on a series of investigations aimed at limiting the hepatic elaboration and secretion of triglyceride-rich lipoproteins.

A number of agents (e.g. nicotinic acid and the fibrates) capable of achieving this effect and of proven efficacy already exist but new modalities are currently under study. One promising candidate target is microsomal triglyceride transfer protein, whose role is to integrate lipid into the nascent lipoprotein particle within the hepatic endoplasmic reticulum, and several pharmaceutical companies have a range of lead compounds under intensive investigation at the time of writing. If they realize their promise, they will offer important lipid-lowering capability which will complement that achievable with statin monotherapy.

LOST OPPORTUNITIES FROM INEFFICIENT PRESCRIBING

Many organizational and psychological barriers impede the initiation of risk-factor management in hospitals and primary care. These obstacles are evident in numerous surveys, which, despite compelling evidence of benefit,[5–11] have revealed that statins are dramatically under-prescribed in primary and secondary care.[12–14] Hospital cardiologists are more focused on treating the acute coronary event with diagnostic and therapeutic procedures than on long-term therapy. Cardiologists are also frequently too short of time to initiate such a plan, especially as patients are in hospital for only a short time while the acute event is being treated. Secondary prevention is thus often referred to the primary-care setting. However, the lack of urgency by the cardiologist in initiating a risk-factor reduction plan signals to the primary care physician that this is not a high priority. Furthermore, a delay in communication often means the impetus to instigate a follow-up plan is lost, which further widens the therapeutic gap. Primary care physicians also have a

limited awareness of the benefits of risk-factor modification,[15] which leads to further obstacles in initiating statin therapy for high-risk patients. The problem is further compounded by the lack of information passed on to patients with existing coronary heart disease (CHD) about the need to lower 'normal' as well as elevated cholesterol with pharmacological therapy rather than dietary measures, which often fail to work. In addition, even when patients are treated, many do not achieve their goals because of incomplete information, which leads to non-compliance with preventive strategies.[16] Thus, the primary care physician and cardiologist need a better understanding of each other's needs and concerns to ensure the message of secondary prevention is reinforced throughout medical care.

Conclusive evidence has been documented showing impressive benefits of several interventions in reducing recurrent infarction and mortality after an acute coronary event. This applies, for example, to aspirin treatment,[17] blood pressure control,[18] statin treatment,[5–11] and, in selected patients, beta-blockers[19] and ACE inhibitors.[20] However, the wide therapeutic gap in implementing these evidence-based approaches seen in the early surveys of secondary CHD prevention[12,13] still exists. Recent reviews reveal there is still a lack of urgency by the cardiologist in addressing management of cholesterol and, to a lesser extent, blood pressure, which results in a shortfall in patient rehabilitation within primary care.[12,13]

Physician perceptions

Preventive strategies have been shown to be haphazard in primary care.[21] Primary care physicians are often uncertain about screening and treating hyperlipidaemia.[22] They may correctly assess the relative risk of CHD in individual patients but over-estimate the absolute risk of CHD risk factors, including the benefits of lowering cholesterol and blood pressure, and stopping smoking.[23] An audit of 95 practices in the Netherlands found that primary care physicians had a critical attitude to integrating prevention into clinical practice and few were organized well enough to provide preventive services.[24] Thus, there is a wide therapeutic gap in implementing the prevention of CHD using the multifactorial approach advocated in the European Task Force recommendations,[16] even among high-risk patients with established CHD.

A recent, large-scale, pan-European, market research survey of primary care, Cholesterol Monitor,[25] found that rates of cholesterol screening for primary and secondary CHD prevention varied widely across Europe, from only 50% in the UK and Sweden to over 80% in France, Italy, Germany and Spain. Across Europe, the average cholesterol level was 6 mmol/l (232 mg/dl) and the intervention level was 7.5 mmol/l (290 mg/dl). In a subset of nearly 7000 patients with CHD treated for more than six months, the average reduction in total cholesterol achieved across Europe was less than half of that required to attain the recommended cholesterol level of below 5 mmol/l (193 mg/dl). In all six countries, this goal was achieved by fewer than 10% of CHD patients.

A further study in the UK of secondary CHD prevention treatment and behaviour among 1921 patients in primary care found that aspirin was prescribed in 63% of patients and in 85% of those with a recent history (less than five years) of myocardial infarction (MI).[26] Within three years, 92% of patients had received a blood pressure check, nearly all of whom received appropriate management in accordance with the guidelines. However, only 25% of these patients had their cholesterol checked during the three years. Furthermore, of the patients with cholesterol levels above 5.2 mmol/l (200 mg/dl), less than one-fifth were receiving cholesterol-lowering therapy and less than one-third of the total population received beta-blockers. This study concluded that nearly all patients in this study had at least one aspect of their medical management that would benefit from change and half had at least two modifiable risk factors. Furthermore, only 7% of respondents were receiving all the medical management available for the optimal secondary prevention of CHD. Infrequent use of beta-blockers may be because of a lack of awareness of their efficacy, as they

have not been as widely promoted as calcium antagonists, which may actually be harmful in acute MI.[27]

A follow-up of participants in the landmark WOSCOPS trial, 2.5 years after this study was closed, further exposes a reluctance of primary care physicians to implement evidence-based therapy in CHD prevention (Shepherd, unpublished findings). The WOSCOPS trial of primary prevention of CHD in 6595 men had earlier reported one-third fewer fatal and non-fatal MIs in patients receiving pravastatin, compared with placebo, over five years. Pravastatin was also extremely well tolerated and led to a reduction in all-cause mortality with no increase in morbidity and mortality from non-cardiovascular diseases over the study period. A follow-up of the study participants after approximately 2.5 years revealed that the pravastatin-treated patients continued to benefit from a reduction in cardiovascular mortality, while non-cardiovascular mortality remained unaffected compared with the placebo group. Yet, paradoxically, less than two-thirds of event-positive patients in either group were still receiving statin treatment. These results echo the findings of a recently reported survey[28] which, disappointingly, showed that only half of the primary care physicians who participated believed that aspirin, beta-blockers and lipid-lowering drugs were of proven clinical value. No wonder, then, that only half of all patients discharged from hospital with a confirmed diagnosis of MI are actually receiving appropriate statin therapy one year later.[13]

Patient compliance

Patients perceive that premature parental death from a coronary event and cigarette smoking carry greater risk than high cholesterol and blood pressure. In a survey in primary care of 3725 middle-aged men and women who were screened as part of the British Family Heart Study, more patients were optimistic (37%) than pessimistic (21%) about their risk of developing CHD.[29] Over-optimistic perceptions of risk and indifferent attitudes to change may explain why health promotion campaigns have had only a modest effect in changing attitudes about prevention of CHD.[30]

Even post-MI patients have been reported to be more concerned about the risks of non-cardiovascular diseases.[14] The recent pan-European Heart European Leaders Panel (HELP) study was designed to provide more information about awareness and attitudes towards reducing CHD. The investigators interviewed over 10 000 patients in five European countries. The study population comprised members of the general public ($n = 5013$), high-risk individuals (based on specific risk factors, $n = 2500$), patients who had suffered a MI ($n = 1256$) and their relatives ($n = 1249$). This study found that individuals had a reasonable knowledge of the risks involved in triggering an acute coronary event, yet many, even those who had suffered a previous MI, displayed indifference to reducing this risk.

Both the general public and high-risk groups in the HELP study identified cancer and heart disease as the two major causes of death.[14] In describing their attitude to their own lifestyle, 21% of the general public and only 4% of the high-risk group said they lived a healthy lifestyle but both of these groups expressed equal levels of worry of experiencing a heart attack. Surprisingly, 72% of the general public claimed to have had their cholesterol checked, compared with only 51% of the high-risk group. However, more patients in both of these groups said they had received information about cholesterol reduction from friends and magazines rather than from their doctor. Despite this, both groups rated the cardiologist, primary care physician and hospital as the three most credible sources of information.

Although post-MI patients said that they were not overly worried about experiencing another heart attack (5.1 on a scale of 1–10 compared with 4.1 for the high-risk group and 4.5 for relatives of post-MI patients), 80% reported making spontaneous changes to their lifestyle after the heart attack.[14] More post-MI patients received information from the medical profession than from television, magazines and newspapers, compared with the general public (primary care physician/cardiologist: 58%

Table 17.1 Proportion of the general public and post-MI patients who obtain their heart health information from healthcare professionals and from various media sources

Source	Percentage (%) of patients	
	General public	Post-MI patients
Television	20	5
Newspapers	18	4
Magazines	14	2
Doctor	16	30
Cardiologist	2	28
Consultant	2	13
Family	6	2
Friends	5	1
Don't know	6	3
Other	11	12

Adapted with permission from ref. 14.

post-MI patients vs 18% general public; media: 11% post-MI patients vs 52% general public) (Table 17.1). However, only 23% of the post-MI group had been warned that their cholesterol level was too high and, of these patients, only 21% could recall their cholesterol level, while 16% of the post-MI patients reported being advised to lower their blood pressure. Of the post-MI group, 53% claimed to have followed all of their primary care physician's advice, while 27% reported to have followed most of it. All groups also returned a very high level of satisfaction with the advice given by the primary care physician.

The HELP study concluded that although patients had access to many sources of heart health information, which in the case of the medical profession were perceived as highly credible, this had only a limited impact on their adherence to preventive treatments and advice.[14] This study also highlights the fact that once the information is provided, little is performed to ensure it is implemented. It seems that where lifestyle changes fail to be carried through, the use of cholesterol-lowering statin therapy is less than adequate.[25] In post-MI

Table 17.2   Physicians' perceptions about which messages regarding CHD prevention are succeeding and those which are failing to get through to post-MI patients

'Messages' to post-MI patients regarding preventive measures	
Getting through	*Failing*
Diet and health	Cholesterol lowering
Exercise	Therapy compliance
Smoking	Weight reduction
Regular screening	Family screening
Stress management	

Adapted with permission from ref. 14.

patients, in particular, the medical profession believes that only certain messages such as diet, exercise, smoking, regular screening and stress management are getting through to patients, whereas messages of cholesterol lowering, therapy compliance, weight reduction and family screening are not (Table 17.2).[14]

BARRIERS TO IMPLEMENTING CHOLESTEROL-LOWERING STATIN THERAPY

Many barriers have been identified which obstruct the implementation of evidence-based therapy in the secondary prevention of CHD. This treatment gap may result from one or more weaknesses in the chain of opportunities to provide risk-reduction care. These include the formulation and implementation of a risk-reduction plan by the hospital, the effectiveness with which the plan is communicated into primary care follow-up, the formulation of a new plan or implementation of the hospital-recommended plan and finally patient compliance with the treatment plan.[31–33]

Within hospital, lines of responsibility may be ambiguous and few healthcare providers have received formal training in the behavioural aspects of risk-factor management; neither is there a standard of performance that

is expected of these professionals. In addition, the hospital may not institute a risk-reduction plan, in the belief that this will be initiated in primary care.[31] The hospital, therefore, often does not provide the systematic follow-up of patients that is essential for ensuring continuity of any advice given by the cardiologist.[34]

Primary care physicians are in a favourable position to take on the task of secondary CHD prevention because they have an on-going relationship with the patient, which offers them the chance to monitor the patient's progress,[35] motivate the patient to make lifestyle changes and ensure long-term compliance with pharmacotherapy.[16]

Like cardiologists, however, primary care physicians lack time but, unlike cardiologists, they report limitations in their training, skills and experience to implement preventive strategies. Many primary care physicians are aware of the guidelines but many have gaps in their knowledge, which leads to inconsistencies between the guidelines and clinical practice.[36] Primary care physicians are often unaware of key advances in the secondary prevention of CHD.[12,13,28] The prescribing practices of cardiologists and primary care physicians therefore differ, though the treatment recommendations of cardiologists have been reported to be a strong influence on motivating primary care physicians to prescribe new therapies in CHD management.[37]

Despite the potentially positive impact of the cardiologist, preventive medicine is often disrupted at the interface between primary and secondary care, where patients are discharged from hospital with limited recommendations to modify risk factors such as cholesterol levels in the 'normal' range. This suggests to the primary care physician that preventive strategies are unimportant.[38] Where risk-reduction recommendations are given by the hospital, they are frequently delayed so that the impetus to instigate a follow-up plan in primary care is lost.[31]

The lack of clear national or local guidelines for implementing secondary prevention is reported to be a shared barrier for both cardiologists and primary care physicians in taking any preventive action.[29] Cardiac rehabilitation after a coronary event plays an integral role in secondary prevention by assuring the application of available knowledge and avoiding complications and the progression of CHD.[39] However, adherence to national rehabilitation guidelines is poor[12,13] and few primary care physicians play an active role in this crucial component of preventive care.[12,13,31,33]

Conflicting guidelines issued by various professional bodies coupled with their perceived complexity[40] dilutes the effectiveness of applying evidence-based policy in practice. Non-evidence-based factors, such as historical, cultural or ideological influences, create further barriers to the implementation of evidence-based guidelines. National guidelines should ideally be tailored to local circumstances, a process that requires commitment from cardiologists to develop sound policies in balancing research evidence with clinical circumstances. Clearly, the cardiologist and primary care physician need to support each other's efforts and be aware of each other's needs in reinforcing preventive advice and providing consistent and strong recommendations for risk-factor management.

Successful programs of health education must be tailored to attitudes and capabilities of the patients they are designed to help. During hospitalization for an acute coronary event, patients are often in pain or undergoing multiple procedures and may not fully absorb preventive advice that is given at that time. Apart from problems in recalling health-related advice,[41] the practical problems in achieving lifestyle change may be perceived by patients as arduous, unpleasant and not worth the effort. For example, the Good Hearted Glasgow Project found that of 77% of 266 patients who were advised to stop smoking, only 11% succeeded after one year.[42]

Patients consistently report that preventive healthcare is important and want appropriate advice, yet physicians frequently perceive patients as non-compliant or not motivated. Conversely, patients cite physicians' failure to order tests, give information or communicate results as reasons for not requesting preventive services.[31] The lack of commitment to optimizing patient compliance that exists in primary care reduces the effectiveness of risk-factor management.

Patients are not followed up systematically after leaving hospital because cardiologists often do not provide preventive follow-up advice for patients and primary care providers.[16] If patients are to be active participants in decisions about their care, the information they receive must accord with available evidence. Consultants often have little time to provide this information and there is much evidence to show that patients do not receive the information they want and need from hospitals.[43] As a result, non-compliance and non-adherence by patients to lifestyle recommendations and pharmacological therapies is widespread. In the USA, for example, of the three billion prescriptions written, only 50% are thought ever to be filled and the medication taken.[44]

TEMPER THE APPLICATION OF GUIDELINES WITH CLINICAL JUDGEMENT

Risk management for the prevention of CHD is based on global risk assessment as enshrined in the latest set of Joint European guidelines;[16] these enlightened practices have now been adopted and promulgated in the USA by the Expert Panel on Detection, Evaluation and Treatment of High Blood Cholesterol in Adults, a group within the framework of the National Cholesterol Education Program (NCEP ATPIII).[45] Their report, although still focusing on LDL cholesterol as the primary target of treatment, expands its horizons to include other lipid and non-lipid risk factors within a management portfolio for prevention of vascular disease on the basis of absolute risk for the patient. The basic principles of the European and US coronary prevention guidelines are fundamentally the same, promoting use of global risk assessment and treatment strategies, which broaden choice for the clinician and expand options for the at-risk patient.

There is strong emphasis on the importance of achievement of targets for both blood pressure and lipids – the ideal concentrations of total and LDL cholesterol are 5 mmol/l (193 mg/dl) and 3 mmol/l (116 mg/dl), respectively, in Europe. However, does treatment to reach these target

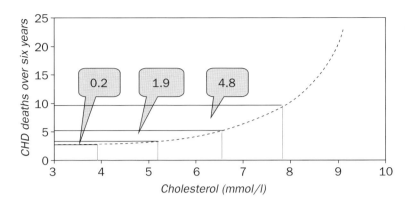

Fig. 17.1 Estimate of number of events avoided for every 1.29 mmol/l (50 mg/dl) reduction in cholesterol concentration in 1000 patients.

values make best use of restricted healthcare resources?

In 2001, prescription of statins in the UK cost £469 million,[46] and this figure is predicted[47] to rise to £2.1 billion by 2010 even if only 80% of Britons with a coronary risk equivalent to that of the WOSCOPS cohort (1.5% per annum) are given the drugs. Staggering figures like these feature strongly in the current discussion to limit expenditure on statin therapy in the primary prevention of coronary disease to those whose annual risk of an event is 3%, i.e. twice as high as that of the WOSCOPS and 50% higher than the accepted level for intervention in the rest of Europe.[16] However, is this approach doing a disservice to our patients by rationing the prescription of statins to those at the highest level of risk (i.e. 3% in the UK), who hardly comprise the majority of first-time admissions to our coronary care units?

The curvilinear relation[48] between cholesterol concentrations in plasma and risk of coronary death is well established but poorly appreciated. If this relation holds in individuals who have their cholesterol level lowered, then a 1.29 mmol/l (50 mg/dl) fall in cholesterol, from 7.8 to 6.5 mmol/l (300 to 250 mg/dl), will produce a substantially greater reduction in events than will a closely similar fall from 6.5 to 5.2 mmol/l (250 to 200 mg/dl) (Fig. 17.1). This hypothesis provides a credible explanation for findings of investigators from the WOSCOPS[49] and CARE[50] studies that as cholesterol and LDL cholesterol concentrations in plasma are lowered further by statin treatment, vascular risk reduction becomes increasingly attenuated. By impli-

cation then, strenuous efforts to drive LDL cholesterol concentrations further downwards could be excessively zealous, since for most mildly hypercholesterolaemic individuals, a reduction in this concentration of about 25% seems to yield all the benefit expected from intervention.[49]

The economic importance of the argument becomes even clearer when we remember[51] that doubling of the dose of a statin will only reduce plasma cholesterol concentration by a further 5–6%. That is, two-thirds of the maximum lipid-lowering benefit of a statin is realized at the starting dose. Hence, clinicians face several conflicting dilemmas in the management of hypercholesterolaemia to prevent first heart attacks.

Behind all these facts there is a disquieting sense that chosen target concentrations do not have a sound scientific basis, and that heroic attempts to reduce cholesterol concentrations in most patients (except familial hypercholesterolaemics) by more than 20% might gain little. Consideration of the experiences of the WOSCOPS participants might offer interim advice on how to proceed.[52] At baseline, the average LDL cholesterol concentration in participants of WOSCOPS was 4.96 mmol/l (192 mg/dl), and if we assume that treatment for all is an appropriate option, the European guideline target would be 3.0 mmol/l (116 mg/dl). As it happened, on an intention-to-treat basis, only one-fifth of the pravastatin-treated group in WOSCOPS actually reached the target (Fig. 17.2). On average, LDL cholesterol in the group was 3.67 mmol/l (142 mg/dl) and individuals in the highest quintile (whose compliance was in

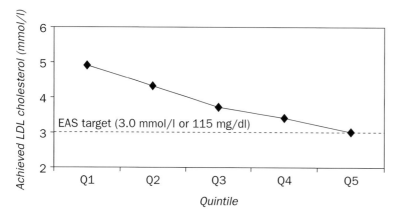

Fig. 17.2 Concentration of LDL cholesterol achieved with pravastatin in the WOSCOPS cohort. Only one-fifth of the group (Q5) achieved target European guideline LDL cholesterol values.

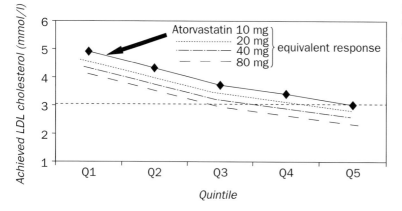

Fig. 17.3 Concentration of LDL cholesterol achieved with different doses of atorvastatin.

serious doubt) showed little improvement from baseline concentrations.

The treatment strategy of WOSCOPS used the maximum recommended dose of pravastatin (40 mg/day). To achieve greater LDL reduction would have needed a change to a more powerful statin than pravastatin, such as atorvastatin, in which a 10 mg/day dose seems to achieve the same reduction in LDL cholesterol concentration as 40 mg/day of pravastatin.[51] If we then assume that the LDL response curve to pravastatin in WOSCOPS would have been achieved in practice with 10 mg of atorvastatin, i.e. including non-compliers in a real-life clinical scenario, and that further reductions of 6% were obtained every time the atorvastatin dose was doubled (Fig. 17.3), then even at the highest 80 mg atorvastatin dose, only about 60% of the WOSCOPS cohort would have reached European guideline targets.

On the basis of these considerations, does statin deployment, targeting individuals at highest risk in primary coronary prevention, make best use of limited resources? Consider two alternative scenarios, which we will call the treat-to-target strategy (Box 17.1) and the fire-and-forget approach (Box 17.2).

For the same cost it is possible to avoid twice as many events by prescribing starting dose statin therapy more liberally, but less intensively, to individuals at lower vascular risk rather than by attempting, in those at highest level of risk, to drive LDL cholesterol values downwards to the 3.0 mmol/l (116 mg/dl) target currently recommended in Europe.[16,53]

Finally, although statins are among the safest drugs used in clinical practice, experiences with cerivastatin remind us that – at high doses and in certain combinations – they can lead to severe, even life-threatening, complications. That said, all available data from clinical trials show that benefit in prevention of cardiovascular disease far outweighs risks of myopathy which the hydrophobic, cytochrome P450-

---

Box 17.1   The treat-to-target strategy

- Treat 10 000 middle-aged WOSCOPS equivalent individuals with atorvastatin to reach European LDL cholesterol guideline targets.
- From Fig. 17.3, even in a best-case scenario of good compliance:
    20% would need 10 mg of drug per day
    20% would need 20 mg of drug per day
    60% would need 40 mg of drug per day *or more.*
- Total daily drug outlay would be 30 000 mg.
- If we ascribe to the group a global coronary risk of 3% per year (equivalent to the limit set by the Scottish Intercollegiate Guidelines Network),[53] the number of vascular events avoided over five years will be, according to the statin trial evidence, one-third of 1500 or 500 events.

Box 17.2   The fire-and-forget approach

- Deployment of atorvastatin at a dose of 10 mg per recipient per day will treat 30 000 individuals for five years.
- Assume, pessimistically, that risk reduction achieved with the 10 mg dose changes proportionally with LDL response to treatment. Then, the risk reduction achieved by the 20% of the cohort who reach their guideline LDL cholesterol target value will be in line with the statin trials, i.e. one-third. In a worst-case scenario, the reduction in the remaining 80% of patients who do not reach target would be at least 20%.
- These assumptions would then result in avoidance of 300 events over five years in 6000 patients who achieved European guideline targets and 720 events in 24 000 individuals whose reduction in LDL cholesterol concentration was more modest. The total number of events avoided for the same expenditure would be 1020, or more than twice the number who benefited by the treat-to-target approach.

---

metabolized reductase inhibitors seem to possess. Nevertheless, in addition to the economic arguments presented above, safety considerations should caution clinicians to choose statins that are not metabolized via cytochrome P450, and to apply dose escalation cautiously in an attempt to achieve target concentrations whose clinical validity still awaits confirmation from continuing trials.[54]

STATIN PRESCRIBING: TODAY AND TOMORROW

Despite the tardiness with which the medical profession espouses new treatments of proven benefit and discards yesterday's often anecdotal habits, the appropriate prescription of lipid-lowering statin therapy is growing rapidly, spurred on no doubt by the publication of new and authoritative evidence-based guidelines.[16,45] The one remaining barrier to full implementation is fiscal. Many economists, health professionals and governments remain concerned over the impact that this will have on healthcare budgets. Consequently, old, unproven, albeit cheaper therapeutic approaches remain in place despite evidence of the clear benefits of cholesterol lowering with statin drugs. This is poor medicine and of questionable benefit to society. The problem is most acute in countries where the prevalence of atherosclerosis is high. Under such circumstances, full and immediate implementation of approved guidelines may be unfeasible and a staged approach to implementation may be required.[55] The loss of statin patent protection, which has occurred for some drugs and will continue over the next few years, will lead to the introduction of lower-priced statin generics and eliminate the significance of the cost-containment argument. Indeed, in the future, and subject to the longer-term proven safety of these drugs, statins may receive widespread over-the-counter status, thereby transferring the cost consideration of their use from health authorities to the individual.

REFERENCES

1. Yamamoto A, Sudo H, Endo A. Therapeutic effects of ML-236B in primary hypercholesterolemia. *Atherosclerosis* 1980; **35**: 259–66.
2. Mabuchi H, Sakai T, Sakai Y et al. Reduction of serum cholesterol in heterozygous patients with familial hypercholesterolemia. *N Engl J Med* 1983; **308**: 609–13.
3. Roberts WC. The underused miracle: the statin drugs are to atherosclerosis what penicillin was to infectious disease. *Am J Cardiol* 1996; **78**: 377–8.
4. Davies M. Stability and instability. Two faces of coronary atherosclerosis. *Circulation* 1996; **94**: 2013–20.
5. Long-Term Intervention with Pravastatin in Ischemic Disease (LIPID) Study Group. Prevention of cardiovascular events and death with pravastatin in patients with coronary heart disease and a broad range of initial cholesterol levels. *N Engl J Med* 1998; **339**: 1349–57.
6. Sacks FM, Pfeffer MA, Moye LA et al., for the Cholesterol and Recurrent Events Trial Investigators. The effect of pravastatin on coronary events after myocardial infarction in patients with average cholesterol levels. *N Engl J Med* 1996; **335**: 1001–9.
7. Scandinavian Simvastatin Survival Study Group. Randomised trial of cholesterol lowering in 4444 patients with coronary heart disease: the Scandinavian Simvastatin Survival Study (4S). *Lancet* 1994; **344**: 1383–9.
8. Heart Protection Study Collaborative Group. MRC/BHF Heart Protection Study of cholesterol lowering with simvastatin in 20,536 high risk individuals: a randomized placebo-controlled trial. *Lancet* 2002; **360**: 7–22.
9. Serruys PWJC, de Feyter P, Macaya C et al., for the Lescol Intervention Prevention Study Investigators. Fluvastatin for prevention of cardiac events following successful first percuta-

neous coronary intervention: a randomized controlled trial. *JAMA* 2002; **287**: 3215–22.
10. Shepherd J, Blauw GJ, Murphy MB et al. Pravastatin in elderly individuals at risk of vascular disease (PROSPER): a randomised controlled trial. *Lancet* 2002; **360**: 1623–30.
11. Sever PS, Dahlof B, Poulter NR et al. Prevention of coronary and stroke events with atorvastatin in hypertensive patients who have average or lower-than-average cholesterol concentrations, in the Anglo-Scandinavian Cardiac Outcomes Trial – Lipid Lowering Arm (ASCOT-LLA): a multicentre randomised controlled trial. *Lancet* 2003; **361**: 1149–58.
12. EUROASPIRE Study Group. A European Society of Cardiology survey on secondary prevention of coronary heart disease: principal results. *Eur Heart J* 1997; **18**: 1569–82.
13. EUROASPIRE II Study Group. Lifestyle and risk factor management and use of drug therapies in coronary patients from 15 countries. *Eur Heart J* 2001; **22**: 554–72.
14. Shepherd J, Alcalde V, Befort PA, for the HELP Study Group. International comparison of awareness and attitudes towards coronary risk factor reduction: the HELP study. *J Cardiovasc Risk* 1997; **4**: 373–84.
15. ASPIRE Steering Group. A British Cardiac Society survey of the potential for the secondary prevention of coronary disease: principal results. *Heart* 1996; **75**: 334–42.
16. Recommendations of the Second Joint Task Force of the European and Other Societies on Coronary Prevention. Prevention of coronary heart disease in clinical practice. *Eur Heart J* 1998; **19**: 1434–503.
17. Antiplatelet Trialists' Collaboration. Collaborative overview of randomized trials of antiplatelet therapy. I. Prevention of death, myocardial infarction, and stroke by prolonged antiplatelet therapy in various categories of patients. *BMJ* 1994; **308**: 81–106.
18. Cruickshank JM. Beta-blockers: primary and secondary prevention. *J Cardiovasc Pharmacol* 1992; **20** (Suppl 11): S55–S69.
19. Yusuf S, Wittes J, Friedman L. Overview of randomized clinical trials in heart disease. I. Treatments following myocardial infarction. *JAMA* 1988; **260**: 2088–93.
20. Konstam M, Dracup K, Baker D et al. *Heart Failure: Evaluation and Care of Patients With Left Ventricular Systolic Dysfunction. Clinical Practice Guideline No. 11.* Rockville, MD: Agency for

Health Care Policy and Research, Public Health Service, US Department of Human and Health Services, 1994.

21. Bradley F, Morgan S, Smith H, Mant D. The Wessex Research Network (WreN): preventive care for patients following myocardial infarction. *Fam Pract* 1997: **14**: 220–6.

22. Tannenbaum TN, Sampalis JS, Battista RN et al. Early detection and treatment of hyperlipidemia: physician practices in Canada. *Can Med Assoc J* 1990; **143**: 875–81.

23. Grover SA, Lowensteyn I, Esrey KL et al. Do doctors accurately assess coronary risk in their patients? Preliminary results of the coronary health assessment study. *BMJ* 1995; **310**: 975–8.

24. Hulscher MEJL, van Drenth BB, Mokkink HGA et al. Effects of outreach visits by trained nurses on cardiovascular risk factor recording in general practice: a controlled trial. *Eur J Gen Pract* 1997; **3**: 90–5.

25. Shepherd J, Pratt M. Prevention of coronary heart disease in clinical practice: a commentary on current treatment patterns in six European countries in relation to published recommendations. *Cardiology* 1996; **87**: 1–5.

26. Campbell NC, Thain J, Deans HG et al. Secondary prevention in coronary heart disease: baseline survey of provision in general practice. *BMJ* 1998; **326**: 1430–4.

27. Wilcox RG, Hampton JR, Banks DC et al. Trial of early nifedipine in acute myocardial infarction: the Trent Study. *BMJ* 1986; **293**: 1204–8.

28. Piwonski J, Pytolak A, Kurjata P. Prevention of ischaemic heart disease. General practitioners' views. Part II. Secondary prevention. *Kardiol Pol* 2000; **539**: 223–8.

29. Marteau TM, Kinmonth Al, Pyke S, Thompson SG. Readiness for lifestyle advice: self-assessments of coronary risk prior to screening in the British Family Heart Study. Family Heart Study Group. *Br J Gen Pract* 1995; **45**: 3905–8.

30. Pharoah PDP, Sanderson SP. Health promotion in primary care: modelling the impact of intervention on coronary heart disease and stroke. *J Public Health Med* 1995; **17**: 150–6.

31. Pearson TA, Peters TD. The treatment gap in coronary artery disease and heart failure: community standards and the post-discharge patient. *Am J Cardiol* 1997; **80**: 45H–52H.

32. Martinez M, Agusti A, Arnau JM et al. Trends of prescribing patterns for the secondary prevention of myocardial infarction over a 13-year period. *Eur J Clin Pharmacol* 1998; **54**: 203–8.

33. Pearson TA, Laurora I, Chere H, Kafonek S. The lipid treatment assessment project (L-TAP): a multicenter survey to evaluate the percentages of dyslipidemic patients receiving lipid-lowering therapy and achieving LDL cholesterol goals. *Arch Intern Med* 2000; **160**: 459–67.

34. Pearson TA, McBride P, Houston-Miller N, Smith SC. Organization of preventive cardiology service. 27th Bethesda Conference. Matching the intensity of risk factor management with the hazard for coronary disease events. *J Am Coll Cardiol* 1996; **27**: 1030–47.

35. Editorial. Preventing recurrent coronary heart disease. *BMJ* 1998; **316**: 1400–1.

36. Shea S, Gemson DH, Mossel P. Management of high blood cholesterol by primary care physicians: diffusion of the National Cholesterol Education Program Adult Treatment Panel Guidelines. *J Gen Intern Med* 1990; **5**: 327–34.

37. Pryce AJ, Heatlie HF, Chapman SR. Buckling under the pressure: influence of secondary care establishments on the prescribing of glyceryl trinitrate buccal tablets in primary care. *BMJ* 1996; **313**: 1621–4.

38. Boekeloo B, Becker D, Yeo E et al. Post-myocardial infarction cholesterol management by primary physicians. *J Am Coll Cardiol* 1995; **27**: 77A (abst).

39. Gohlke H, Gohlke-Barwolf C. Cardiac rehabilitation. *Eur Heart J* 1998; **19**: 1004–10.

40. Hayes B, Haines A. Barriers and bridges to evidence-based clinical practice. *BMJ* 1998; **317**: 273–6.

41. Kravitz RL, Hays RD, Sherbourne CD et al. Recall of recommendations and adherence to advice among patients with chronic medical conditions. *Arch Intern Med* 1993; **53**: 1869–78.

42. Cawston P, McEwen J. Three-year follow-up survey of smokers who attended 'Good Hearted Glasgow' screening sessions. *Public Health* 1990; **108**: 185–94.

43. Audit Commission. *What Seems to be the Matter: Communication Between Hospitals and Patients.* London: HMSO, 1993.

44. Berg JS, Dischler J, Wagner DJ. Medication compliance: a health care problem. *Ann Pharmacother* 1993; **27** (Suppl): S2–S22.

45. Executive Summary of the Third Report of the National Cholesterol Education Program (NCEP) Expert Panel on Detection, Evaluation and Treatment of High Blood Cholesterol in Adults (Adults Treatment Panel III). *JAMA* 2001; **285**: 2486–97.

46. Moore W. 21st century heart solution may have a sting in the tail. *BMJ* 2002; **325**: 184.

47. Wanless D. Final report on NHS financial review. www.hm-treasury.gov.uk (Accessed 30 September 2002).

48. Stamler J, Wentworth D, Neaton JD. Is the relationship between serum cholesterol and risk of premature death from coronary heart disease continuous and graded? Findings in 356,222 primary screenees of the Multiple Risk Factor Intervention Trial (MRFIT). *JAMA* 1986; **256**: 2823–8.

49. West of Scotland Coronary Prevention Study Group. Influence of pravastatin and plasma lipids on coronary events in the West of Scotland Coronary Prevention Study. *Circulation* 1998; **97**: 1440–5.

50. Sacks FM, Moye LA, Davis BR et al. Relationship between plasma LDL cholesterol concentrations during treatment with pravastatin and recurrent coronary events in the Cholesterol and Recurrent Events Trial (CARE). *Circulation* 1998; **97**: 1446–52.

51. Jones P, Kafonek S, Laurora I, Hunninghake D. Comparative dose efficacy study of atorvastatin versus simvastatin, pravastatin, lovastatin and fluvastatin in patients with hypercholesterolemia (the CURVES study). *Am J Cardiol* 1998; **81**: 582–7.

52. Shepherd J. Resource management in prevention of coronary heart disease: optimizing prescription of lipid-lowering drugs. *Lancet* 2002; **359**: 2271–3.

53. Scottish Intercollegiate Guidelines Network. *Lipids and the Primary Prevention of Coronary Heart Disease*. Sign Publication No. 40. Edinburgh: Royal College of Physicians, Sept 1999.

54. LaRosa JC. Unresolved issues: unanswered questions. *Eur Heart J* 1999; **1** (Suppl): 18–23.

55. *Standing Medical Advisory Committee on the Use of Statins*. NHS Executive. London: Department of Health, 1997.

Index

Page numbers in *italics* indicate figures or tables.